OUTSMARTING CANCER

Outsmarting Cancer

**Risk Reduction
and the Power of Prevention**

Adam Barsouk, MD

JOHNS HOPKINS UNIVERSITY PRESS
Baltimore

This book is not intended as a substitute for the medical or healthcare advice of physicians or other licensed professionals. Readers should consult healthcare providers in matters relating to their health, particularly with respect to any symptoms that may require diagnosis or medical attention.

Johns Hopkins University Press
2715 North Charles Street
Baltimore, Maryland 21218
www.press.jhu.edu

Library of Congress Cataloging-in-Publication Data is available.

ISBN 978-1-4214-5385-9 (hardcover)
ISBN 978-1-4214-5386-6 (paperback)
ISBN 978-1-4214-5387-3 (ebook)

A catalog record for this book is available from the British Library.

Special discounts are available for bulk purchases of this book. For more information, please contact Special Sales at specialsales@jh.edu.

EU GPSR Authorized Representative
LOGOS EUROPE, 9 rue Nicolas Poussin,
17000, La Rochelle, France
E-mail: Contact@logoseurope.eu

To my grandparents Boris and Natalya, whose light shines on to illuminate my path, long after their passing

To my wife and parents, who provide my life with love, warmth, and meaning

To my mentors and patients, who've graciously given their time and bodies to my practice of the art of medicine

Contents

Online Supplement

The author has prepared an expanded version of *Outsmarting Cancer*'s bibliography. It can be found by visiting the specific book page on press.jhu.edu.

OUTSMARTING CANCER

Introduction

There is no glory in illness. There is no meaning to it.
There is no honor in dying of it.
—John Green

An ounce of prevention is worth a pound of cure.
—Benjamin Franklin

They warn you about many things when you rotate through the Veterans Administration (VA) hospital. The health records system is bare-bones, the staffing is unpredictable, and the cafeteria hours leave much to be desired. What they don't prepare you for is the stoicism of some patients.

When a middle-aged father of three learned he had glioblastoma, a rare and deadly cancer of the brain, he soldiered on silently. I had seen tears, prayers, even wails from patients before, but his silence was harrowing. While "oncology" means the arm of medicine concerned with cancer, "onc" means "mass" in ancient Greek, but it also translates as "burden." My patient's glioblastoma was a burden that he could shoulder in silence, but it was not his to shoulder alone. His wife, rejecting the silence, demanded answers. I knew all about the limited treatment options and dismal prognosis (predicted outcome; one common statistic gives a five-year survival rate of less than 5%) because I had published research on glioblastoma management. What I couldn't answer was why it had to be *her* husband.

Later that night, I started sifting through a different kind of oncologic research, not on the mechanisms or treatments of glioblastoma, but on risk factors. I learned that countless young veterans of wars in Iraq and Afghanistan, like my patient, have been recently diagnosed with brain cancer, and only now had we uncovered a likely culprit: burn pits. For decades, the US military had disposed of its trash on bases by incinerating it at high temperatures, releasing cancer-causing agents (carcinogens) straight into the lungs of their soldiers. At bases like Camp Lejeune, they dumped toxic waste into the water our soldiers and their families drank. Veterans returned from war carrying indelible trauma in their psyche (or "flak happiness" as the airmen called it) and the harbingers of cancer deep within their cells.

My patient had risked his life for a country that failed him because it didn't care to put more thought into something as simple as disposing of trash. If the medical community didn't do everything in our power to prevent deadly cancers like his, we would be failing him, too.

In 1775, Percivall Pott described the first example of preventable cancer. He noted that chimney sweeps, often orphans or children of poor families, no older than 11 (the only ones small enough to fit), would develop a black ulcerated growth on their scrotum. Dr. Pott realized the soot, mixed with sweat and caught in their trousers for years on end, was actually to blame for scrotal cancer.[1]

We've come a long way since (in medicine and in child labor). Today we know that nearly half of global adult cancer deaths are preventable,[2] and research is revealing new risk factors every day. At the same time, cancer is afflicting more people, earlier in life, and is predicted to soon surpass heart disease as the leading cause of death. Preventing cancer is more possible, and more imperative, than ever before.

CANCER: ENFEEBLED OR EMBOLDENED?

As recently as a century ago, cancer was only the eighth leading cause of death. Tuberculosis, pneumonia, and gastrointestinal infections like cholera made up the top three. As revolutions in sanitation and sterility and the discovery of antibiotics have made these infections much less common and deadly, cancer and heart disease have risen through the ranks. Although we've also made remarkable strides in the prevention and treatment of both, the pace has been much slower.

As long as there's been a written record of medicine, we've known that cancer kills. An ancient Egyptian papyrus dating back to 3000 BCE (over 5,000 years ago) is the first preserved mention of cancer, describing tumors of the breast. The papyrus reports that while the tumors could be shrunk (very painfully) with a "fire-drill," a technique known as cauterization that's still in use, even the ancient Egyptian doctors recognized the breast tumors as ultimately "incurable."[3]

Thankfully, that is not always the case anymore. Survival rates for some cancers, including breast cancer, have more than doubled over the past four decades. Today's 10-year survival rate for breast cancer is 83%, and for tumors caught before they spread from the breast (metastasize), that figure jumps to 99%. For the first time in medical history, we are regularly conducting research not just on cancer patients, but cancer *survivors* (who, for instance, are still at a heightened risk of COVID-19 infections even decades after being cured). Building on a century of research, we now use breast-conserving surgery; radiation; therapies that stimulate the immune system; targeted therapies that block specific receptors essential to cancer growth; and even lab-engineered chimeric antigen receptor thymus (CAR-T) cells harvested from a patient, genetically modified, and then re-infused to fight cancer (and this list is *far* from exhaustive). Because of our advancements, a smaller percentage of patients are dying of cancer, and far more people are *living* with it. Yet even with CAR-T and immunotherapy, for the first time in history, my generation will live shorter lives than our parents, fueled by a roiling epidemic of young adult cancer.

For many patients, we are winning the battle. But what about the war? Chemotherapy and radiation can wreak havoc on the heart and lungs decades down the line, and even cause new "secondary" cancers to arise. Immunotherapies, which are much better tolerated, result in autoimmune targeting of the thyroid or adrenal glands. Even CAR-T is largely only administered in a hospital, because most patients developed a powerful immune response that can land them in the intensive care unit, and some have even died. Other tumor types, like glioblastoma or pancreatic cancer, have retained their dismal prognoses despite the billions of dollars in research funding that we've thrown at them.

And while countless dollars and hours are funneled toward cutting-edge therapies, we remain utterly clueless about what's causing the cancer epidemic afflicting our young adults. Is it skyrocketing rates of obesity, processed foods, microplastics, COVID-19, or something else entirely that we haven't yet discovered? These are questions seldom raised and seldom answered. While extending lives, we're ignoring the origins of a brewing crisis. In our era of mind-boggling, exorbitant therapeutic advancements, prevention remains the best medicine, and yet it's the aspect of oncology for which we devote the least time and money.

DEEP IN OUR CELLS AND MINDS

Cancer has been a domineering force in my life since childhood. When the grandparents who raised me got diagnosed with rare blood cancers, I had a front-row seat to their losing battle. I was with them in the park when they couldn't walk any farther. I was with them in the clinic, interpreting in Russian the doctors' questions. I was with my grandfather in the hospital when he died, and a few years later, I was back there with my grandmother. I had stumbled my way into the world of medicine as their translator and advocate, and after they passed, I found myself wanting to stay. I started volunteering with cancer patients and working in a translational research lab in high school, and quickly realized medical communication had become my passion. I could offer explanations to families like mine, constrained by language or literacy. I authored newspaper articles sharing my findings from the lab, and that became my foray into public health education. All the while, working with patients, I got to translate not just from Russian or Spanish, but also from science to English. I remember one of my patients kept smoking because all her friends with lung cancer had been diagnosed *after* they'd stopped. When I took the time to explain latency periods and cancer development, she agreed to try to quit.

My path led me to graduate summa cum laude from an accelerated medical program, graduate top of my class in medical school, and begin internal medicine training at the Hospital of the University of Pennsylvania. But the more I saw how much I could teach patients, the more I realized how much the field of medicine still had to learn.

Nowhere was this more evident than on my night shifts. There's a certain delirium that sets in late at night in the hospital, for insomniac patients and providers alike. Covering dozens of patients on the dark, eerie wards, deprived of daylight and social interaction, I've faced my most shaking existential crises. What was I doing here? Admitting the same people, with the same problems, only to discharge them and see them back a week later through the revolving door we call health care. In those quiet, wee hours I most starkly appreciated our ineptitude, our utter failings in making progress on chronic disease. Like many of my patients, I yearned for change, for the opportunity to make meaningful differences in the public's health, but I had no idea where to start. I knew one thing for sure: change would not start at 3:00 a.m. in the emergency department.

Over decades of training and practice, doctors often begin to see patients as mere diseases and treatment plans. As a newly minted member of the medical community, I have endeavored to see patients through the life stories and circumstances that lead them to make decisions, scattered with opportunities to intervene and prevent disease. In tandem with doctors across the country, I began publishing a series of epidemiology reviews in medical school, exploring prevention strategies for all the most common cancer types. The more I learned about the risk factors behind cancer for my research, the more I saw them pop up in all my patients' stories. I only started learning about cancer prevention (of my own accord) *after* I was taught about oncological management. This education should occur the other way around, with prevention coming first.

With ballooning health care costs and consistently dropping life expectancy, we are missing the forest for the trees. We invest billions in new therapies, which have indeed doubled survival over the past decades, and even made certain cancers curable. But many of these therapies come with life-long risks of immunosuppression, heart disease, or even secondary cancers, and some have side effects that have proven fatal. In oncology, as in most of medicine, *prevention is better than cure*. And yet, our spending on research, education, and evidence-based public health initiatives for cancer prevention has been virtually *non-existent*. There are billions to be made in treating cancer, but relatively few incentives to prevent it. The $500,000 price tag of *one* CAR-T therapy (the enigma of pharmaceutical pricing warrants a whole book unto itself) could, for instance, improve the diet of hundreds of Americans or reduce liver cancer–inducing aflatoxin exposure for thousands of farmers in Asia or Africa. Prevention can occur on scales large and small. On an individual level, there are numerous evidence-based lifestyle modifications that each of us can make to lower our cancer risk (and as many, if not more, supplements and recommendations that are unfounded).

We are living through a new era of medical uncertainty. In many countries and US states, cancer has overtaken heart disease as the leading cause of death. Racial disparities in cancer risk and survival continue to worsen. We're seeing an "epidemic" of cancers in those under 50, with obesity believed to be the chief, but not sole, culprit. Early studies hypothesize that the inflammation and mutations brought about by COVID-19 may increase our long-term cancer risk. Now is the time to understand and target not just the molecules but also the risk factors that lead to cancer.

Unfortunately, we are also living through an era of unprecedented distrust in doctors and the health care system. Much of this distrust has been duly earned by doctors, who have for centuries ignored women and experimented on patients of color, and administrators, who have prioritized profit over people. But this distrust has also significantly hindered good doctors and public health initiatives that are paramount for cancer prevention, like human papillomavirus (HPV) vaccination or cancer screening. These issues have been exacerbated by the echo chambers of the internet, and the leaders who foment division and propagate lies for political gain. In this chaotic world, it can often be difficult to appreciate a light at the end of the tunnel. But I know it's there. In a bizarre way, growing up in a family of doctors humbled me. I wasn't taught to see doctors as an unquestionable paragon of truth; rather, they were my fallible, human mom and dad. Consequently, I've never cared for hierarchy or authority when it came to my interactions with patients, nor do I insist on using fancy, inaccessible terminology with patients just to pretend I know all the answers. I've found that treating patients like colleagues, rather than clients, and meeting each person at their level has been my most successful tool against medical distrust. I hope to share with you what I've learned from listening to medical pioneers and patients alike.

In the pages to come, I break down the most common risk factors for cancer worldwide, sharing historical anecdotes, the latest epidemiological statistics, and studies on the best lifestyle and public health interventions. Some cancer risk factors, like smoking, are well known, but others—such as a bladder-dwelling parasite, an addictive nut with psychostimulatory properties, and an invisible gas found in most of our basements—may surprise you. I address the social aspects of cancer prevention, like stigma against smokers (which interferes with optimal counseling on smoking cessation) and racial disparities in cancer risk and treatment. I also tackle the rising threat of misinformation and the billion-dollar supplement industry that has fueled and profited from it. Through it all, I share the stories of family members and countless patients that give cancer prevention the urgency it deserves. All of us have lost someone to cancer. I believe we can channel that grief to help others avoid the same fate.

CHAPTER 1

Why Us? Cancer Risk and Prevention

Why you? Why us for that matter? Why anything? Because this moment simply is. Have you ever seen bugs trapped in amber?
—KURT VONNEGUT, *SLAUGHTERHOUSE-FIVE*

In Vonnegut's novel *Slaughterhouse-Five,* Billy Pilgrim, a World War II veteran stricken with post-traumatic stress disorder, is left questioning the cruelty of his reality. Like many of my VA patients, he had experienced horrors that no human being should see, and he finds himself asking the omniscient aliens of his imagination: "Why me?" I've heard mothers, fathers, grandparents, even children diagnosed with cancer ask me the same question: "Why me?" What did they do wrong to deserve such a fate?

Cancer is as old as life itself. On display in the Carnegie Museum of Natural History in Pittsburgh is a leg bone of a 200-million-year-old sauropod (a large herbivorous dinosaur) with a now-crystalized tumor eating away at it. Whether or not it ultimately died of the cancer, the behemoth had roamed for years with a bowling ball–sized tumor growing on its thigh. The ancient Egyptians described a case of breast cancer in the oldest preserved medicinal text; for this ailment, there "was no treatment."[1] As long as multicellular organisms have existed, there have been cells that go awry, subjecting their host to an ancient curse. The older you get, and the more divisions your cells undergo, the greater your risk. Even in the present day, as modern medicine has curtailed mortality from infections and heart diseases, cancer has remained stubbornly difficult to treat and cure. Certainly, survival rates have risen with the latest immuno- and targeted therapies, but so have the rates of diagnosis. Today, every other man, and one in three women, can expect a cancer diagnosis in their lifetime. And in many countries and regions of the US, cancer has surpassed heart disease as the leading cause of death.[2] The better we get at medicine, the more cancer patients we leave with the age-old question: Why me?

As Vonnegut puts it, "Well, here we are, trapped in the amber of this moment. There is no why."[3] Like bugs in amber, we are victims of our random circumstances, the universe's cruel trick upon beings that have evolved to recognize the frailty of our mortality but have not evolved far enough to escape it. My patients feel similarly duped by fate. Many have risk factors that increased their chances of developing cancer, and some do not. I've heard all sorts of regrets voiced and faced difficult questions, like "Was it the cigarettes that caused this?" and "Are my children doomed to get cancer, too?" Nobody, regardless of what they did in life or who their parents were, *deserves* their diagnosis, and we can never say for certain whether any one decision made the difference. Risk and chance offer little reassurance to patients and families diagnosed with cancer. But for those of us looking to prevent further tragedies, discussions of *why* cancer happens can be prescient, and even life-saving.

A GAME OF RISK

Cancer is an umbrella term for hundreds of different disease processes caused by thousands of different mutations. Historically, we classified cancer by the organ in which it spawned. With the advent of the microscope and many special stains, and more recently genomic testing, we have started to classify cancers by their molecular "fingerprints." We've found patterns that transcend organs, patterns that reflect *how* a cancer arises, rather than *where*. I ask you, while reading this book, to abandon the age-old notion of cancer as an organ-based disease; instead, we will classify cancers by their many catalysts: pathogens, toxins, radiation, medicines, genes, and bodily processes gone wrong. The seed behind the original cancer cell determines how it evolves, and only years later do we see the end result in the unlucky affected organs. To prevent cancer, we must understand its many causes, that is, risk factors.

Cancer is a matter of risk, like any casino game. No individual outcome can be predicted with certainty. No risk factor, whether smoking or even radiation exposure, guarantees cancer. It merely *increases* risk. Anyone who's done sports betting, bought stocks, or played poker knows there are many ways to quantify odds or risk. For simplicity's sake, I've chosen to present the "relative risk" from the studies I encountered (unless I specify otherwise). Relative risk refers to the risk of getting cancer if you perform a certain action (like smoking) or belong to a certain group (such as women), compared to *not* performing the action or *not* belonging to that group.

The average person's lifetime risk of developing *any* cancer is around 40%, and the risk of dying (or mortality) from it is around 20%.[4] However, the risk of any individual cancer is far lower; for instance, the lifetime risk for nonsmokers of getting lung cancer is 1.5%.[5] The relative risk for smokers is 600%, which means smoking increases your risk by 7 times,[6] increasing lifetime risk to 10% for smokers. Additional factors, such as sex, race, and number of cigarettes smoked modify that risk further.

Nearly every risk factor we discuss in this book will be a weaker risk factor than smoking. When I say obesity carries a relative risk of 30% for colorectal cancer, that means you are 30% *more likely* to develop colorectal cancer if you are obese.[7] Bear in mind, the absolute risk (the actual chance you get colon cancer), may be exceedingly low. If the average absolute risk of getting colon cancer is 0.3% every year, a 30% relative risk would only increase it to 0.4%. The difference may seem negligible. But when you tally up all the years you live, all the risk factors you may have, and all the cancer types affected by a given risk factor (obesity increases the risk of over a dozen cancers), the absolute risk begins to add up. With obesity, your lifetime risk of *any* cancer ends up closer to 10%.

Equally important is the language we use when describing risk. I use the term "risk factor" because, without prospective studies, it is hard to say for certain whether an action *causes* cancer. Sure, for something like tobacco, the preponderance of evidence from laboratory and observational studies are enough for us to label it cancer causing, or a "carcinogen." But for most products, we simply don't have that level of evidence, so we label them "risk factors," meaning they have been shown to increase the risk of cancer. The most scientifically accurate description of any risk factor would be, "X risk factor is associated with a Y% increased risk of Z cancer in a given patient population." To improve readability and not bore you to sleep, I have opted to sometimes shorten this statement to "X risk factor increases cancer risk by Y%." This does **not** mean that X risk factor has been experimentally proven to cause that cancer; rather, it has been associated with increased risk in observational studies. To summarize, "risk" refers to real-world data on the likelihood of getting cancer, while "carcinogenicity" refers to laboratory data about whether a compound can cause mutations that lead to cancer in a test tube or animal model.

CARCINOGENESIS

When it comes to carcinogenesis, or the process by which cancer arises, the science is even more complicated. We are all made up of trillions of cells, each of which has instructions to follow (written in deoxyribonucleic acid, or DNA) to make sure it's fulfilling its purpose within the body. Fundamentally, cancer is a cell disobeying its instructions and instead, replicating (multiplying) nonstop. If left unchecked, that cell grows into a tumor and then spreads to other sites in the body (known as metastasis, pronounced "muh-TA-stuh-sis"). Cancer is, in its essence, a cell that only cares about its own replication and prioritizes this drive over the well-being of its host. While cancers can arise in nearly every organ in the body, the overall process by which cells become cancerous is fairly consistent throughout.

To succeed as a cancer, a cell must develop over a dozen "hallmarks of cancer"—skills like avoiding the immune system, disobeying internal limits to cell division, extracting limitless energy to power its ceaseless replication, and creating a blood supply to grow and spread. Any risk factor that affects any of these hallmarks increases cancer risk—for instance, any drug that suppresses your immune system will increase your risk of cancer. But at its root, the original cancer cell arises because of numerous defects in its instructions, mutations in its DNA.

A mutation is simply a change in the DNA's code, and it can happen in many ways. Our DNA is three billion letters long and must be copied in full every time a cell multiplies. While the

DNA replication machinery is over 99.99% accurate, no system is perfect, so random errors still occur in the code, resulting in mutations. With every division, our cells run the risk of accruing and accumulating mutations. External players like ultraviolet rays from the sun or high-energy particles created by metabolism can randomly strike the DNA and deposit their energy, also leading to mutations. Toxic chemicals, drugs/medications, and viruses can also mutate DNA, as can damage from our immune cells (yes, you read that right) as they try to fight these viruses. Because of the ever-present risk, all our cells harbor numerous, redundant safeguards, such as DNA repair mechanisms and cell division checkpoints, which prevent cells from dividing if their DNA is corrupted. These safeguards are collectively labeled "tumor suppressor genes," because they suppress cancer development. In contrast, mutations that lead to cancer are called "oncogenes."

In order for a cancer to arise, a cell must develop hundreds, sometimes thousands, of mutations to bypass all the body's safeguards. Anything that disrupts the safeguards, like hormones that turn off cell division checkpoints, or inherited defects in DNA repair proteins (like BRCA1/2), increases cancer risk. Particularly harmful are mutations that arise in crucial regions of DNA, like mutations in telomeres, the ends of chromosomes, which function to limit cellular divisions. Any external exposure that promotes these mutations contributes to cancer risk. For instance, compounds like those formed by the burning of tobacco, by processing meats, or in industrial pollution can all cause mutations in DNA. If these mutations turn off one of those vital safeguards or turn on one of those pernicious oncogenes, a cell can go barreling toward cancer. In the coming chapters, you will note time and again that any process or chemical that mutates DNA, the fundamental code that keeps our cells in check, culminates in cancer risk. Statistically, the most common perpetrators of DNA damage are inflammation, metabolism, and radiation—each of which can take many shapes and come from many sources, as we will explore in the chapters to come.

However, there are probably other causes of cancer that we haven't even recognized yet. We are witnessing a harrowing new trend: the ballooning diagnosis of cancer in young adults. I've treated several 20- and 30-year-olds diagnosed with cancers that were previously considered exclusive to retirees. Over the past decades, the average age of a cancer clinic patient has drifted from the 70s to the 60s and may soon reach the 50s. Whether this tragedy is a function of the obesity epidemic, the ubiquitous microplastics and toxins in our air and water, stress, the microbiome, or something we don't even know about remains to be seen. Whatever the cause, medicine is armed with a deepening knowledge of carcinogenesis and growing appreciation for epidemiology (the study of the causes of disease) to face the crisis head on.

Preventing cancer is a constant game of risk on both a cellular and social level. Deep inside our bodies, millions of cells develop mutations and start to head down the path of cancer every single day. Thankfully, our safeguards are so numerous and robust, they stop almost all of them. The minuscule risk that any of these cells breaks through all of the barriers and becomes cancer is then influenced by our choices as individuals and as a society. Many of our actions give that aspiring cancer cell an infinitesimally slight edge, which over a lifetime of lotteries, may create just the right circumstances for that cell to break out and wreak havoc and death. This numbers game is played out on such microscopic but inordinately large scales that it is impossible for our minds to conceptualize. But that doesn't make it any less real for the countless lives and families affected by cancer.

EPIDEMIOLOGY AND PREVENTION

Nearly all of the studies I will discuss in the coming pages are *retrospective*, which means they are looking back at patients with or without a certain risk factor. Other terms to describe this approach are "real world" or "observational" data. Unlike the prospective trials we conduct to evaluate new therapies, where we randomly assign participants to receive different treatments and then compare how they do over years of follow-up, retrospective trials have a lot of inherent "confounders." Confounding means when variables *other than* the one we are studying affect our results. When we see that alcoholics get more lung cancer, are we sure that's because of the alcohol, or is it because people who drink are also more likely to smoke? Human lives are complex, and countless "confounding variables," many of which we may never discover, occur in retrospective studies. Therefore, all data on cancer risk factors that we discuss should be taken with a grain of salt.

Other statistical terms you may hear include "incidence" and "prevalence." Incidence is the number of people who get a disease, like cancer, in any given year, while prevalence is the overall number of cases of a disease in a population. With better treatments and earlier detection, the prevalence of certain cancers has increased even while the incidence has gone down, and that's a good thing—it means people are living longer with that cancer! Unfortunately, overall incidence of cancer around the world has only gone up over the past decades. Statistical values have to be put into context, evaluated for bias, and interpreted as trends in order to fully appreciate what they mean. The study of all these risk factors and how they play into a population's rate of diseases is called epidemiology.

Why does all this evidence even matter? Couldn't we just all follow the advice we hear from friends, or online, about living healthy, come what may? I've worked with many doctors (especially old-school ones) who practice medicine similarly, based on personal and anecdotal experience, prescribing medicines they've seen work, even if large-scale trials say they don't. Sometimes it can be therapeutic, for both patient and provider, to know that something is being tried. But we can't optimize outcomes and costs in large, billion-dollar health care systems on the whims of individual doctors. Similarly, we can't optimize cancer prevention on the whims of individual influencers, and in fact, certain unscientific suggestions may actually *increase* cancer risk. Data brings objectivity and stability, order to the chaos of medicine. Or as Joseph Stein put it in the eponymous quote, "Without our traditions, our lives would be as shaky as a fiddler on the roof!"

The crux of prevention is action. When we identify evidence-based risk factors in a population, we find ways to minimize them. Epidemiology is theory, and prevention is practice. Prevention can be further broken down into categories. Primary prevention is avoiding the risk factors in the first place, like avoiding smoking or radiation exposure, or getting vaccinated. In our game of risk, avoiding these risk factors is like getting dealt a better hand in a card game, but it guarantees nothing. Hence comes secondary prevention: minimizing the risk of poor outcomes in those who've already been exposed, which often takes the form of screening. For smokers, we screen with low-dose computed tomography (CT) scans to detect lung cancer early, so we can cut it out before it spreads. In all women, but especially those diagnosed with HPV, we screen for cervical cancer via Pap smears and HPV tests. Many cancer screenings are based solely on sex and age, which are by themselves some of the largest risk factors. All of these screening tests have been studied across thousands of patients and proven to decrease mortality or morbidity (suffering from disease), but obviously they cannot decrease the actual rate of disease (in fact, they often increase incidence because we detect more early-stage cancers). Some, like prostate cancer tests, have not been shown to significantly impact mortality or morbidity, and are therefore falling out of favor (more on this later). Finally, tertiary prevention involves screening those with disease for worsening of the disease. For instance, in patients with lung cancer, we often suggest brain imaging every year to try to catch metastases to the brain early. This book focuses mostly on primary prevention, that is, minimizing risk factors that lead to cancer, but we will discuss the other forms of prevention in later chapters.

We should be careful not to associate preventable factors with blame. For instance, lung cancer has historically had far less fundraising than breast or prostate cancer, despite being the most fatal cancer, because of its association with smoking. When we hear someone has lung cancer, we subconsciously blame them for smoking, perhaps to reassure ourselves that we won't suffer the same fate. However, some 10%–20% of lung cancers are unrelated to smoking, and that figure is climbing.[8] Moreover, we now know smoking is an addiction that could grip anyone, regardless of willpower or discipline. As for the other causes, people can't control the nefarious genes they inherited or whether they must live in a polluted area for access to work. When we ascribe blame to others' misfortunes, we make false assumptions, and we miss opportunities to help those in need. We should aim to avoid the many preventable cancer risk factors, like smoking, as individuals; but more importantly, we must structure our societies with public health in mind, with economic incentives and cultural support to lead healthy lives. It was not shame or moral brow-beating that helped us turn the corner on tobacco, but rather targeted taxation and regulation, as well as cultural shifts and greater education. These same lessons should be applied to all the other causes of cancer I will outline in the pages to come.

NEGLECTING PREVENTION

We notoriously neglect prevention in health care. Of the $4 trillion we spend on health care in the US annually, only about 3%–5% is devoted to public health and prevention efforts. This includes initiatives like disease screenings, immunizations, health education, and early intervention programs. However, spending on prevention has the highest return on investment, both economically and in terms of patient life expectancy. Every dollar invested in childhood immunizations is estimated to save $16 in health care costs.[9] Smoking cessation programs yield a $2–$3 return per dollar spent, and programs to prevent cardiovascular diseases, like diet or exercise interventions, have shown returns of $4–$6 per dollar invested. Greater spending on prevention is part of the reason why people residing in other developed nations, like Japan, France, and Australia, live an average of 10 years longer than we do in the US,[10] but spend a fraction of what we do on health care.

Prevention in health care is a Cassandra's truth: While public health experts raise the alarm, doctors and patients alike balk at the suggestion of taking money away from "real" treatments to fund the promise of preventive care. The underutilization of prevention is a consequence of economics, the medical-industrial complex, Western civilization, and most fundamentally, human psychology. We value that which is scarce. When diagnosed with metastatic cancer and given months to live, each day becomes treasured. People are willing to spend tens to hundreds of thousands of dollars, sometimes bankrupting themselves and their families, for mere additional months. American health care expenditure is, on average, $80,000 in the last year of life. The entire field of oncology is predicated upon the innate desire for incremental life extension. But in the years prior to their diagnosis, many bristle at the thought of paying $30 for a monthly gym membership or an extra $5 for a salad. Prior to disease, life and health feel abundant and expendable; after diagnosis, life becomes scarce and treasured. We all conceptually understand that we're going to die, but often do not act as though we're mortal until it's too late. Study after study has shown that young people wish they had more money, while older people regret the amount of time they spent pursuing money, and instead wish they had more time with friends and family. When money is scarce, we pursue it blindly; when time becomes scarce, our priorities flip in an instant.

In youth and in old age, we are left disappointed, longing for that which we lack. It would therefore seem wise to outwit our own psyche, to live with a "death-conscious" rather than a "death-denying" mentality. As individuals, we could invest more time in healthy hobbies and friendships while young, knowing that money comes with age, while health dwindles. As a society, we could invest in our youth, providing them with tax breaks and supplemental income to eat and live healthfully and enjoy life. Given that Americans routinely describe college as their happiest time, we could design cities like college campuses, where walkability and public transport allow for close communities and spontaneous friendships unimaginable to our alienating, low-density suburban lifestyle. We would evolve past the idea that, in a world of eight billion plus humans, everyone needs to become special, famous, and successful, and instead focus on doing meaningful work in our small circles. With more investment in a healthy, stress-reduced youth, we would ideally also develop a healthy acceptance of growing old. We would learn to take pride, and even see beauty, in gray hair and wrinkles. Having lived wildly and well while young, we would enjoy the maturity that comes with age. We would gladly pay forward the wealth of old age, donating to our children and communities so they can enjoy their youth rather than taking coffers of cash to the grave. We would have discussions with family about death, what kinds of medical interventions we'd want, and which we wouldn't. We would live out our lives peacefully and healthily, content to take those medicines that extend our quality of life, while avoiding "heroic" medical interventions that would add days to weeks to a pitiful, subhuman existence in a cold, empty hospital room. We would then die at peace, hopefully in the comfort of our home surrounded by loved ones, as humans have done for millennia. This scenario may seem alien compared to our current way of living and dying, yet it is entirely possible, and psychologically far healthier.

All of our most basic fears and maladaptive habits are further exacerbated by our rapidly evolving world. Technology has connected people like never before, empowering miraculous innovation, but also envy, spite, greed, and misinformation. We are bombarded with images of others appearing to be much happier and more successful than ourselves. We are fed the information we seek, creating a crowd mentality that shuts down dissenting opinions and echo chambers that parade blatant falsehoods as facts. Public health has been particularly endangered by erosion of trust in medical expertise and recommendations. In fact, public trust in doctors and hospitals has never before been this low. Hovering around 70% before the COVID-19 pandemic, trust in health care among all demographic groups dropped to 40% with the pandemic, and never recovered.[11] The rhetoric of some of our leaders, who are willing to deny truth for political gain, has emboldened other charlatans and exacerbated these issues. I recognize that this book may not be appreciated, or even read, by the people who need it most. But the direness of the status quo cannot be an excuse not to try, either to write the truth or to read about it.

I am as guilty as anyone of perpetuating our current nightmare. I have spent too much time seeking money and accolades and too little time building friendships and hobbies. I live and work with people like me and rarely venture into foreign social circles. I have prescribed treatments that probably would not help at the insistence of patients and their families. In doing so, I have cost society millions of dollars. In writing this book, I cannot absolve myself of all my mistakes, but I can share them to try to prevent others, and society at large, from making the same mistakes over and over. Today, the US spends around $15,000 a person on health care each year, more than any other country.[12] As health care costs balloon and health disparities widen, our current neglect of cancer prevention is becoming simply unsustainable. As was stated in the opening of the Nuremberg trials, "Civilization cannot tolerate [these wrongs] being ignored, because it cannot survive their being repeated." Our health care system simply cannot survive cancer prevention being ignored.

In summary:

- Cancers arise due to genetic changes (mutations) that disrupt DNA repair, cell division, and immune surveillance.

- Half of cancer deaths are attributable to preventable risk factors: lifestyle or environmental factors that increase the risk of mutations.

- Only 3%–5% of health care spending goes toward prevention, although money spent on prevention has the highest yield in reducing cancer deaths.

CHAPTER 2

What Goes Around

Viruses, Bacteria, and Other Microbes

Support bacteria—they're the only culture some people have.
—Unknown

*I was hoping I was going to get an ulcer. I was hoping
to boost my research career by developing a bleeding ulcer.*
—Barry Marshall

Barry Marshall held a vial of bacteria that he had cultured from the gut of an ailing patient. He looked at the cloudy liquid and sniffed the putrid scent to confirm the bacteria were alive and well. Marshall believed the bacteria he had grown had the potential to cause stomach cancer, and in doing so, rewrite modern medicine. Then, without hesitation, he drank the bacteria in the name of science. Now he just had to wait.

He and his mentor, Robin Warren, working at the Royal Perth Hospital in Australia, had finally grown the elusive *Helicobacter pylori* (*H. pylori*) bacteria in 1982. Since the late 1800s, pathologists looking at autopsies of those with stomach inflammation (gastritis) or stomach cancer had identified these comma-shaped bacteria under the microscope when stained with silver. But while the bacteria happily sat right upon the stomach lining, irritating the cells underneath, nobody could find a way to grow them in the lab. While most bacteria grow quite readily on standard agar plates, *H. pylori* is a fastidious microbe, requiring very particular conditions to grow outside the body. As no one could grow it, the bacterium was forgotten for almost a century. That changed in 1982, when after years of unsuccessful attempts to grow *H. pylori*, Marshall and Warren inadvertently left a plate out for triple the time specified in the protocol, only to come back and see it chock-full of the elusive microbe. Much like Alexander Fleming's discovery of penicillin, a fateful accident resulted in a momentous discovery.[1]

But even with their success, the medical community still refused to recognize *H. pylori* as a major cause of gastritis. So, what if the bacteria were seen in patients with stomach disease? Over half the world suffers from gastritis. There are more bacteria cells in a person than there are human cells. Who was to say that *H. pylori*, *specifically*, was the root cause of stomach inflammation and cancer? For centuries, stomach ulcers had been attributed to stress, not bacteria. "To gastroenterologists, the concept of a germ causing ulcers was like saying the Earth was flat," Marshall quipped. He was convinced he had found the real culprit, but he didn't have a smoking gun. "It was so frustrating to see ulcer patients having surgery, even dying, when I knew a simple antibiotic treatment could fix the problem."[2]

But how to prove it? To give the bacteria to patients as part of an experiment would be clearly unethical. In 1985, with nowhere else to turn, Marshall had only one choice to prove his hypothesis beyond the shadow of a doubt: He drank the *H. pylori* himself. Sure enough, within weeks he started developing symptoms of gastritis (reflux, heartburn, burping), and when his fellow doctors went to get a sample from his stomach, they found the *H. pylori* replicating like wildfire. The evidence was indisputable. *H. pylori* causes stomach inflammation, ulcers, and ultimately, cancer. Thankfully, Marshall was able to cure his infection with antibiotics and went on to win the Nobel Prize in Medicine in 2005 for the discovery, alongside his mentor Warren.[3]

Marshall was, without a doubt, brave to choose to drink the flask of bacteria. But he was also privileged to have the choice in the first place. We now know that over half the world's people are infected with *H. pylori*.[4] Most people in developing nations live with some baseline level of stomach inflammation due to these bacteria. Why some of them develop stomach cancer, and others do not, remains unknown. But when Marshall pinched his nose and swallowed the vial of *H. pylori* for science, he was unwittingly actually joining the ranks of most of humankind.

Viruses, bacteria, and fungi have existed alongside humanity for our entire history. They even played a central role in creating us! Viruses replicate by using the host's DNA replication machinery. In the process, they can spread pieces of DNA between the individuals they infect, almost akin to how bees pollinate flowers. In fact, nearly one-tenth of our DNA comes from viruses that left their mark on our genomes over millions of years. While 99% of this viral DNA is "junk" that does not do anything, on rare occasions, these viruses can change the course of evolution. Evidence suggests that 160 million years ago, a virus enabled our mammalian ancestors to develop a placenta and thus give live birth.[5]

Viruses aren't the only microbes we've learned to live with. Millennia before the discovery of penicillin, Neanderthals may have been eating fungi for their antibiotic properties, or at least so we think from analyses of their teeth.[6] Common diseases of the blood like sickle cell anemia and thalassemia (another type of anemia) evolved multiple times, across continents, and served to improve our ancestors' survival against one nasty parasite: malaria. Clearly, microbes have been part of us forever. And yet, we've learned that nearly 20% of global cancers are caused by viruses, bacteria, and other microbes. From hepatitis causing liver cancer and lymphoma to HPV causing cervical and head and neck cancers to a Middle Eastern parasite called *Schistosoma* causing bladder cancer, the examples are endless. Anywhere in the body that microbes establish a base, driving our immune system wild and causing inflammation, cancer can follow.

Thankfully, in the developed world, the proportion of cancers caused by microbes is diminishingly small, only around 3%.[7] Public health initiatives like vaccination and sanitation have significantly improved our quality of life over the past century and are imperative in developing nations to reduce global cancer burden. However, a wave of misinformation, mistrust, and austerity threatens to undermine our progress and reverse some of the greatest health achievements of our species.

H. PYLORI AND STOMACH CANCER

Like Warren, Rudolf Virchow was a pathologist, a doctor who studies disease. Working at Humboldt University in Berlin in the 1850s, he dissected thousands of cadavers, searching for clues to account for the deaths. In his time, autopsy was a very imperfect science, but Virchow was seeking to standardize it. He would come to be known as the "father of modern pathology" and among his peers, the "pope of medicine."

One of the discoveries he is best remembered for is "Virchow's node," known medically as the left supraclavicular lymph node. Lymph is the fluid collected in the tissues all around the body and returned to the blood through the thoracic duct above the heart. On its way back to the heart, lymph passes through multiple clusters of nodes housing immune cells, which filter the fluid, searching for bacteria. The lymph is also how most cancers travel through the body. Cancer cells often get deposited in the nodes along the way, stimulating the local immune cells and causing the nodes to grow. As such, swollen, firm, painless, or fixed lymph nodes are considered high-risk physical exam findings for cancer. In many cases, these lymph nodes are cut out so they can be evaluated under a microscope.

Virchow, our nineteenth-century pathologist, identified a specific lymph node in the groove above the left clavicle (collarbone) that was enlarged in many of the cadavers he studied. When he probed further, he recognized that all of these individuals had died of stomach cancer. Thirty years later, French pathologist Charles Emile Troisier would correlate this lymph node with many other cancers, including breast, colon, prostate, bladder, and kidney, as well as syphilis and tuberculosis. Because most of the body's lymph passes through that same duct in the left side of the chest, it seemed that cancers from all over the body would deposit cells in that group of lymph nodes along the way.[8] However, it is important to note that Virchow originally described the node as related to stomach cancer, which was probably far more common in Germany in his time. The culprits, as we've discussed, were the microscopic, ubiquitous bacteria *Helicobacter pylori*.

These bacteria have been infecting human stomachs long before even Virchow's time. In fact, the temple of Asclepius from the fourth century BCE, dedicated to the ancient Greek god of medicine, mentions stomach ulcers probably caused by *H. pylori*. Quite fittingly, Asclepius's rod with a snake wrapped around it, which has now become a universal symbol of medicine, may have derived from the practice of threading parasitic Guinea worms out of the skin—another reminder of the diminished role such infections play in many of our lives today.

Today, despite the near eradication of *H. pylori* in many developed nations, gastric cancer is still the fifth most common and third most deadly cancer worldwide.[9] Among cancers of the lower stomach, 90% are still associated with *H. pylori*.[10] Meanwhile, gastric cancer of the upper stomach seems to arise by a different mechanism, associated with reflux and obesity. Overall, untreated *H. pylori* appears to increase one's odds of developing gastric cancer in the next 10 years about sixfold.[11]

The vast majority of people infected with *H. pylori* pick up these bacteria within the first year of life. For most people, they lie dormant, never causing trouble. The bacteria colonize the lining of the stomach, aggravating the immune cells underneath in certain individuals. The stomach boosts its acid production to fight off the bacteria, causing heartburn and stomach ulcers (which themselves may become cancerous). Our inflammatory cells, in an attempt to clear the infection, dump pro-inflammatory signaling molecules, wreaking havoc on the neighboring stomach stem cells. These stem cells, responsible for regenerating the ever-sloughing lining of the stomach, are deliberately hidden away in crypts to avoid damage from all the acids and toxins of the stomach. But when the *H. pylori* response goes into overdrive, even their little alcoves get caught in the crossfire. All it takes is one of these stem cells, which by design can replicate indefinitely, to sustain enough mutations to start cloning itself uncontrollably. That's how we get gastric cancer from *H. pylori*. The bacteria can also drive the inflammatory cells themselves to become cancerous, resulting in what's called mucosa-associated lymphoid tissue lymphoma. Thankfully—amazingly—this lymphoma (that is, cancer of the lymph, or immune, cells) actually tends to resolve on its own when the *H. pylori* is treated and inflammation subsides.

What's also fascinating is that while over half the people living all over the world have *H. pylori*–associated stomach inflammation, fewer than 0.1% of them develop gastric cancer. Different strains of *H. pylori*, some more irritating to the stomach than others, account for part but not all of the variability. For instance, while nations in East Asia, where *H. pylori* is common, have a gastric cancer risk up to 10 times that of the US, the cancer rate in India, where *H. pylori* is *even more common*, is actually around the same as in the US. Apparently, the interaction of genetics, diet, and lifestyle choices (like alcohol, smoking, and physical inactivity) *with H. pylori* accounts for the discrepancies in gastric cancer risk. For example, East Asians and Indigenous people of the Americas[12] have the highest rates of stomach cancer worldwide. What they have in common (besides *H. pylori*) is a high consumption of smoked and preserved meats in their diet. As we will discuss in a later chapter, unsurprisingly, diet plays a large role in the development of gastric cancer. Epstein-Barr virus (EBV), the virus that causes mononucleosis, or the "kissing disease," also seems to account for 5%–10% of gastric cancers, and the risk of cancer is compounded in those with both infections. While the virus is prevalent (endemic) around the world, East Asians also seem to have higher rates of EBV-associated cancers.[13]

Interestingly, while *H. pylori* causes almost all lower stomach cancers, some studies suggest that it actually *protects against* gastric cancer of the upper stomach. This type of cancer has grown more than sevenfold in developed nations like the US, coinciding with increasing obesity and the eradication of *H. pylori* due to better hygiene.[14]

H. pylori infection is also associated with lower rates of esophageal cancers, asthma, and obesity, leading to what has become known as the "hygiene hypothesis." The thinking goes that growing up with a small, baseline amount of inflammation, such as from *H. pylori* infection, may help regulate the immune system and prevent it from going into overdrive later in life. However, this hypothesis is largely based on comparing rates of disease between developed and developing nations. Because there are so many variables to control for, it is impossible to know whether *H. pylori*, or something else entirely, contributes to the differences we've noted. What we can say for certain is that *H. pylori* contributes to stomach inflammation, ulcers, and cancer, and should be treated with antibiotics and acid-reducers when diagnosed. It is safer to develop children's immune systems in other ways than not treating an *H. pylori* infection, as we will discuss in later chapters.

H. pylori is not just a problem due to its cancer-causing properties. *H. pylori* accounts for over 80% of all stomach ulcers;[15] besides creating a risk of cancer, ulcers can be excruciatingly painful or can bleed profusely. My parents trained as doctors in the Soviet Union. They've told me many stories of how, when they finally fled to the US and had to retake their exams here, they realized that so much of the medicine they had been taught was flat-out wrong. Dismissing Marshall's and Warren's discoveries about *H. pylori* in 1985 as "imperialist, capitalist propaganda," the Soviet Union did not teach its doctors to treat the infection with antibiotics (at least during my father's time). Instead, a common treatment for stomach ulcers was the vagotomy—a surgical procedure that involves cutting one of the largest nerves in the body to reduce stomach acid production. I knew several of my grandparents' friends, all burly Russian men, who had this procedure done. The complications of such a major operation are numerous, from diarrhea to gallstones to vomiting.[16] To this day, Russia and Eastern Europe have some of the highest rates of *H. pylori* and gastric cancer, in part due to their government's failure to trust and disseminate scientific results. As we shall see throughout this book, our society, too, suffers its fair share of mistrust of scientifically established facts.

Anyone with recurring upper abdominal discomfort, acid reflux, or belching should discuss their symptoms with their primary care provider. They will likely prescribe a class of antacids known as proton pump inhibitors. Untreated stomach acidity and inflammation, in and of itself, is a leading cause of stomach and esophageal cancers. If the acidity does not respond to the medicines, and especially if you or anyone in your household is from a developing nation or high-risk community, consider undergoing testing for *H. pylori*. While much of the world coexists with these bacteria, for those who didn't grow up with it, *H. pylori* is often more than we can stomach.

A URINARY PARASITE AND BLADDER CANCER

H. pylori is not the only globally prevalent microbe contributing to cancer risk. *Schistosoma* is a group of protozoa, or microscopic animals, that we colloquially label "parasites." Technically, a parasite is any organism that depends on another and often directly or indirectly causes harm to the other. Some parasites are more horrifying than others, and some are the stuff of nightmares.

Schistosoma larvae are released from snails that live in fresh water in warm climates. Upon contact with the water, these larvae penetrate our skin and irritate our bladder and intestines. The larvae mature and release their eggs in our urine and feces, which hatch in fresh water to repeat the cycle over and over. Makes you think twice before going for a swim, huh? Today, over 250 million humans worldwide are infected with

Schistosoma, though only about 75 million of them (30%) are receiving treatment.[17]

After malaria, *Schistosoma* is probably the second most deadly parasite worldwide. Some scientists estimate that globally, nearly 30 million years of disability-free life are lost due to this parasite, which is also called a blood fluke.[18] Particularly affected are people in developing nations, living in poverty and without access to clean water.[19] We take for granted blessings like clean water and sanitation, while the billions of people living without them are under constant threat of infection and death.

Untreated infection with *Schistosoma* (schistosomiasis) has two main medical consequences: bladder cancer and portal hypertension. *Schistosoma haematobium* (its scientific name) remains in the bladder, triggering immune cells known as eosinophils to go haywire trying to eliminate it, but to no avail. First one may notice blood in the urine (hence the name "haematobium"); after decades, the irritation results in scarring or cancer of the bladder and urinary tubing. Similarly, another group of *Schistosoma* affects the intestines, causing abdominal pain, diarrhea, and retained fluid; this ultimately puts too much pressure on the liver (the organ tasked with filtering blood from the intestines), resulting in liver failure.[20]

Bladder cancer is the sixth most common and ninth most deadly cancer worldwide. Today, 90% of cases arise from urogenital, or "transitional," cells, and these cancers are most commonly associated with tobacco smoking and occupational exposures to toxic chemicals. However, the remaining 10% are squamous cell cancers of the bladder, which are all caused by one nasty culprit: *Schistosoma*. In areas of the Middle East and Africa where *Schistosoma* are endemic, bladder cancer due to the parasite is the *second most common* cancer diagnosed. Liver cancer is the most commonly diagnosed cancer in these areas of the world, and it is also caused by endemic microbes, which we will discuss next.[21]

Disinfection of drinking and bathing water and avoidance of freshwater swimming and wading in areas where *Schistosoma* is endemic could help prevent thousands of cases of bladder cancer worldwide. As with many other parasites, the ecological range of *Schistosoma* has broadened due to global climate change. Travelers should seek professional guidance before entering or consuming fresh water in developing nations, and if exposed (or planning to get exposed) consult a health care provider about preventive medication. Thankfully, the oral antiparasitic medicine praziquantel is highly effective, although is not yet readily available in many of the developing areas where it is needed most. Vaccines against the parasite are currently under development. However, even without vaccines, there is hope. As it relies on humans to reproduce, the parasite has been successfully eradicated by mass drug administration campaigns in many countries, including Japan, Tanzania, and most of the Caribbean.[22] Unfortunately, sometimes in public health, it seems as though no good deed goes unpunished.

LIVER VIRUSES AND CANCER

Until recently, schistosomiasis was the greatest public health hazard in Egypt. In 1918, British physician John Brian Christopherson discovered that a combination of toxins—antimony salt and tartar emetic—could be injected into the bloodstream to kill the parasite. Incidentally, Christopherson would later become famous as one of the pioneers of another infusible toxin: chemotherapy for cancer. By the 1950s, the Egyptian authorities decided they had had enough of the schistosomiasis menace, and they decided to implement a massive campaign to eradicate the parasite with Christopherson's formula. Over the next 30 years, over 36 million intravenous infusions were given to nearly 5 million patients. Unfortunately, little did they know that in the process of combatting schistosomiasis, the authorities were actually fanning the sparks of Egypt's newest public health crisis: hepatitis C virus.[23]

The sterilization techniques employed in Egypt's campaign were inadequate, since at the time the dangers of viruses and sharing needles were not realized. With millions of needles to keep track of, and six to nine injections indicated per person, many needles were reused between patients.[24] It didn't help that in over 80% of cases, hepatitis C has no acute clinical symptoms, meaning patients can carry the virus for decades without knowing they have it.[25] All these factors combined led to an explosion of cases of hepatitis C in the decades following the public health campaign. Ironically enough, hepatitis C has now replaced schistosomiasis as the leading cause of liver disease in Egypt (though those infected with both have the worst risk, with nearly half developing liver cirrhosis).[26] In some areas, over 40% of blood samples test positive for hepatitis C. Thankfully, the development of oral medicines against *Schistosoma* began to replace the injections in the 1970s, and more recently, we've developed successful oral treatment for the previously incurable hepatitis C as well.[27]

There are now five main types of hepatitis virus, named A, B, C, D, and E. These viruses have next to nothing in common with one another, except that they all infect the liver. Hepatitis A and E cause nasty acute symptoms like profuse vomiting and diarrhea, but after several days, the body usually successfully heals (clears) the infection. Hepatitis C, on the other hand, is stealthy. The body fails to clear the infection in nearly all people infected; in fact, over 80% don't know they even have the virus, until it's too late. Hepatitis B falls somewhere between the two, with most patients clearing the infection but about 10% going on to develop chronic liver disease. Lastly, hepatitis D is hepatitis B's dependent little brother, as it cannot infect anyone without hepatitis B by its side. The two have evolved to help one another while destroying the liver.

As the hepatitis viruses unwaveringly replicate in the liver cells, they draw the ire of the body's immune system surveillance. T cells begin to recognize the viral particles and attack them, destroying the liver cells harboring the virus in the process. This is the inflammation of viral hepatitis. If the immune system defeats the infection, as is the case in hepatitis B over 90% of the time, the inflammation stops and the liver regenerates. If the infection cannot be eliminated, as in most cases of hepatitis C, the inflammation becomes chronic, and the liver is slowly destroyed from within. As fewer liver cells are available to fulfill their function, the liver fails, with harsh consequences. Several of the liver's primary jobs include filtering toxins from the blood from our intestines and eliminating metabolic byproducts like bilirubin into the stool. When the liver begins to fail, patients' skin may get yellowed (jaundiced) and itchy from bilirubin, which begins to accumulate throughout the body. One of the worst-case scenarios is when the liver fails much like a water filter in your home's plumbing, resulting in a backup of blood in the gastrointestinal tract. The blockage results in a high-pressure buildup that stretches the already-thin blood vessels of the esophagus, resulting in swollen blood vessels or lymph vessels. These can rupture and cause life-threatening blood loss or even result in a patient choking on their own blood.

Chronic liver disease, most commonly due to excess alcohol use, obesity, and viral hepatitis, exists on a continuum. On the very end of the continuum is cirrhosis, which is irreversible scarring leading to liver failure. The only cure for cirrhosis is liver transplant. The other steps along the way, such as steatosis (fatty liver) or steatohepatitis (fatty and inflamed liver), are likewise irreversible. But with treatment of the underlying cause, the progression to cirrhosis can be delayed or halted. At any point along this continuum, a rogue liver cell, mutated by the virus or the body's caustic immune response, may go off the rails and begin to replicate uncontrollably. If the cell and its progeny overcome all the body's immune defenses, the patient will eventually be diagnosed with hepatocellular carcinoma (the scientific word for cancer), or "primary" liver cancer ("secondary" liver cancer due to metastases, usually from the colon, is more common, but it is treated like the original cancer as opposed to liver cancer). Liver cancer can arise from any stage of liver damage, but the risk is greatest when a patient has reached cirrhosis. In fact, cirrhosis due to the hepatitis C virus causes the greatest risk of liver cancer, with as many as 30% of cirrhosis patients developing cancer over the next five years.[28] People with hepatitis C, many of whom have no symptoms and are unaware of their disease, may compound their cirrhosis risk with further injury to the liver, through alcohol use and obesity (which, as we will discuss later, causes the release of pro-inflammatory signaling molecules from fat cells). In order to prevent this fatal cascade, all adults aged 18–79 in the US are recommended to receive screening for hepatitis C; many older adults may have contracted the virus from a blood transfusion decades ago, before blood products were thoroughly tested.[29] Targeting the three main causes of liver failure—viral hepatitis, alcohol consumption, and obesity—would prevent the vast majority of liver cancers.

Primary liver cancer is the sixth most common and fourth most deadly cancer globally. Because it is prevalent across most of Asia, hepatitis B remains the leading cause of liver cancer worldwide. In developed nations, thanks to mandatory neonatal vaccinations, alcohol has surpassed hepatitis B as the dominant cause of liver cancer. In the US, hepatitis C, with an estimated 2.4 million cases, remains more common than hepatitis B, with estimates ranging from 730,000 to 2.2 million. Both viruses claim more lives in the US than HIV (human immunodeficiency virus) but garner significantly less attention. Since hepatitis C was not discovered until the 1990s, it was primarily spread by unsafe blood transfusions in the years prior. In fact, the US Centers for Disease Control and Prevention (CDC) now recommends that all adults born from 1945–1965 get tested for hepatitis C, since their risk of having the disease has been estimated as high as 3%.[30] Today's targeted antiviral agents, first approved in 2014, can cure hepatitis C with a 95% success rate, but they cannot undo the liver damage, and subsequent cancer risk, from the virus. Unfortunately, today only one in three Americans receive timely treatment for hepatitis C, largely due to under-diagnosis or poor insurance coverage.[31] Thus, it is estimated that universal testing for hepatitis C could save upward of 120,000 lives per year, constituting a very successful example of secondary prevention.[32]

Hepatitis B, meanwhile, is more varied in its transmission and disease course. It can be spread by blood, semen, childbirth, and even oral secretions (like kissing). It can cause acute symptoms upon infection, but it doesn't have to. Similar to hepatitis C, as many as 70% of people with the virus do not know they carry it. While only 15% of those with chronic infection progress to liver cirrhosis, about 25% develop liver cancer, with many by-passing the cirrhosis altogether. Hepatitis B is clearly more un-predictable, and that's part of what has made it so dangerous. In the US, the primary source of hepatitis B is immigration from nations where the virus is common. Some countries even re-quire proof of negative hepatitis B testing to visit or immigrate. Asian Americans and Pacific Islanders represent about 6% of all US citizens but over half of all hepatitis B patients.[33] However, when it comes to new infections, the rate for Black Americans is actually double that of Asian Americans.

Unlike hepatitis C, hepatitis B could be entirely eradicated with a comprehensive, global vaccination program. And unlike the $24,000 price tag of the cheapest hepatitis C treatment,[34] the hepatitis B vaccine retails for less than $100 in the US. In fact, vaccination at birth prevents 90% of transmissions of the virus from mothers who have hepatitis B. Public health initia-tives to vaccinate in middle- to low-income nations have saved an estimated 38 million lives and $81 billion, constituting one of the greatest public health successes in modern history. And yet, over half of all babies born today are not receiving the hep-atitis B vaccine. If they did, twice as many lives could be saved.[35] For patients infected with chronic hepatitis B, antiviral drugs like those used for HIV can help control the disease and prevent the development of liver cancer, but they must be taken one's entire life (unlike hepatitis C, hepatitis B is unlikely to be cured). Additionally, patients with hepatitis should undergo regular liver cancer screenings, beginning at age 40 for women and 50 for men, to catch liver cancer early, before it spreads and be-comes incurable.[36]

While infant vaccination in the US has been widespread and successful, the current vaccine rate for those 19 and older is only 30% in the US, and adult-onset hepatitis B has actually been increasing. Many patients and even providers are unaware of the latest recommendations. As of 2022, the CDC now recommends that health care workers and all adults aged 19–59 receive additional vaccination, as well as adults over 60 with risk factors such as recent travel or diabetes. Most of us in medicine are already required by our employers to test our levels of hepatitis B antibodies regularly to prove that we still have vaccine protection, and if it has waned, get a booster. Considering that hepatitis B vaccination is far more effective before the onset of chronic liver disease, and liver disease cannot be undone, the CDC estimates that universal vaccination against hepatitis B would actually pay for itself many times over.[37] Unfortunately, these recommendations come at a time when vaccine hesitancy is at an all-time high, particularly among Black Americans, who have the highest rates of hepatitis B infection.[38] As we will discuss in later chapters, engaging groups culture-consciously is crucial to any successful public health intervention.

At your next annual visit, discuss adult hepatitis B vaccination and hepatitis C testing with your health care provider, especially if you've got any underlying chronic medical conditions, are immunocompromised (meaning your immune system is not working normally), have any international travel plans, or are otherwise high risk, such as experiencing homelessness or using injection drugs. Any individual who meets these criteria, as well as all men who have sex with men, are also recommended by the CDC to receive the hepatitis A vaccine as an adult. Make sure to get tested for hepatitis B before starting any immunosuppressive medications. Patients with hepatitis or any history of cirrhosis should get screened for liver cancer with ultrasound and blood tests every six months. Lastly, although unsafe blood transfusion practices were largely to blame for the hepatitis C and HIV epidemics of the past decades, today's blood donations undergo rigorous testing, and your risk of transmission of either of these viruses via transfusion is under one in a million.[39]

AFLATOXINS

Hepatitis B and C, however, are not the only infectious source of liver cancer. While we've already covered bacteria, parasites, and viruses in this chapter, there's one more class of infectious organisms to consider: fungi.

By the sheer number of deaths, the most dangerous fungus, worldwide, is probably the mold *Aspergillus*. In patients who are immunocompromised or have chronic lung diseases like asthma, *Aspergillus* can cause life-threatening infections. However, by and large, *Aspergillus's* cancer risk and death toll come not from infection but from what *Aspergillus* produces. This fungus grows in warm and humid climates in the soil, below crops such as wheat, corn, peanuts, and cottonseed. While it grows in the soil, it produces a family of poisonous, cancer-inducing toxins called aflatoxins, which can contaminate the crops above. If those crops are fed to animals, for instance, their meat can also get contaminated. The disease was first discovered in the 1960s, when over a hundred thousand turkeys around the London area died from contaminated peanuts in their feed. The toxin can also spread through the skin, typically of farmers handling crops.

Overall, aflatoxins are estimated to account for some 3%–20% of all liver cancer cases. The wide variation comes from the fact that areas high in aflatoxin, such as East Asia, also have a hefty prevalence of hepatitis B, and these risk factors work synergistically to increase liver cancer risk over 30-fold. In many areas of sub-Saharan Africa, aflatoxins are, by and large, the greatest cause of liver disease and cancer.[40]

Thankfully, the US and other developed nations have strict regulations to monitor aflatoxin levels in our crops. However, climate change has made conditions for the fungus more favorable. As much as 25% of food waste around the world is now due to aflatoxin contamination.[41] Besides the cancer risk, the sheer loss of food is responsible for millions of deaths.

Even in the US, not all crops are tested rigorously. Many rural farmers do not have access to the latest testing equipment, and outbreaks and recalls are increasingly common. The damage of aflatoxins to the liver is cumulative, and even though they may be unavoidable in our food, minimizing intake is the best means of liver cancer prevention. Children and adults who are immunocompromised (from, for example, HIV/AIDS [acquired immunodeficiency syndrome]) or malnourished are at highest risk. Avoiding moldy foods and washing all fruits and vegetables for at least five seconds with water is recommended.[42] Meanwhile, soap, detergent, and bleach are currently *not* recommended, as regular consumption of these harsh agents comes with its own risks. Rinsing with water also helps wash away pesticides, which are toxic; among the most commonly bought produce, including strawberries, lettuce, nectarines, spinach, and peppers, over 90% test positive for pesticides.[43]

Aspergillus may not be quite the apocalyptic fungus shown in horror movies, but it is slated to contribute to thousands of liver cancer deaths across the globe.

TO CATCH A VIRUS

The microbes we've discussed so far are the most commonly implicated in carcinogenesis, but the list is far from exhaustive. Countless microbes are so obscure that their cancer risk has not been studied, and countless others still wait to be discovered. But perhaps the more fascinating ones are the microbes that are exceedingly common.

Epstein-Barr virus, or EBV, is the virus that causes mononucleosis, the "kissing disease." It belongs to the same family of viruses as herpes and chickenpox. An estimated over 90% of the world population has been infected with EBV. And yet, most of us recover without any consequences. Many aren't aware they've ever had it at all. However, decades later, an unlucky minority will get a vast array of cancer diagnoses associated with the virus.

EBV infects the liver, the oropharynx (mouth and throat), and the B cells, antibody-producing immune cells. With this in mind, the initial symptoms of EBV make perfect sense: sore throat, abdominal fullness, and immunosuppression. The spleen, which houses many B cells, swells as it gets infected, and is at risk of rupture; this is why athletes are advised to avoid contact sports for at least three to four weeks following infection. For patients who are not immunocompromised, the infection gets cleared by the body's immune system and symptoms vanish without a trace—or so we thought.

Studies have since implicated EBV in the development of liver, gastric, and nasopharyngeal cancer (cancer of the nose and pharynx), most commonly in East Asians, and the development of Burkitt lymphoma in Africans. The mystery of how the same virus causes such different cancers, in different groups of people, is still being elucidated, but one hypothesis is that it has to do with its interaction with other microbes. In East Asia, EBV seems to synergistically collaborate with hepatitis B to cause liver cancer and with *H. pylori* to cause gastric cancer. In Africa, EBV in combination with malaria or HIV results in the greatest risk of lymphoma.[44] Strangest is the case of nasopharyngeal carcinoma, which seems to occur almost exclusively among EBV-infected patients in southern China. Even when people emigrate from the region, their risk of this elusive cancer follows them. It seems that something about their immune response to EBV specifically predisposes them to this niche cancer. Thankfully, screening for EBV and nasopharyngeal cancer are becoming increasingly common in southern China; providers all around the world should be aware of this rare disease if they treat southern Chinese patients.[45]

Sometimes awareness is the hardest part for a health care provider. I recall one time in medical school when I was seeing an elderly woman in the hospital with advanced brain lymphoma. Like most patients with the disease, her cerebrospinal fluid had tested positive for EBV, though she had no recollection of ever having the disease. As the cancer spread in her brain, and we tried various drugs and radiation to stop it, the adjacent parts of her brain got swollen and compressed. Every day, she complained of a new symptom: headaches, dizziness, pain, pressure. Nothing seemed to help. After she had spent weeks in the hospital, her ever-evolving complaints were dismissed by the doctors and residents, who were drowning in patients to see. But I, as a medical student, had the time to sit and listen to her and her family. It felt fitting then that one morning, of all the providers who saw her, I was the first to notice that her left side was weaker than her right. Admittedly, I also questioned and even dismissed my findings as another case of "the boy who cried wolf." But when several minutes later half of her face began to droop, the team quickly mobilized a stroke alert and moved her into a scanner. Ultimately, she was found to have worsening swelling, and even bleeding, of the brain, and she passed away in the subsequent days. At first, I beat myself up for not having addressed the weakness sooner, knowing full well it probably would not have changed anything. But when her daughter reached out to thank me for the attention I had shown them, I was reminded of the value I could provide to patients and their families just by listening. She was a victim of EBV-induced brain cancer and of the aggressive chemo and radiation used to treat it. But she didn't have to be a victim of a heartless medical system, too.

On that same rotation in medical school, I remember seeing a patient who had an aggressive case of advanced T-cell lymphoma. Like my previous patient, he also had a cancer of immune cells, but in this instance, it involved T cells instead of B cells. His was also a cancer caused by a virus—the esoteric but aptly named human T-cell lymphoma virus 1, or HTLV-1 for short. For unknown reasons, this virus predominantly infects patients in Japan, the Caribbean, Central Africa, and the Pacific Islands. In Australia, it infects predominantly Aboriginal people, with as many as one in every two people in this group testing positive. Overall, some 5–10 million people are known to be infected, though the real value is probably much higher.[46] As with EBV, it seems that something about the immune system of people with certain ethnic backgrounds makes them more susceptible, in the same way that a lack of diversity of immune complexes (due to a small population of founders) among Native Americans made them particularly susceptible to smallpox. But when it came to my unconscious patient, whose body was shutting down as cancer cells overtook each of his organs, the virus at the root of it all hardly seemed to matter.

As the situation grew bleak, we arranged a family meeting to discuss next steps, such as trying a new experimental drug or discontinuing treatment altogether. This patient's only relative in the US was his sister, who came with their pastor. At first, they were shocked to learn of just how dire his situation was. But as they came to terms with the reality, they both spoke of an option we had never considered. When asked what he would want if he were awake, they both confidently said to go back home to Liberia and pass away in his village, with his family. Given the condition he was in, we recognized this as an unrealistic request, but said we would try our best nonetheless. The next day, almost miraculously, our patient regained consciousness. His sister had known him well. When she explained his situation, he concurred that he did not want any further treatments—only to board a plane and return home. Despite the objections of insurance companies, administrators, and even airlines, the doctors were able to get him enough supplies, pain meds, and steroids that he could safely board an airplane. We never heard what happened to him afterward, but I would like to think he died surrounded by his loved ones in the land he pined for. In retrospect, it seems a much better place to go than a cold, sterile, lonely hospital room in the dead of winter in Philadelphia.

Medicine should be all about listening, collaborating, and compromising to allow our patients to best live the lives they desire. Prevention should be much the same; to be successful, we must embrace human nature and go with peoples' natural tendencies, not against them. Telling high school or college students to abstain from kissing or other forms of intimacy is an unrealistic, and overly prudish, means of trying to lessen the spread of mono. But advising them not to share water bottles, or to quarantine while sick, or to avoid contact sports for a few weeks (down from previous recommendations of *months*) all seem perfectly realistic.

Microbes exist all around us, in quantities unfathomable. To avoid all of them we would have to live in a bubble, and even

then, we would probably prove unsuccessful. Public health interventions aimed at mitigating or eliminating the specific
pathogens responsible for the bulk of human disease have been
some of the best success stories of the past century. In 1900, the
life expectancy in the US was 47 for white men and 33 for Black
men, and the top three causes of death were pneumonia, tuberculosis, and gastrointestinal infection—cancer was eighth on
the list, not far above diphtheria. Today, infectious causes don't
even crack the top 10 causes of death, and most developed nations have life expectancies around 80 years.

We often attribute our "defeat" of infectious disease to antibiotics, but by the time penicillin became widely available in
1945, US life expectancy had already risen to 66 years. The bulk
of the progress had been made before penicillin by improvements in sanitation, filtration and chlorination of drinking
water, and improved nutrition.[47] The revolution against infection began not with Alexander Fleming's discovery of penicillin in 1928 but with John Snow's tracing of cholera to the Broad
Street water pump in London in 1854.[48] In the retelling of infectious disease history, as in oncology history, we have neglected prevention in favor of cure.

Some of these histories are humanity's most remarkable
success stories, which we should be striving to replicate. The
original meaning of "vaccine" comes from the Latin for "cow,"
because British physician Edward Jenner had described in 1796
how inoculation with cowpox could prevent the much more
deadly smallpox. Funnily enough, George Washington had already made a similar discovery some 20 years earlier and inoc-
ulated his troops against smallpox to help stave off a pandemic.
While the Americans won the Revolutionary War, the British
got credit for the first vaccinations. Fast forward two hundred
years to 1980, when the World Health Organization officially

declared smallpox—the disease that had decimated the hundred million plus people of the Americas—eradicated.[49]

This feat was not achieved by vaccinating every individual on Earth; that would have been impossible. Instead, public health workers painstakingly tracked down every new case of the disease, and vaccinated anyone who could have been exposed (known as contact tracing). They formed bonds with local leaders to ensure cooperation in surveillance. After two centuries of scientific development, and two decades of committed contact tracing, smallpox died not with a bang but a whimper. The last person to contract the disease, in 1978, got it from a lab conducting virology research. There haven't been any such missteps since.[50] One can imagine that if the same funding and commitment were applied toward hepatitis B, we could rid the world of millions of cases of cancer for decades to come.

Prevention can be difficult and often lacks the same glory as a cure. The surgeon gets to cut a tumor out of a person's lung; the oncologist gets to see a tumor shrink with her chemotherapy. But cancer prevention requires acknowledging and appreciating all of the disease and suffering that *could* have been but *didn't* appear, thanks to our efforts.

While infectious disease may often feel like a battle that we've largely won, the past few years have humbled our pride. COVID-19 swept across the world like a wildfire as our attempts at quarantine and prevention fell short. Infectious diseases that belong in history books, like tuberculosis, syphilis, and measles, have all created more cases than expected over the past years. Homelessness, crowding in prisons, and lack of safe-sex education and resources (as we'll discuss in the chapters to come) are creating the same conditions, ripe for infectious disease, that plagued the US a century ago. The frightening reality is that, in many aspects of public health, we may actually be plunging backward. It was public investment in sanitation and clean water that overcame cholera. It was a $1 million investment by John D. Rockefeller in shoes, public bathrooms, and antiparasitic medications that eradicated hookworm across the American South.[51] It must be investment in schools, communities, science, and health care, across the world, that will overcome the ever-lurking microbes of our time.

In summary:

- The bacterium *Helicobacter pylori* increases the risk of stomach ulcers and cancer, but it can be easily treated with antibiotics if diagnosed.

- *Schistosoma*, a freshwater parasite in North Africa, causes bladder cancer.

- Hepatitis B and C, viruses spread by blood, sexual activity, and childbirth, are a leading cause of liver cancer worldwide; infants should be vaccinated and adults screened with blood tests.

- Aflatoxin, produced by the fungus *Aspergillus*, causes thousands of liver cancer deaths, mainly among farmers in developing nations.

CHAPTER 3

You Are What You Eat

Foods and Toxins

*Eat an apple on going to bed and you'll keep
the doctor from earning his bread.*
—Earliest recorded version of "An apple a day,"
Wales, United Kingdom, 1866

I say let the world go to hell, but I should always have my tea.
—Fyodor Dostoevsky, *Crime and Punishment*

Food is life. At its most basic, food provides the nutrients and energy necessary for the body to function. It fuels growth, repairs tissues, and supports the immune system, making it essential for health and survival. Beyond mere sustenance, food is deeply intertwined with culture and tradition. It reflects heritage, identity, and the history of a community or nation. Meals often serve as social rituals that bring people together, fostering a sense of belonging and shared experience. Holiday feasts, family recipes, and communal dining are examples of how food transcends mere sustenance to become a source of connection. Food is foundational to economies and livelihoods, from farming and fishing to restaurants and food industries. We've organized civilizations around food, discovering hundreds of animals, plants, and fungi that can be eaten, and innovating thousands of ways to prepare and enjoy them. But some of these meals are better for our health than others. Everything we eat spends an average of 42 hours passing through our body, and over that time, faces numerous opportunities to be absorbed into our bloodstream or affect the millions of cells lining our stomach and intestines. The foods we ingest affect each of our organs on a molecular level, including their risk of becoming cancerous. Fundamentally, we *are* what we *eat*.

MEAT AND CANCER

It's early in the afternoon, you've just gotten home from work, and your wife asks you to pick up some groceries for dinner. She plans to serve meat and potatoes, and she needs you to swing by the store to pick up some ketchup. You make your way down the bustling sidewalks to the local corner store and ask the clerk for some ketchup, only to realize you have no idea what kind. Mushroom? Anchovies? Alcohol? As a nineteenth-century ketchup consumer, you've got many options. However, you must choose wisely. These are the days before Heinz invented the glass bottle, so you can't really see what you're buying. Your ketchup is probably made of all sorts of leftover, or even rotten, ingredients, such as juice from pickled mushrooms or last season's tomatoes. Nonetheless, you know ketchup is essential! Like many nineteenth-century women, because the refrigerator has not been invented, your wife is cooking with rotting meat, and she needs the ketchup to mask its putrid smell and taste. In fact, it's a common belief that tomato ketchup, invented by a doctor named James Mease in 1812, actually prevents gastrointestinal disease from meat.[1] Today we know there may even be some truth underlying the hype: the acidity of the ketchup neutralizes certain bacteria in the meat, such as *H. pylori,* a stomach-cancer-causing bacterium. But unfortunately, even tomato ketchup won't help you dodge the many health dangers of the typical 1800s diet.

During the nineteenth century, populations were riddled with stomach cancer. We've already discussed the leading contributor, *H. pylori,* which has been experimentally *proven* to cause stomach ulcers, that over decades develop into stomach cancer. We are now learning of a myriad of other dietary risk factors that may have caused gastrointestinal cancers throughout history, and many are still relevant today.

In the days before refrigeration, processed, pickled, and even rotting foods were commonplace. Meat could be made to last longer by curing (think salami or pepperoni), which involves processing with chemicals called nitrates and nitrites. These additives help retain color and flavor, improve shelf life, and prevent bacterial growth. While the techniques have changed over time, the concept of preparing meat so it doesn't go bad is ages old. Centuries ago, meat was preserved through ancient curing techniques with salt, which made salt more valuable than gold in the ancient Roman empire (workers were paid in salt, hence the word "salary" comes from "sal," the Latin root for salt). These salts naturally contained nitrates and nitrites, which helped to preserve the meat. In the nineteenth century, scientists isolated the nitrates, then nitrites, and started using them in isolation to preserve and flavor meat. Along with ketchup, this novel technique for curing meat became the next great innovation for food during this time. Unfortunately, we now know that through the same mechanisms these compounds kill bacteria, they also damage the human cells lining the stomach, leading to stomach and colon cancers. Along with *H. pylori,* smoked or processed meats became a leading contributor to gastric cancer, which for a few decades reigned as the most common form of cancer.[2]

Today, the International Agency for Research on Cancer (IARC) classifies processed meats as Group 1 carcinogens, the highest (worst) ranking possible.[3] This ranking is well deserved. Experiments have shown that the compounds in meat processing, like nitrites and nitrates, cause mutations in cells that ultimately lead to cancer. These nitrogen compounds have been shown to reduce telomere (the end of a DNA molecule) length and drive cells into senescence, which is when cells shut down and stop dividing. However, a few unlucky cells prove contrarian, gaining a mutation that flicks the switch to lengthen their telomeres and overcome the body's safeguards. Mutated and ravenous, these cells don't know when to stop dividing—the definition of cancer.[4]

France, one of the leading consumers and producers of cured meats in the form of *charcuterie*, announced in 2022 regulations to limit these additives in processed meats, and many countries and companies have since followed suit.[5] Nitrate- and nitrite-free salamis are becoming more common in stores, and are a good option for reducing cancer risk (although the salt, saturated fats, and numerous other chemicals in these meats still make them a source of protein that is less than ideal). All deli meats, even those advertised as nitrate free, will inevitably contain more chemicals than freshly prepared meats. When it comes to processed meats, you really *don't* want to know "how the sausage gets made."

In contrast, nonprocessed red meats, such as beef, pork, and lamb, are classified by the IARC as Group 2A, or "likely" carcinogens.[6] These meats appear red because they contain more myoglobin, a protein in muscle, than poultry or fish. But more muscle and fat in the meat also means more inflammatory signals that our bodies absorb, and more rich tissue that our metabolism has to process, creating cancer-causing byproducts.

Red meats have been associated with an increased risk of stomach and colon cancer in many observational trials, but experimental results have not been enough to *prove* that red meat causes cancer (and given the diversity of types of red meat and their prevalence in global diets, it would be rather difficult to study in a clinical trial). There are also many confounding variables. High red meat consumption is associated with the classic "Western" diet rich in refined sugars and alcohol, which themselves increase cancer risk. In other words, we can't know whether it's the steak, or the wine and mashed potatoes that go with it, that's truly causing cancer. It is also difficult to parcel out how much of the likely cancer-causing effect of red meat is due to preservatives such as nitrites and nitrates, versus other mechanisms, such as pro-inflammation signaling molecules. Lastly, the preparation of the meat further muddies the picture. Grilling and frying at high temperatures create carcinogenic compounds, which may increase cancer risk independent of the actual meat. In summary, while processed meats are very likely to cause cancer, the data around red meat is less certain. Nonetheless, the American Institute for Cancer Research (AICR) recommends limiting red meat to 12–18 ounces per week, which equates to about 1 small serving every other day.

Many people have taken to cutting red meat out of their diet entirely for health reasons. India, composed of predominantly Hindus who do not eat beef (and some who eat no meat at all), and Muslims who do not eat pork, has some of the world's lowest rates of colon cancer.[7] In the US, some have labeled eliminating red meat the "pollotarian" ("pollo" means "chicken" in Spanish) diet—with chicken, fish, cheese, and plants replacing beef and pork as sources of protein. Without a doubt, cutting out red meat is good for cholesterol and overall caloric intake, and thus reduces risk of heart attack, stroke, and obesity (although certain cuts of lean pork may be no more caloric than chicken). The evidence around the cancer preventative benefits of abstaining from eating red meat, however, remains controversial (bear in mind, it would probably take decades of red-meat avoidance to see the benefit). Nonetheless, today around 10% of Americans have rejected meat entirely, and now identify as vegetarian or vegan. Observational studies have found a 31% reduction in prostate cancer and a 43% reduction in colorectal cancer rates among vegetarians (although consider that other factors may explain some of these differences—for example, vegetarians are more likely to be highly educated, drink and smoke less, and exercise more).[8]

The data supporting veganism is the most robust. One study of biological twins, which controlled for genetics and many of the other "confounders," found that the twin who adopted a strict vegan diet saw reversals in signs of cellular aging within just 8 weeks—with an average "age reduction" of about 0.6 years.[9] Admittedly, these estimates are based entirely on a type of DNA modification called methylation, which has *not* been clinically correlated with actually living longer. Eight weeks of a vegan diet was also found to reduce cholesterol and fasting insulin (which, in the long term, means lower risk of heart attack and diabetes), as well as facilitate weight loss.[10] Veganism and vegetarianism make our cells appear healthier. We can even look back (retrospectively) and see that vegans, on average, live longer, but without a forward-looking (prospective) trial that controls for all the variables, we can't *know* whether it's because of the veganism or because of all the confounders that come with veganism. Such a large-scale trial would take decades and cost millions of dollars, so the chances we'll ever have a definitive answer are slimmer than a rib of celery.

Even with vegetarianism at record highs, on average, Americans still consume more meat per capita than any other nation: 250 pounds per person per year.[11] Setting aside cancer risk, lowering meat consumption (particularly red meat) is proven medical advice for heart health and obesity, as well as the environment (producing meat creates far more greenhouse gas emissions than growing vegetables). While chicken or lean pork are better than beef, the AICR still recommends limiting any meat to three ounces per plate—making meat more of a condiment than star of the dish. Replacing meat with protein-rich plant products like tofu, tempeh, and legumes has added benefits, such as cancer-protective fibers, which support our microbiome to suppress inflammation. We will explore this further in future chapters.

PICKLED FOODS

As a medical student in an oncology clinic in South Philadelphia, I recall meeting an elderly Japanese woman, accompanied by her granddaughter. The grandmother would always come early, and never alone. I remembered my own experience as a high schooler, accompanying my grandmother to her oncology clinic appointments to translate. I related to the girl at her grandmother's side, and perhaps that's why I still remember her. At first glance, the patient looked far younger than the age of 85 written in her chart, but she was gaunt, weak, and wheelchair bound. She had metastatic gastric cancer, and it was eating her alive. She could no longer eat without vomiting, and she and her family did not want a PEG (percutaneous endoscopic gastrostomy) tube, an onerous surgical feeding tube for nutrition (a decision I agreed with wholeheartedly). Like many of my elderly patients who were from East Asia, she was stoic, offering one-word answers and denying any pain, even as the cancer out-stripped her internal organs. Her family wanted her to try an-other line of therapy, but she seemed resigned to her fate. She had outlived her husband and many of her children and rela-tives, and was left tired and alone in a facility trying to build back strength that she no longer had. Extrapolating from her age, she had lived through a war that left her country in ruins, a painful national reconstruction, an arduous immigration process, and now a new cancer diagnosis and two lines of toxic chemotherapy. I couldn't blame her for wanting to stop.

We ultimately agreed to transition to hospice care, and she was able to live out her remaining weeks at home, with her grandchildren, nurses, and ample pain and nausea medicine. At the conclusions of our visits, she would always try to prop her-self up from her wheelchair to give a bow as she said "Arigato" ("Thank you"). At the final visit, she no longer had much strength, but she summoned all she had left to bow her head. I bowed back and wished her farewell, knowing this was likely to be our last.

This patient was but one of countless East Asian patients I have taken care of who developed gastric cancer, which is a rel-atively rare cancer in the US. But in Japan and Korea, the rate is over four times higher, and it is the most common cancer.[12] Many Japanese figures, from esteemed author Mitsugu Saotome to the most famous samurai, Miyamoto Musashi, have fallen to the disease. Even East Asian immigrants to the US continue to have a much higher rate of gastric cancer as compared to other Americans. Without a doubt, the cancer-causing stomach bug *H. pylori* explains some of this disparity, but not all of it. For one thing, about two-thirds of the world's population is infected with *H. pylori*, but Japan and Korea, specifically, bear the brunt of gastric cancer diagnoses. The other major factor is probably pickled and salted foods.

Pickled vegetables and noodles are staples of the Japanese and Korean diets. The process of pickling, which involves fermentation with high concentrations of salt, is common in many colder climates to preserve produce through the winter. Even soy sauce is produced through salty fermentation with certain molds of the family *Aspergillus*. While the Japanese diet, typically high in vegetables and fish and low in meats, likely contributes to lower rates of obesity and longer life expectancy than in the US, it does come with the nasty side effect of gastric cancer risk. It seems that salt, especially in a fermented liquid, wears away at the lining of the stomach, causing something called "atrophic gastritis." Over decades, this destruction of the stomach lining leads to mutations and stomach cancers. Observational studies of East Asian populations reveal about a 50% increased risk of stomach cancer associated with high intake of pickled foods.[13]

Interestingly, as many East Asian nations adopt more components of the "Western" diet, it seems their rates of gastric cancer are falling, while their rates of obesity are climbing.[14] With globalization, many nations find themselves trading one evil for another.

Thankfully, Japan and Korea have implemented standard gastric cancer screening with endoscopy every 2–3 years for all adults above 40–50 years old, allowing for earlier detection of cancers and increasing the chance of curative surgery. In the US, our relatively low rates of stomach cancer do not make endoscopic screening "worthwhile" for all patients (and thus it is not regularly prescribed or covered by insurance). However, some doctors suggest that immigrants of Japanese or Korean origin might still benefit, especially if they are having any symptoms, such as heartburn, abdominal pain, or weight loss.

These screening programs constitute secondary prevention, or an attempt at detecting disease early to intervene and prevent some of the problems associated with the disease. Primary prevention, that is, preventing stomach cancer in the first place, would be best achieved with decreasing intake of pickled and high sodium foods. Substitutes such as low-sodium soy sauce and fresh vegetables give many health benefits besides decreasing cancer risk—namely, reducing high blood pressure and kidney disease (although recent studies implicate insulin resistance and obesity in high blood pressure, rather than salt).[15] Today, we even have sodium-free salt substitutes such as potassium chloride, which provide the same or more "saltiness" to food without the negative impacts on blood pressure. Whether these new salts affect gastric cancer remains to be seen, but I regularly recommend salt substitutes to my patients who have high blood pressure, as long as they don't have bad chronic kidney disease. Unfortunately, these sodium-free substitutes are expensive; a small 3-ounce *potassium* chloride salt shaker sells for $6–$10. Curing meats and pickling vegetables are age-old adaptations that served our ancestors well, but in the era of global food production, refrigeration, and even salt substitutes, we are finding new ways to enjoy our favorite recipes without harming our health.

AFLATOXINS

While we are fortunate to often know and choose the toxins we eat, many under-resourced farming communities worldwide are exposed to foodborne toxins without even eating the food, just by virtue of their jobs. The most common and deadly of these are aflatoxins, which is produced by a fungus species called

Aspergillus that grows on stores of peanuts, corn, and grains. Aflatoxins account for anywhere from 25 to 155 thousand cases of liver cancer globally each year, 40% of which occur in sub-Saharan Africa. These toxins are breathed in, absorbed through skin, or consumed on foods and processed by the liver, resulting in powerful toxic byproducts that accumulate in liver cells and cause mutations that lead to cancer. Even in countries where aflatoxins are prevalent, workers who do not deal directly with the crops, such as those in paper mills, waste management, or textiles, have been shown to have increased risk of aflatoxin-induced liver cancer, probably due to airborne exposure. To further complicate the picture, many developing nations with high rates of aflatoxins also have high rates of hepatitis B, which work synergistically by two different mechanisms to cause liver cancer.

The burden of aflatoxin-induced liver cancer falls upon the impoverished, often equatorial nations we rely upon to produce our cheap and year-round produce. We benefit from the food, and they suffer from the consequences of food production. Consequently, these nations often do not have the resources to mount large public health initiatives to wipe out the fungus. We should take responsibility for our food's production and invest in resources and education on safe farming practices, which have been shown to decrease aflatoxin risk.

ARECA NUT

Caffeine is America's most popular drug. Ninety-four percent of Americans get their daily caffeine fix, mostly through coffee, tea, and sugary energy drinks. For many, the hustle and bustle of twenty-first-century life demands more energy than we can naturally muster. In Southeast Asia and Polynesia, a different abundant stimulant—but a deadly one—is commonly used: the areca nut.

Commonly known as betel quid, areca nut is a plant that has been used for centuries, both recreationally and as part of rituals. A compound in the nut creates stimulating and psychoactive effects by antagonizing the gamma-aminobutyric acid (GABA) receptors, which is the exact opposite mechanism of alcohol. As expected, chewing these nuts makes you more alert, causes euphoria, and even helps suppress appetite, a welcome side effect in a region with prevalent food insecurity. On many islands, while food is scarce, areca nuts are indigenous and plentiful. Polynesian nations such as the Solomon Islands have some of the highest usage, with as much as 77% of the population regularly partaking.[16] Unfortunately, these nuts also account for over half of oral, head, and neck cancer cases in Southeast Asia and Polynesia.[17] Besides the compounds that stimulate the brain, the nuts contain numerous other toxic compounds, which probably evolved to keep animals like us from eating them. Over time, the irritation they cause to our mouth and throat lead to cancer. To add insult to injury, many people worldwide add tobacco to areca nuts to increase their stimulatory properties, which in turn increases the cancer risk. In combination, chewing tobacco and areca nut increase throat cancer risk far more than either alone, as much as 10-fold.

Fortunately, public education and health initiatives have succeeded in curbing areca nut usage. For instance, in northern Thailand, head and neck cancer rates dropped 200%–300% after a concerted campaign to educate young adults about the danger.[18] While highly addictive, areca nuts are still less addictive than tobacco, requiring an average of 5 attempts before successful cessation (compared to 11 attempts for tobacco smoking).[19]

In the US, certain refugee communities have continued to import and use areca nuts. Programs to improve health literacy, in particular by engaging community leaders, have proven most successful at stopping their use.[20]

HOT BEVERAGES

As the child of Soviet immigrants, I am no stranger to hot tea. In fact, tea is the most popular beverage around the world. It was developed originally in China as far back as four thousand years ago. Legend has it that emperor Shen Nung asked his servants to boil water under a tree, when the wind blew and some of the tree's leaves fell into the water.[21] The emperor tried the water with boiled leaves, and tea was born. From China, it spread across the globe, with countries that received it by land trade, like Russia and India, naming it "chai," and nations that obtained it by sea trade, like England and Spain, naming it "tea." Thousands of years later, around the 1400s, goat herders in Ethiopia learned to boil coffee beans to stay awake, and Muslin, Jewish, and even Viking traders soon spread coffee across the Middle East and Europe.[22] Together, these two hot beverages allowed millions to avoid waterborne bacteria through boiling, while also providing stimulatory processes that enabled workers to keep up with the demands of the industrial revolution. However, as with nearly all pleasurable things in life, there is a dangerous side to hot beverages: esophageal cancer.

Observational studies of populations that drink copious amounts of scalding hot beverages have uncovered a twofold increased risk of a certain type of upper esophageal cancer, called esophageal squamous cell carcinoma.[23] This cancer appears distinct from esophageal adenocarcinoma, the much more common esophageal cancer in the US, which is associated with obesity and acid reflux. Instead, esophageal squamous cell cancer is associated with chronic irritation of the esophagus, and has been mostly observed in nations that smoke tobacco and/or drink very hot beverages. Chief among them are Turkey and Iran, where tea is traditionally drunk hot, above 158°F (above 70°C).[24] In fact, Turkish coffee is traditionally served taken directly off coal embers. Consequently, Turkey has the highest rate of esophageal squamous cell cancer. If the beverage is hot enough to burn your mouth, it's hot enough to burn your esophagus, and the repeated cycle of burning and healing creates ample opportunity for mutations to develop and cancer to form. It is important to note, however, that coffee and tea at slightly cooler temperatures are considered completely safe, and still very pleasant, or even more pleasant. All things considered, if unsweetened coffee or tea replace drinks like soda and sugary juices, they're probably preventing cancer (we will discuss the link between caloric intake and cancer in the chapter to come). In fact, most Americans already prefer drinking their hot beverages at cooler temperatures, between 120°–140°F, which are much safer for the esophagus. So next time you're served a piping hot cup of joe, let it cool for a few minutes, if not for your tongue, then for the sake of your esophagus.

FALSE FLAGS

By the same token of repeated irritation and reflux exacerbation, some researchers hypothesized that carbonated beverage consumption, such as soda, would also increase the risk of esophageal cancer. However, a large study run by the National Cancer Institute actually found the opposite: Soda consumption was associated with *fewer* cases of esophageal cancer.[25] This finding was attributed to the fact that most participants drank diet soda, and thus actually had lower risk of obesity, compared to their counterparts who drank sweet juices and other sugary non-carbonated drinks. Ultimately, soda, particularly diet soda, is completely safe, from an esophageal cancer perspective. But it does raise the interesting point that health today may depend less on what you eat, and more on how much you eat.

Another similar "false flag" culprit that has been somewhat exonerated is the artificial sweetener aspartame. Since its introduction in the 1980s, evidence of aspartame causing cancer in animal models was glorified as clear evidence of its carcinogenic properties in humans. But the latest studies suggest the amounts that caused cancer in rats far exceed what an average person would consume. The IARC has deemed aspartame to have "limited evidence" as causing cancer, and the World Health Organization has affirmed a safe daily intake of 40 mg/kg, which would constitute 9–14 cans of diet soda a day for an average adult. While diet beverages are not without risks, they remain better for your health than nondiet options (with plain water, tea, or black coffee still the healthiest options—at a reasonable temperature, of course).

Although often credited to Mark Twain, it was actually British satirist Jonathan Swift who said, "A lie can travel halfway around the world before the truth can get its boots on."[26] Many of the facets of modernity have been unfairly implicated in causing cancer. For instance, there is no evidence that microwaves, power lines, or cell phones cause cancer (although heating food on plastic may leech chemicals into your food). Despite some worrying laboratory studies, no evidence in people suggests that aluminum and other chemicals in antiperspirants increase the risk of breast cancer.[27] Similarly, despite rumors that soy "mimics" estrogen and can lead to breast cancer, studies have actually found that people who eat more soy products like tofu and soymilk have a *lower* risk of cancer (probably because plant foods have less fat and thus cause less inflammation than animal products, as we'll discuss in the next chapter).[28] Early studies suggested that a compound in burned foods and dark roast coffee, called acrylamide, may have caused certain cancers, but more recent studies have called these findings into question as well.[29] Of course, it's impossible to *prove* a negative, so researchers have trouble saying with certainty that something does *not* cause cancer.

There are far too many myths about cancer-causing foods to debunk in one book, let alone one chapter. Your best bet to answer any specific question would be—believe it or not—to search for it online, and to trust only reputable websites like award-winning professional news outlets (NPR, CNN, *The New York Times,* etc.), prestigious hospitals and universities (University of Pennsylvania, Mayo Clinic, Harvard, etc.), and legitimate organizations (American Cancer Society, National Institutes of Health, National Women's Health Network, etc.). Any food sold on the shelves of reputable stores will not "cause cancer" in isolation. But the excess calories and high-risk chemicals that are prevalent in the typical Western diet certainly increase our chance of developing cancer.

PROCESSED FOODS

Aside from the few examples discussed above, most foods are not specifically linked to cancer, nor proven to prevent cancer. Celebrities like Tom Brady may flaunt their diet, restricting everything from dairy products to tomatoes, but such ascetic choices have no basis in evidence. Instead, diet ought to be viewed holistically and foods considered in major groups rather than singled out as individual "junk foods."

In particular, high consumption of ultra-processed foods that have copious added sugar, salt, and preservatives has been associated with 23% increased risk of head and neck cancer and 24% increased risk of esophageal cancer in observational studies.[30] Besides adding chemical preservatives of doubtful safety, ultra-processed foods usually reduce or eliminate the natural ingredients (protein, fiber, and healthy fats) that make food nutritious and filling and replace them with shelf-stable added sugars and salts. When we take grains, fruits, or vegetables and "process" them (even something as simple as blending fruit into a smoothie), we destroy some of the nutritional value of the fibers. Now consider your average cookie or cake sold in American grocery stores; there's basically nothing natural of any nutritional value left. Unfortunately, such ultra-processed foods (e.g., chips, white bread, cookies, cereals) are becoming increasingly common, now accounting for 71% of the American food supply! In fact, the rise of ultra-processed foods is believed to be one of the factors underlying the rising epidemic in early-age cancers.

Where does this leave American consumers? Avoiding 7 out of 10 items in the grocery store is unrealistic, especially on a budget. While ultra-processed foods may seem ubiquitous, all are not equally bad. For instance, sparkling water and air-popped popcorn are technically ultra-processed, but have relatively little added sugar, salt, or calories. The same goes for whole-grain granola, hummus, guacamole, and Greek yogurt. Consumers should seek foods that contain natural ingredients and are nutritionally valuable, meaning they're high in proteins, unsaturated fats, and/or fiber (which help keep you feeling fuller for longer) while low in added sugars and salt. While still controversial, added preservatives pose less of a danger to long-term health than obesity due to added sugars. Obesity promotes cancer, as we'll discuss in the next chapter.

Of course, the best way to guarantee nutritious food is to cut out the middlemen (the processing) and go straight to the source. For each packaged and one-year shelf-stable snack, healthier alternatives exist. Replace white bread and cookies with whole-grain breads and fresh pastries, potato chips with dried vegetables or nuts. Instead of snack bars or fruit-based treats, which hide copious amounts of added sugars, consider unprocessed snacks like nuts, fresh fruits, and dark chocolate. As a rule, the fewer processing steps there are between a food source and your mouth, the healthier the food. Even foods classically demonized, like cheeses and meats, can be relatively healthy (in moderation) when opting for a less processed option (think fresh mozzarella ball over "American" cheese, or lean cuts of chicken and pork over deli meats). After all, the French and Italians routinely eat pastas, cheeses, and pastries, and yet live on average a decade longer than their American counterparts. While dietary recommendations can be changeable and difficult to keep track of, whenever in doubt, just google it! Most major newspapers, magazines, and medical institution websites will offer reputable dietary advice, but be wary of anyone selling you particular diets or products. It doesn't take a medical degree, nor an overpriced kale smoothie, to eat healthfully.

In science, particularly when it comes to dietary recommendations, we must always remain humble and keep an open mind toward change. Recommendations have changed drastically over the last decades. In the 1970s, doctors began to disparage fats and cholesterol, recommending that people avoid foods such as butter and eggs, and instead opt for fat-free alternatives like margarine. Today, we've learned that sugars and processed foods contribute far more to obesity, cholesterol (heart attacks and strokes), and even cancer risk than fat does.[31] Fructose, a sweetener derived from corn, is particularly harmful but ever present in our diet due to the legacy of corn subsidies.[32] Meanwhile, protein from eggs and unsaturated fats from plant sources, like olive oil and avocado, have come full circle, and are now key components of a healthy diet. Dietary recommendations need to evolve with science, and we must avoid confusing the pursuit of truth with blindly following dogma. The medical community's decades of advocacy against fat, despite obvious holes in the data, was probably responsible for millions of early deaths. Today, I'd like to think we know better. We rely on organizations like the aforementioned IARC and AICR, who hire world experts to analyze and evaluate all the data before issuing their recommendations.

We've discussed how smoked and red meats, pickled foods, piping hot beverages, and ultra-processed foods are all associated with cancer risk. But what *to* eat is as important as what *not* to eat. The latest science in nutrition suggests that the optimal diet for reducing cancer risk is one high in fiber, such as found in fruits, vegetables, and grains. When eaten, that fiber is difficult to digest and absorb; instead, it hangs around in our intestines, where it sustains a whole ecosystem of bacteria called the microbiome. Perhaps most importantly, fiber helps us feel full, but unlike simple sugars, it does not get quickly absorbed into our bloodstream and consequently into fatty tissue. The less processed the grains—such as quinoa, brown rice, and whole wheat, the greater the concentration of fiber relative to excessively caloric simple sugars. As a rule, the closer a food is to its original state, the lesser the concentration of added sugars or cancer-causing artificial compounds. Besides grains and vegetables, poultry, fish, and other lean meats are important sources of protein, but they should be eaten in moderation—less than three ounces per meal. Substitutes like tofu and beans may be even better for our health and for environmental sustainability. Equally important is trading sugary (or artificially diet) beverages for water, tea, coffee, or whatever other low-sugar or no-sugar alternative you prefer. Our ancestors on the African plains evolved scavenging scraps of marrow from bones and subsisting on vegetables, tubers, and unprocessed grains, and these are the foods groups that remain healthiest, even in the modern day. As we will discuss in the next chapter, total calorie consumption affects cancer risk far more than any individual food by modulating obesity, and in turn, inflammation. But making broad modifications to diet, by optimizing proportions of food groups and opting for "whole foods," can reduce calorie consumption while also minimizing exposure to carcinogens in our food.

Ultimately, the age-old adage "You are what you eat" holds true in more ways than one. Our ancestors used innovations like smoking, curing, and pickling to preserve their foods, and these techniques became part of our cuisines and cultural identities. Today, we are learning to make subtle substitutions in their famed recipes, utilizing modern scientific findings to reduce toxin consumption in our diet. Our diet reflects our priorities as a society, with nearly every culture having developed some form of stimulant, whether tea, coffee, tobacco, or areca nut, to keep up with the demands of work and life. But in a broader sense, our diets reflect our ways of life. In importing foods from around the world yearlong, we have optimized our lives while subjecting the planet to greater greenhouse emissions and exposed impoverished farmers to the inherent dangers of aflatoxin (as well as the near-slavery working conditions rampant in the production of many crops, like chocolate and coffee). We are able to eat gluttonously and have grown accustomed to addictive, sugary foods with no nutritional value, fueling a raging obesity epidemic, as discussed in the next chapter. Food is fundamental to human history, culture, daily life, and even cancer prevention. We truly are *what* and *how* we eat.

In summary:

- Cured and processed meats (like deli meat) are known to increase gastrointestinal cancer risk; you should minimize consumption of these foods.

- Red meat, like beef and lamb, probably increases colorectal cancer risk; limit it to 12–18 ounces a week.

- Pickled foods are associated with gastric cancer, particularly in East Asian populations.

- Very hot (greater than 150°F) beverages increase the risk of throat and esophageal cancer.

- Ultra-processed foods (chips, cookies, cereal, etc.) may increase gastrointestinal cancer risk by about 20%; opt for whole grains, nuts, beans, fresh fruits and vegetables, and unprocessed meats and dairy products.

- If uncertain, google your foods, but stick to reputable institutions and newspapers.

CHAPTER 4

The Gift of Living Well
Diet, Exercise, and Obesity

*God gave us the gift of life; it is up to us to
give ourselves the gift of living well.*
—Voltaire

*Now you will not swell the rout
Of lads that wore their honours out,
Runners whom renown outran
And the name died before the man.*
—*To an Athlete Dying Young*, A. E. Housman

The other night I caught myself chowing down on chicken tenders and fries while listening to a didactic lecture on the obesity epidemic. The irony no longer struck me; tenders and fries are a staple (and often the only option) on night shifts in hospitals around the world. I remember hearing my mom's stories about how she subsisted entirely on french fries through her four years of residency, and I had promised myself I would do better . . . I had not. Tenders and fries, I soon learned, are the *only* option in the hospital cafeteria at night—that is, if it's even open. We often joke about how all our efforts in helping people live longer in the hospital are outdone by the cafeteria's facilitation of an early death. Whether it be the person with diabetes guzzling down juice until their blood sugar level flies off the charts, or the patient who recently had a heart attack ordering

71

KFC using Uber Eats to be delivered to their hospital room, food and health are intimately intertwined on the wards and in the clinic.

Hospital cafeterias are not unique in promoting a poor diet. My young cousin recently immigrated from Ukraine as a refugee, and almost immediately started gaining weight rapidly. Despite your preconceptions, she had not been starving back home, and actually enjoyed a healthy diet of grains like barley and fresh vegetables. But upon trying the pizza and nuggets that were staples of her school lunch, she started refusing the whole foods she'd previously enjoyed. My aunt would find sweets hidden in couch cushions, and hear from teachers how her daughter was begging for more money to buy cookies at lunch. These are scenarios experienced by concerned parents around the nation. If you ask most foreigners, they'll tell you American white bread tastes sweet like a dessert, our beverages are all sugary beyond compare, and our portion sizes at restaurants are comically large. After decades of corn and sugarcane subsidies, we are a nation hooked on sugar and artificial sweeteners, which some consider as addictive as cocaine.[1]

We are in the midst of an epidemic, with over 40% of Americans, and 1 in 8 worldwide, suffering from obesity. Obesity is defined as a body mass index (BMI) greater than 30, or the level at which excess fat is most likely to cause chronic health issues. When you include patients who are overweight (BMI greater than 25), you find that a whopping 75% (!) of Americans are above their ideal body weight.[2] Except for some well-intentioned immigrant grandmothers, we all know that obesity is bad for your health, especially when it comes to heart disease and strokes. It used to be thought that excess cholesterol from poor diet deposits itself in your blood vessels and cuts off blood flow to your heart or brain, leading to lifelong disability or death. Today, we know the process is much more complex; saturated fats, carbohydrates, and inflammation play a larger role in the cholesterol plaque deposits that lead to heart attacks and strokes.[3] However, drugs called statins that affect cholesterol transport can slow down this process. In the clinic, we often joke that adding statins to the water supply would prevent more deaths than anything we do as doctors. But the hazards of excess body weight far exceed just heart attacks. More and more, we are learning how fatty cells lead to a spiral of inflammation, which damages healthy cells and sets them on the path to becoming cancerous. Experts now believe obesity to be the primary risk factor behind the growing epidemic of early-age colorectal cancer, which has been increasing by about 2% every year.[4] It has claimed the lives of young celebrities such as Chadwick Boseman. Obviously, not all these individuals are obese, and much is unknown about why some people develop certain cancers while others don't.

It's not just colon cancer, and obesity is not the only life-threatening epidemic; we've seen a 79% increase (near doubling) in early cancers of all types over the past 30 years,[5] particularly breast, lung, stomach, and colon. One investigation found that 17 out of 34 types of cancer studied have become more common, and deadly, in millennials and Generation X, as compared to prior generations.[6] Obesity can't explain all of it, and this alarming phenomenon has scientists scrambling for answers, examining everything from pollution to ultra-processed foods. Regardless of the other causes, the rising rate of early-onset cancers is one of many lesser-known consequences of the obesity epidemic, afflicting celebrities, athletes, and everyday people, with no thought to the families it tears apart.

FAT AND INFLAMMATION

Fatty tissue is a means of storing excess energy, and this mechanism has evolved across animal species. On average, humans have 14%–31% body fat, compared to 9% in other primates, which speaks to our ancient ancestors' long periods of hunger as they made their way across the African plains.[7] The fat they carried allowed them to save excess energy from times of plenty for times of famine, facilitating our vast migration through different climates and across continents.

Fat has an important evolutionary role, but today it's gotten too big for our britches (literally). Excess fat has become a leading cause of cancer. Fat cells and the cancers they cause may be on opposite ends of the body, and separated by decades, but the two are inextricably linked. The prevailing theory is that as fatty tissue accumulates, it outgrows its own blood supply, leading to cell stress and death. This recruits immune system cells such as macrophages, which are tasked with cleaning up debris. They release further cytokines, or signaling molecules, that lead to a cascade of immune system changes that we collectively call inflammation.[8]

Inflammation comes from the same root as "flame," and it often refers to joints that have arthritis or gout or red, warm skin injuries that appear as though they have been "set aflame." This process is mediated by the very same cells and signaling molecules as the inflammation in fat cells. Yet unlike with our skin and joints, we do not see or feel the chronic inflammation brewing within our fatty tissues. The more fat an individual has, the more inflammatory molecules their body produces. These inflammatory molecules, meant to recruit our immune cells to reproduce to help clear out the debris, go into overdrive. Unable to distinguish friend from foe, they attack and kill healthy cells, leaking more debris that just perpetuates the cycle. Like Anakin Skywalker in the *Star Wars* series, or the soldiers of the Fourth Crusade during medieval times, the immune cells become like what they wanted to destroy: in this case, cellular dysregulation (impairment). The damage that results inadvertently creates the perfect environment for cancer development; cells leak hormones that fuel cancer and cause metabolic stress that damages DNA, creating more mutations. Mutations, defects in the blueprints that cells must follow, create faulty cells that turn cancerous when they can no longer understand their own instructions. Many years later, when the cancer that rose from these ashes spreads around the body, the fingerprints of the original inflammation remain. Studies of people with breast cancer have found that the more signs of inflammation are seen under a microscope in their breast tissue, the worse their overall prognosis (estimate of recovery) will be, regardless of their BMI.

Not all body fat is created equal. Brown fat, named based on its color under a microscope, gives off anti-inflammatory signals and helps mobilize our metabolism to produce body heat and burn calories. Brown fat is the "good" fat that evolved to help us survive long, harsh winters in northern latitudes in the eons before central heating. White fat, in contrast, is the true "excess fat." It accumulates when daily caloric intake far exceeds caloric expenditure, and white fat is what causes dangerous inflammation.[9] For various reasons, the fat stored around the waist is more likely to be white fat, while brown fat is more likely to be stored in the hips. This dichotomy is becoming increasingly appreciated in our evaluation of weight. Some doctors are now replacing BMI altogether with body roundness index (BRI) (questionably named, in my opinion), which is calculated based on waist size (instead of weight) compared to your height. BRI has been shown to correspond to poor cardiovascular outcomes better than BMI does. BRI also seems to better account for the racial bias of BMI; Black people seem to carry the same heart attack or cancer risk at a higher BMI than white people, largely because Black people (on average) carry more weight around the hips. BRI helps to adjust for that and provide a more accurate and achievable target for people of all races/ethnicities looking to get to a healthy weight (or perhaps a healthy "roundness").[10]

Obesity-related cancers like colorectal and breast are increasingly claiming the lives of those age 50 and below, shifting cancer away from just an old person's disease. In the hospital, we often say it's not the older, chronically sick patients who die first. It's usually the young mother or father who arrived relatively healthy who ends up on the brink of death the next day. In the emergency room (ER), they call this the "nice guy sign": being a young, kind patient, with a caring family, seems to increase their risk of dying astronomically. Although part superstition, it does bear some truth. The cancers that afflict young people tend to be the most aggressive, like acute leukemia, T-cell lymphoma, and testicular cancer. A young person's cells are full of replicative potential, with longer telomeres, allowing cancer to divide unchecked. Even among cancers that historically afflicted the old, such as colon or breast, when diagnosed in younger patients, these people die more quickly.[11] Anecdotally, I have seen octogenarians live for years with cancers that struck down 40-year-olds in months. When these young patients die of cancer, it can be particularly devastating, depriving young children and spouses of treasured loved ones. Families like my wife's grow up motherless. As Abraham Lincoln put it in the Gettysburg address, it's left "for us the living"[12] to mend the broken pieces.

With every birthday, this macabre realization worsens my generational anxiety. But it also lends urgency to the need to mend the obesity crisis. As innovative medicines for heart failure and evolving stenting techniques for heart attacks have drastically reduced the rate of heart disease deaths, cancer has quickly become the new frontier of death for the young and overweight. Curing cancer is not as easy as opening up a clogged blood vessel (and your cardiologist will be first to tell you that's no easy feat, either). Curing cancer means identifying tumors early enough to cut them out, and then often giving multiple cycles of toxic chemotherapy and/or unpredictable immunotherapy to help stamp out any surviving cells. Curing cancer means pouring millions into research to identify specific driver mutations, then millions more into creating molecules that inhibit those precise receptors, then millions more into organizing clinical trials to try to prove that the drug actually works (97% don't[13]).

But *preventing* obesity-driven cancer is much simpler. It can be as easy as revising school menus or opening grocery stores that serve fresh foods in underserved communities (and allowing food stamps to be used for healthy, cooked meals). Preventing obesity can take the form of disclosing calories and taxing certain ultra-caloric, ultra-processed food groups, or providing folks with low incomes with access to gym membership and the ever-prevalent weight loss medications. Prevention is, by far, the low-hanging fruit when it comes to obesity.

DIET AND EXERCISE

When it comes to weight loss, our society disproportionally focuses on exercise. Without a doubt, exercise has a myriad of health benefits. It keeps your heart strong and builds skeletal muscles, which consume sugar, staving off diabetes and thus reducing your risk of heart attack or stroke. But when it comes to strictly weight loss, over 60 studies have shown that diet is superior to exercise by 3 to 1 (with high-intensity, interval training outperforming slow and steady workouts, in terms of weight loss).[14] One's basal metabolic rate, or the calories you burn just by being alive, accounts for about 80% of all calories burned, leaving only 20% for exercise.[15] And if you've ever followed the calorie count on your treadmill or bike, you'll notice that the 300 calories you burn from an hour-long workout can be easily gained back with one pastry or avocado. The most effective way to lose weight is, unsurprisingly, to eat less. A recent study found that sustained calorie restriction of 12% led to an average 20-pound weight loss, reduction in inflammatory markers, and even improvement in muscle strength.[16]

How much you eat is often affected by *how* you eat. Our fast-paced, dopamine-craving lifestyles have made many people forget how to simply sit and enjoy food. Every day at work, I see people chow down on their lunch while staring at a computer screen, and at home I'm equally guilty of watching TV during dinner. When we pay attention to other things, we fail to pay attention to the actual act of eating, and we lose our body's own cues on hunger and satiation (being full). Many of us were taught from childhood to eat all the food on our plate. We've since forgotten how to hear that signal from our stomach telling us we're full, and we find ourselves eating so much we feel tired and bloated afterward. Instead, eating more slowly, chewing thoroughly, and paying attention to the food we're eating, without distractions, have all been shown to increase satiation and reduce hunger. Likewise, interspersing bites of food with sips of water, tea, or any other unsweetened beverage, can help our stomach get full faster. I've found that when I follow these recommendations, pause, and wait 5 to 10 minutes after finishing a modest portion, I actually start to feel full and lose all desire to eat more. It doesn't happen overnight, and it takes time to unlearn decades of bad habits and learn to listen to your body. Nobody knows this better than a person trying to get back into an exercise routine.

Even though diet is the largest contributor to weight, exercise is still lifesaving. Exercise works in synergy with calorie restriction; muscle growth results in greater calorie expenditure and thus less fat deposition. Muscle growth also causes reduced insulin resistance; this means that the insulin our bodies produce is able to do its job of moving sugars from our blood into our cells. If someone is insulin resistant, their insulin is not able to move sugars into their cells, and instead the sugars are deposited as fat. The US Centers for Disease Control and Prevention recommends at least 150 minutes of moderate-intensity physical activity for adults each week, with muscle-strengthening activities performed on at least 2 days per week.[17] Along with diet, physical activity can also facilitate weight loss. Exercising after eating stimulates muscles to take up sugar, reducing the spike in blood sugars and thus decreasing deposition of these excess calories into fat. Rather than focusing on the calories burned on the treadmill, the more accurate way to lose weight would be to use an online daily calorie calculator. These calculators factor in your age and exercise levels to estimate how many calories you should consume to meet your weight loss goals. Whether calorie restriction and weight loss can truly prevent cancer or increase lifespan is currently being investigated, but observations of "Blue Zone" areas around the world, where people routinely live to over 80, reveal some common trends: reduced life stress, physical activity, and natural, moderately restricted eating patterns.[18]

Of course, it's usually not that simple to lose weight, especially in our bustling, stress-ridden society. I have a line of patients out the door of my clinic saying they barely eat and keep gaining weight, and I have a line equally long of those who can't stop losing weight no matter how much they consume. Weight is part genetic, part hormonal, part volitional, and part luck (or at least part unexplained by modern science). Many find diets and exercise regimens to be Sisyphean; as soon as they stop to rest, the rock rolls right back down and the weight comes right back. Studies show that a variety of popular and crash diets do not result in weight loss in the long term, as the body decreases its metabolic rate to adjust to rapid changes in consumption,[19] and most people find they cannot sustain the tough restrictions that many diet and exercise regimens call for.

Fortunately, we are living on the edge of a revolution in weight loss medication. A class of drugs called glucagon-like peptide 1 (GLP-1) agonists, including Ozempic and Wegovy, initially approved for diabetes, have now gained US Food and Drug Administration (FDA) approval for weight loss. They are flying off the shelves, leading to worldwide shortages.[20] These medicines help patients decrease their weight by an average of 10–15 pounds in multiple ways, but chief among them is quite simply by decreasing appetite.[21] GLP-1s also send signals to push our metabolism into overdrive, helping us burn excess calories and reduce blood sugars. Through the various mechanisms that curb obesity-associated inflammation, GLP-1s have been shown to reduce risk of heart attacks and nonalcoholic fatty liver disease. They may even protect against Alzheimer disease. In addition, they've been shown to decrease the risk of 13 types of obesity-related cancers among diabetics.[22] But as anyone who's watched a drug advertisement knows, there are always side effects. Some patients end up getting so nauseated and unable to eat that they lose weight too fast, requiring a lower dose or stopping the drug altogether. Other patients develop "Ozempic face," where rapid loss of facial fat results in sagging and aged-appearing skin. Finally, some studies have noted an increased risk of thyroid cancer, particularly medullary thyroid cancer (a particularly deadly subtype), among patients taking GLP-1s.[23] Anyone with a history of thyroid, parathyroid, or adrenal cancers in their family should discuss their risk with doctors before starting to take the drug. The far-reaching and evolving benefits of GLP-1s testify to the many ways in which we're only now learning that excess weight affects all our organ systems, mostly through inflammation.

While GLP-1s have become the latest fad, capturing masses and celebrities to the point of nationwide shortages, they are far from the only obesity solution in the works. Bio-engineers have designed numerous "fixes" for our sugar addiction, from enzymes that would convert sugar to unabsorbable fiber in our stomachs, to optimized sugar crystals that would taste equally sweet while containing 10% as much of the sugar content as regular sugar. These innovations have not yet hit store shelves, but they have attracted millions in investment from food manufacturers. Whether they prove affordable and accessible to average consumers, or whether they have unintended side effects like diet sweeteners do, or both, remains to be seen.[24]

In some ways, these innovations represent our evolution come full circle. Our ancient ancestors were shaped on unpredictable grasslands, undergoing long periods of hunger. Before we developed the body size and brain to be able to hunt effectively, we subsisted on scraps, like leftover bone marrow or tubers we could unearth with simple stone tools. Our bodies evolved to utilize the bare minimum of calories, creating a finely tuned metabolic machine. Then we grew successful at agriculture, became more sedentary, and became overweight, with an excess of poor-quality food. More fat meant more calories for our metabolism to burn, creating more byproducts called reactive oxygen species. Like exhaust from a car, these oxygen "free radicals" pollute our cells, depositing their excess energy in our DNA and creating mutations. More food meant more metabolism, more oxygen radicals, and more cancer. Now, with weight-loss medicines flooding the market, we've finally developed an overengineered solution to a simple problem: how much junk we eat.

The GLP-1 agonists are an innovative solution for a rudimentary problem, but they are certainly not the only way to eat less. Eating slowly, chewing longer, and drinking water with meals has been shown to help develop the sensation of fullness more quickly. Learning to listen to your body's signals, and knowing when to stop, is a skill many of us have lost. Likewise, consuming foods rich in protein, fiber, and unsaturated fats, as opposed to simple sugars or problematic diet sweeteners (which have been shown to increase appetite and even increase your risk of heart attacks and strokes),[25] can help you feel fuller, longer. Even aerobic exercise has been shown to suppress appetite by the same mechanism as those fancy GLP-1 agonists;[26] I've sometimes stopped to do push-ups to curb hunger during the seemingly endless pre-lunch rounds (which often run as late as 3:00 p.m.) to check on patients in intensive care.

All of these solutions are easier said than done. As a descendant of an impoverished land, I hail from a family that sure knows how to eat. When planning my wedding, my parents were adamant: Forget those tiny, finger-sized hors d'oeuvres and serve some *real* meat and potatoes. They even had the nerve to call dibs on the leftovers. I was taught to live to eat, not eat to live. Consequently, I struggled with my weight, and I got bullied for it. Later in life, I became obsessed with weight in the opposite direction, starving myself and compensating with unhealthy amounts of exercise to the point of injury. Food consumed my life, instead of me consuming it.

Society has poisoned our perception of health and weight to a degree that would take far longer books than this, and far smarter minds than mine, to solve. What I can say, from lived experience, is that easy fixes are not always the best ones. GLP-1 agonists hold great promise for many of my patients, but they are not without risks. I've seen patients become skeletal with drastic weight loss, unable to hold down any food but insisting they must continue taking the drug. Some are so blinded by their pursuit of society's arbitrary "perfect body" that they can't even realize their own self-harm. As more people use drugs or cosmetic surgeries to lose weight, it enables body standards to become thinner, creating a self-fulfilling prophecy of bodily dissatisfaction. As in the Red Queen's race in *Alice in Wonderland,* "it takes all the running you can do, to keep in the same place."[27] Many people who start taking GLP-1s don't recognize that they must rely on these drugs for the rest of their lives, because if they stop taking them, the weight usually comes right back. I've even seen people go bankrupt trying to keep up with a thousand-dollar price tag, having never tried to cut out soda or fast food instead. On the other hand, I've seen patients fail to recognize their obesity even when they can barely move and when they exceed the weight capacity of the MRI table. Perhaps more than discipline or drugs, to get to the root of addressing obesity we need insight into why we want to look the way we do, and what our bodies want from us.

METABOLISM AND AGING

The connection between metabolism, food, and cancer transcends humanity. Some of the longest-living animals on Earth, like the Greenland shark (the oldest recorded at nearly 500 years), have some of the slowest metabolisms, while small, fast-metabolism creatures like hummingbirds and rodents typically live only a measly few years. (The naked mole rat, which maintains a low body temperature and slow metabolism, is the exception, with a 31-year life expectancy.[28]) These observations have led many researchers to target metabolism in the search for a "cure" for aging. But such lofty dreams are not without folly. In search of the "elixir of long life," an ancient Chinese alchemist ironically ended up creating gunpowder, perhaps the worst manmade purveyor of death.[29]

Metabolism and life expectancy are inextricably entwined. Over 40 years ago, in some of the first "anti-aging" experiments, researchers took a tiny roundworm called *C. elegans*, feeding it less and keeping it in a colder, low-oxygen environment to slow down its metabolism. The worms who got this "special" treatment saw their lifespans double.[30] This experiment paved the way for a whole field of anti-aging research, with numerous compounds and interventions identified in worms and mice being hailed as the next "fountain of youth," only to usually fail in human trials. Metformin, the first and most widely prescribed non-insulin diabetes drug, had been shown to slow down metabolism and increase lifespan in a number of animal models. These results, combined with observational studies of lower cancer rates in diabetics who take metformin, inspired scientists to conduct million-dollar trials studying metformin, specifically for life extension and cancer prevention. So far, none of these trials have shown any benefit in preventing cancer[31] (metformin remains an excellent option for diabetes). Humans are far more complex than worms, and without a controlled environment, like in a laboratory, there are so many confounding variables, like lifestyle and genetics, which will muddy the results of any trial. Nonetheless, the fledgling but far-reaching biological discipline of anti-aging research, as well as the billion-dollar supplement industry it enables, have continued pumping out unproven products.

Imagine metabolism as the aforementioned car engine, burning gasoline (food) to create energy, and polluting the air with the byproducts of combustion (damage to DNA). The simplest way to minimize the damage would be to burn less fuel, for example, by eating less or taking your bike to work. But to many of us, the more intriguing option would be downstream intervention, such as tweaking the engine to be more fuel efficient, or placing a net to catch the pollutants before they cause damage. Therefore, researchers create antioxidants and other supplements that promise to prevent cancer and slow aging.

SUPPLEMENTS, VITAMINS, AND SNAKE OILS

Antioxidants refer to any compound, natural or manmade, that inhibits the production of oxygen free radicals, the nasty cancer-causing byproducts of our metabolism. Thousands of antioxidants exist, and those most commonly found in fresh foods, such as vitamins A, C, and E, copper, zinc, and selenium, have all been shown to eat these free radicals when mixed in a test tube.[32] These compounds started to capture the spotlight in the 1990s, when scientists first connected these free radicals to coronary artery disease, which causes heart attacks. Unsurprisingly, research quickly revealed that people who eat lots of fresh fruits and vegetables, which are rich in antioxidants, have a dramatically lower risk of heart disease and other chronic health problems. These findings inspired a gold rush of supplements and clinical trials of various antioxidants. Unfortunately, the studies did not pan out. Vitamin A, C, or E supplementation failed to prevent heart disease or cancer. Of note, one trial did find that selenium supplements for patients with low levels of this element could decrease lung cancer risk by 44%, but the effect was not seen in patients who had normal selenium levels to start.[33] We now know that the benefits of fresh foods lie more in fiber and weight control than in any one "miracle" antioxidant.

Without a doubt, each of the vitamins (compounds formed by living beings) and minerals (naturally occurring compounds) that fresh foods contain play a necessary role, but very few when given individually have been shown to make any difference, and others may even be dangerous. For instance, many Alaska Natives, who are known for their ingenuity in making the most of every animal they find, have myths warning against eating polar bear meat. We now know that the meat, and particularly livers, of predators such as polar bears is concentrated with vitamin A. Too much vitamin A can cause liver and bone damage, vision loss, and even death.[34]

While most supplements simply pass through the body in urine, some may even increase cancer risk. Beta-carotene, an antioxidant derivative of carrots that gives them their color (and is related to vitamin A), was studied for primary cancer prevention in patients who were heavy smokers, as well as prevention of recurrence in patients already diagnosed with lung cancer. These trials were spectacular failures. In fact, two trials found that beta-carotene supplements *increased* lung cancer risk by 18%–28%. The effect was even worse for active smokers, who suffered an increased risk of 40%.[35] These findings stand in contrast to a recent meta-analysis ("meta" refers to an aggregate of all the reputable studies out there), which found that increased dietary consumption and higher levels of carotenes in the blood was associated with a decreased risk of lung, digestive, prostate, and breast cancers. However, the meta-analysis also found that high carotene *supplementation* (not through food) increased lung and bladder cancer risk.[36] For whatever reason, the natural mix of carotenes we derive from colorful vegetables like carrots may protect against cancer, but taking high doses of beta-carotene alone seems to increase cancer risk, particularly in smokers. Sometimes, less is more, especially when it comes to supplements.

A select few vitamins and minerals have been shown to prevent health problems, and they may even protect against certain cancers in certain individuals. The most notable is vitamin D, which an estimated 42% of Americans are deficient in. Vitamin D is activated in the skin by ultraviolet light, and then goes on to stimulate calcium and phosphate absorption, bone growth, and numerous other health benefits. Unfortunately, most of us these days, especially in northern latitudes, do not get sufficient sun exposure to generate enough vitamin D. Moreover, individuals with ancestors from equatorial latitudes, who evolved darker skin to deflect the sun's rays and prevent skin cancer, have more trouble generating sufficient vitamin D when living in northern, low-sun latitudes. Vitamin D deficiency is particularly prevalent in African Americans and Middle Eastern migrants to Europe.[37] Likewise, the skin of older adults slowly loses the ability to synthesize vitamin D, leading to higher risk of deficiency. In addition, individuals who are obese or who have had gastric bypass surgery have more trouble absorbing vitamin D from foods. In contrast to prevention, prescription of vitamins and minerals to those with proven deficiencies, due to malnutrition, alcoholism, or gastrointestinal issues, is well proven and potentially lifesaving.

While vitamin D levels can be tested, most doctors do not routinely do so. For that reason, some guidelines have begun to recommend supplements for all people at risk of deficiency, such as Black or older individuals. Even so, clinical trials have been fairly unimpressive. Vitamin D has *not* been shown to prevent fractures, muscle loss, or osteoporosis in older people, nor prevent heart disease, diabetes, or depression. However, higher vitamin D levels have been associated with lower rates of multiple sclerosis and even colorectal cancer.[38] The jury is still out on the benefits of vitamin D, especially in people without a proven deficiency, but when taken as recommended, vitamin D is relatively harmless (when taken in excess it can cause kidney failure and even death).

Another vitamin with proven supplement benefits is B12, which is predominantly found in meat, fish, eggs, and dairy products, and is thus routinely recommended for vegans to prevent low blood cell counts. Observational studies have found low B12 levels to be associated with gastric cancer, heart disease, and dementia, although trials have yet to show that B12 supplements make any difference.[39] Meanwhile, vitamin B3, sometimes called niacin or nicotinamide, has been found in observational studies to decrease the risk of common skin cancers, particularly in people who have suppressed immune systems.[40] However, none of these compounds has been studied in rigorous clinical trials (since vitamins, unlike drugs, can't be patented, there's no incentive for companies to invest in testing them). As with many compounds, the most efficient way to absorb vitamin D or B12 is through a balanced diet rich in fruits, vegetables, proteins, and low-fat dairy products (nonfat Greek yogurt is my personal favorite).

As with many things related to health, even natural supplements can be a double-edged sword. Many patients describe the complex assortment of plant- and herb-based supplements they take, much to their doctor's chagrin. It's not that we hate plant-based medicine (or as some of my patients believe, compete with plant and supplement companies for our salaries), but rather that many of these medicinal plants have common and dangerous interactions with other medicines. Most modern-day medicines derive from plants—like aspirin from willow bark, the chemotherapy drug Taxol from the Pacific yew tree, and digoxin from foxglove. But when doctors prescribe medicine, we are backed up by research and pharmacists who have carefully studied how these drugs will interact with other medications and warn us about dangerous interactions. In contrast, medicinal plants can be used by any person, without their doctor's knowing. One common example is St. John's wort, a derivative of a flowering shrub, used to treat depression. While it may have moderate effects on its own, when combined with other anti-anxiety or antidepressant medicines it can cause a life-threatening reaction called serotonin syndrome.[41] Examples of such interactions are a dime a dozen, so I recommend that my patients stay away from most herbal medicines, or at least warn me about exactly what they take. In particular, herbal supplements bought through the internet (often banned in stores), like kava, chaparral, androstenedione, comfrey, and germander, are to be avoided at all costs.[42]

While naturally occurring vitamins line store shelves worldwide, the bulk of the supplement industry's billions in profits comes from lab-synthesized compounds that can be patented and marketed at a profit without any FDA approval of effectiveness (the FDA evaluates supplements for safety only). One of the first anti-aging, metabolism-modifying supplements was resveratrol, a chemical originally derived from red grapes. It was first identified by David Sinclair at Harvard, who observed that activating a metabolism mediator called a sirtuin could extend the lifespans of yeast. Resveratrol sales took off after a highly popularized observational study on elderly people in Europe reported that drinking one to two glasses of red wine daily was associated with longer life.[43] This study has since been questioned, with a common criticism being that people who drink red wine may be more affluent and thus have better health for other reasons. Moreover, newer studies contradict the findings and report that even low alcohol consumption is associated with increased risk of cancer and death.[44] But the damage was already done. With all the hype, Sinclair sold his company marketing resveratrol, called Sirtris, for some $720 million dollars in 2008. Soon after, scientists realized that resveratrol had rather poor absorption, and key studies about health benefits all failed, leading the company to close down less than five years later.[45]

Many similar products have followed in resveratrol's footsteps, each promising to modify metabolism to reduce damage to DNA and prevent cancer and aging. Years ago, I worked as a writer of scientific materials for one such compound, named nicotinamide riboside (NR) and marketed as Tru Niagen. The supplement, now sold for over a dollar per capsule, has several Nobel Prize winners on its maker's scientific advisory board. In addition, over 25 early clinical studies suggest mild improvements in everything from premature infertility to Parkinson's disease to ALS (Lou Gehrig's disease).[46] The studies have all been small and limited in duration and scope. We are very far from being able to conclude that nicotinamide riboside, or the dozen other metabolic, anti-aging supplements like it, have any clinical benefits. Moreover, since the FDA does not evaluate supplements for their effectiveness, supplement companies have no incentive to conduct expensive, large-scale clinical trials like pharmaceutical corporations do. But to NR's credit, it has been shown to reduce markers of inflammation in the blood in a number of chronic disease states, including obesity, which is more than most supplements can say. It is certainly deserving of further study. It is hard to ignore, however, that all these hundred-dollar supplements and thousand-dollar weight loss drugs, promise to prevent cancer by replicating a rather cheap and proven solution: calorie restriction.

THE RED QUEEN'S RACE

Thinking about weight loss, supplements, and cancer, I can't help but return to the Red Queen's race from *Alice in Wonderland*: We are running faster and faster just to stay where we are. On the surface, that's how many aging adults feel about their weight; as our metabolism slows, we must exercise more, and eat less, just to remain at the weight we are. Likewise, in a world of ever-increasing "diet" foods (which are not as healthful as whole foods) and snake oil supplements, it can feel like a full-time job just to figure out how to eat and live healthfully.

Applying the Red Queen's race to weight in a broader sense, our society has medicalized weight loss and metabolism, leading to a body-image goalpost that is always moving and that, like the horizon, can never be reached. We are on a path toward a bimodal society, with the wealthy pressured to use GLP-1 agonists and fat-removing cosmetic surgery to look very thin, while the poor grow larger, having little access to healthy foods, weight medicines, or weight-loss surgery. Collectively, we are now paying billions for medicines, supplements, and fad weight-loss diets that promise to do what the Blue Zone elders in Sicily do for free: eat well, and stress less. It is a roundabout and over-engineered solution emblematic of our twenty-first century social problems. We'd rather spend billions treating obesity than reform our society to promote healthy living.

Strictly from a cancer prevention perspective, GLP-1 agonists like Ozempic may be the most cost-effective intervention to reduce inflammation and early-onset cancers in adults who are overweight. I prescribe these medications regularly, recommend them to family, and would take them myself if I were to develop diabetes or obesity (along with, *not instead of,* dietary modification and exercise).

I wish my career allowed me the free time to expand my physically active hobbies, develop a knack for cooking with fresh foods, or savor all meals instead of rushing through them. Unfortunately, we are all trapped in the same stress-inducing, inflation-ridden, ceaselessly interconnected and impersonal modern world.

Individually, we can only moderately change our circumstances, slow down our lunch breaks, and make responsible decisions. But collectively, we can call upon our legislators and employers to reduce work hours and stress, to provide healthy meals to children and those in need, and to invest in holistic obesity prevention and treatment. Only then will we win the race, and, in the footsteps of our ancestors, learn to eat to live and to live well.

In summary:

- Body fat produces inflammation, increasing the risk of nearly every cancer—particularly breast, colorectal, and prostate.

- Seventy-five percent of Americans are overweight or obese, although criteria vary by race/ethnicity, and waist size (abdominal fat) and heart health matter far more than sheer weight.

- Reducing calorie consumption is more effective than exercise for losing weight, decreasing cancer risk, and likely extending lifespan.

- Trials of antioxidants, vitamins, and other supplements have failed to show reduction in cancer risk.

- New medicines like GLP-1 agonists will probably significantly reduce cancer risk, particularly among younger adults struggling with obesity, but they do carry risks, and they should be used with (not instead of) a healthy diet and exercise.

CHAPTER 5

On and Off the Clock

Occupational Exposures, Pollution, and Plastic

Chim chim cherree, a sweep is as lucky as lucky can be.
—P. L. Travers, Mary Poppins

The fate of these people seems peculiarly hard . . . they are thrust up narrow and hot chimnies, where they are bruised burned and almost suffocated; and when they get to puberty they become liable to a most noisome, painful and fatal disease.
—Percivall Pott (c. 1775)

Only when the last tree has died, the last river been poisoned, and the last fish been caught will we realize we cannot eat money.
—Cree proverb

Since the dawn of the modern economy, workers have faced many occupational hazards. In the eighteenth century, London was rapidly urbanizing, and coal was a primary source of fuel. Chimneys needed to be regularly cleaned to maintain efficiency, and this dirty, dangerous task was often assigned to young boys. Boys as young as 5 years, known as chimney sweeps, would be sent up narrow chimneys to scrape off the soot and coal residue. The lives of these chimney sweeps were far from the depiction in the film *Mary Poppins*. They worked in appalling conditions, were frequently exposed to the toxic soot, and had little protection and poor hygiene. They climbed chimneys with little or no clothing to prevent snagging, and over time, soot would accumulate on their skin, particularly in the folds of their groin area. This practice went largely unchallenged in society, with little concern for the health effects these boys faced.[1]

Percivall Pott, one of the leading surgeons of his time, was known for his keen observational skills. He worked at St. Bartholomew's Hospital in London and treated a wide variety of ailments. In 1775, Pott noticed a disturbing trend among chimney sweeps; many of them developed an unusual form of cancer, which affected the scrotum. This cancer, a type of skin cancer, would first appear as a small wart on the scrotal skin. If left untreated, it would grow and spread, becoming ulcerous and deadly. Pott meticulously recorded the cases he observed, noting that this form of cancer was almost exclusively found in chimney sweeps. He connected their exposure to soot with the disease, marking one of the first instances in history where an environmental factor was linked to cancer. This connection lay the foundation for later developments in epidemiology and industrial hygiene.[2]

The recognition of the link between soot exposure and scrotal cancer eventually led to changes in public policy. Pott's discovery contributed to the passing of the Chimney Sweepers Act in 1788, which sought to regulate the practice of sending young boys into chimneys and improve the working conditions of sweeps. Though the law had limited immediate impact, it was a significant early step toward protecting workers from hazardous environments.[3]

COMMON OCCUPATIONAL EXPOSURES

Many people hate their jobs, but for some, their occupations may be *literally* shortening their lives. Some 4% of global cancers can be attributed to occupational exposure to hazardous chemical elements or compounds.[4] The most common cancers caused by these situations are cancers of the organs (most notably, the lungs) that experience the most exposure to environmental toxins. One might think that skin cancers would be most likely to develop from toxic exposures, but the skin is specifically designed as a barrier to withstand all sorts of hazards. The top layer of skin is composed of cells that are already dead and just waiting to slough off, so the risk of cancer transformation from topical exposure is negligible. The lungs, on the other hand, were not intended to be exposed to the sheer volume of toxins that industrial or polluted air contains, especially when you work close to these toxic compounds.

The most notorious cancer resulting from occupational exposure is mesothelioma. Listening to the radio, you may have heard advertisements asking whether "you or a loved one has been diagnosed with mesothelioma." Mesothelioma is a cancer of the lining of the lungs, and most cases can be attributed to exposure to asbestos.

Asbestos is a naturally occurring fibrous material that does not burn in fire, and its name means "unquenchable" in ancient Greek. The earliest uses of asbestos, dating back nearly 5,000 years, may have been to facilitate the cremation of royalty or the manufacture of ceremonial candle wicks. In the nineteenth century, industrialists began to mine asbestos to use for its fire-retardant properties in everything from clothing to pipes, insulation, flooring, furniture, ships, vehicles, and anything else imaginable. But in the early 1900s, during the peak of the asbestos craze, doctors began to notice its negative health effects. Workers exposed to asbestos were developing serious respiratory diseases, including asbestosis (a chronic lung condition) and a rare cancer—mesothelioma—that affected the lining of the lungs. Today we know that asbestos increases lung cancer risk by over fivefold, especially when combined with cigarette smoking.[5] Asbestos gets breathed in and stuck in the lungs, where the immune system goes into overdrive because it doesn't know what to do with the "unquenchable" compound. After years of inflammation and tissue damage, mesothelioma and other lung cancers arise.

Despite the adverse health effects of asbestos, as many as 50% of older homes still have measurable levels of this hazard.[6] Workers such as insulators, pipefitters, plumbers, electricians, and those involved in demolition and renovation of older buildings containing asbestos are particularly at risk of repeated exposure, and they are now mandated to wear protective masks. Those who were exposed to it on the job before regular safety precautions were implemented and have since developed mesothelioma as a result are often entitled to compensation through class action lawsuits (hence the radio ads). Unlike other types of lung cancer, nearly 90% of mesotheliomas are caused by asbestos exposure,[7] so companies have not been able to blame other risk factors like smoking to avoid compensating their workers. But asbestos exposure is not unique to workers. For example, the BoRit site is a 32-acre dump site in Ambler, Pennsylvania, outside of Philadelphia, where 1.5 million cubic yards of asbestos waste were dumped. The large mound of asbestos-laden waste stands 25 feet high, and for decades, kids used to climb the mound to sled down.[8] Asbestos has also been historically present in talcum powder used for skin, and some studies have suggested a link to ovarian and lung cancer from talc, although the evidence is limited, and today's talcum powders contain significantly less asbestos.[9]

While it is the most notorious, asbestos is far from the only airborne occupational hazard. Silica, a similar compound to asbestos that is found in sand, stones, and concrete, can also get deposited in the lungs, increasing the risk of lung cancer after years of exposure. Workers such as miners have been found to have a 50% increased risk of lung cancer due to silica exposure.[10] Professions such as foundry work, pottery,[11] brick-laying,[12] and sand work[13] are also at increased risk.

Occupational lung cancer risk is not exclusive to those in construction. Truckers are noted to have an increased risk of lung cancer due to exposure to diesel engine exhaust, which has increased by nearly 40% over the past three decades.[14] Exposure to heavy metals, such as arsenic, nickel, and chromium, is also significantly associated with lung cancer. Arsenic, a centuries-old poison implicated in the murder of Napoleon, is the most carcinogenic, increasing lung cancer risk about 65%.[15] Workers who manufacture artificial stone (silica) countertops have also been observed to suffer higher rates of silica lung disease and lung cancer. Chromium, nickel, and cadmium have been estimated to carry about a 30% elevated risk.[16] Many workers in niche manufacturing sectors, such as electronics and computer chips, are at the highest risk of exposure. It comes as no surprise that uranium miners are also at increased risk of cancer in the lungs, as well as in many other organs.

While the lungs are the most commonly affected organ, they are far from alone. Another common organ at risk of cancer is the bladder. Hair stylists are particularly at risk. While the occasional hair dye exposure is safe, repeated exposure to the aromatic amines which give dyes their color and smell can damage DNA; this exposure has been implicated in a ninefold greater risk among hairdressers of developing bladder cancer,[17] or about a 30% greater risk compared to the average person.[18] The bladder concentrates and stores toxins filtered out of the blood into the urine, so is at increased risk of toxin-driven cancer.

Another group of people at particular risk of toxic exposure is those in military service. Across the Veterans Affairs administration, all veterans are now screened for toxic exposures, and nearly 40% report exposure to some toxin during their service.[19] The most common exposures include Agent Orange during service in Vietnam, burn pits during the Gulf Wars, and contaminated water at Camp Lejeune and similarly mired military bases. Each of these exposures has been associated with increased risk of dozens of cancer types for veterans, and sometimes even their families. While it's impossible to prove whether age, toxic exposure, or a combination of both is to blame for a cancer diagnosis, the number of exposed veterans with lung, prostate, or skin cancers I have treated has been staggering. Sometimes, the uncertainty is the worst part. My veteran patients, frustrated by the onerous process to get compensated for their exposure, have felt neglected, even betrayed, by the nation for which they risked their lives. Thankfully, the Sergeant First Class Heath Robinson Honoring Our Promise to Address Comprehensive Toxics Act was signed into law on August 10, 2022,[20] allowing these veterans to qualify for expanded benefits, including no out-of-pocket costs for medical care related to their exposure.

Another occupation that is seldom recognized, but likewise perilous, is being a homemaker, cooking on a poorly ventilated stove. People in this group are typically women living in the developing world. Of all lung cancer cases among nonsmokers in a study from Taiwan, the greatest behavioral risk factor was the "cooking-index," a measure of time spent behind the stove breathing in fumes.[21] The risk is greatest in developing nations where much of the cooking is done on indoor, inadequately ventilated, wood-fire stoves, which produce fumes than contain carcinogenic compounds similar to those in tobacco smoke.

Cooking outside, or at least improving ventilation with a chimney or open windows, is the easiest way to reduce risk, although research on this issue is sparse. Even in the developed world, new data suggests gas stove tops (as opposed to electric) may increase lung cancer for all the same reasons. The poorly studied lung cancer risks of cooking reflect a broader neglect of women and developing nations in medical research. But the injustice of medical neglect may be overshadowed by the deliberate concealment of cancer risk by unscrupulous governments and corporations.

My grandfather spent decades in Ukraine working as a foreman in a factory that manufactured steel and armaments. Although he was never informed, he likely came into contact with nuclear weapons and radioactivity on frequent occasions. In fact, we've since learned that the entire region of Dnipro, where my family lived, is plagued with radioactivity from nuclear power plant leakage (including but not limited to Chernobyl), radioactive waste disposal, and uranium mining, most of which was covered up by the USSR authorities.[22] The human costs of the Soviet Union's various cover-ups, from failed space missions to radiation to biotoxins, may never be fully grasped. We'll never know whether my grandfather's job, or my grandmother's daily exposure, were at the root of their untimely demise.

CLASS ACTION LAWSUITS AND UNIONS

Factory work, construction, and hair styling are among the most common, but far from the only, occupations at increased risk of cancer due to exposure on the job. Thankfully, workers today have more protections and remedies than they ever had in the past.

Some of the earliest lawsuits related to occupational toxin exposure were caused by asbestos and were filed in the 1960s. In *Borel v. Fibreboard Paper Products Corporation*, Clarence Borel, an industrial insulation worker, sued multiple asbestos manufacturers after being diagnosed with asbestosis and mesothelioma. The jury ruled in favor of Borel, marking the first time a court recognized that asbestos companies had a duty to warn workers of the risks.[23] This case set a legal precedent and opened the floodgates for thousands of lawsuits from other victims. As more people were diagnosed with mesothelioma and other asbestos-related diseases, it became clear that individual lawsuits would not be enough to address the scope of the disaster. The number of affected individuals was staggering, and asbestos victims came from various industries, including construction, shipbuilding, and manufacturing. This led to the development of large-scale class action lawsuits.

During the 1980s and 1990s, thousands of mesothelioma victims banded together to file class action lawsuits against asbestos manufacturers. These lawsuits sought compensation for medical expenses, lost wages, and pain and suffering. The sheer scale of these cases led to some of the largest legal settlements in history. *Georgine v. Amchem Products, Inc.*, filed in 1993, involved over 100,000 claimants seeking damages from major asbestos manufacturers.[24] Although the initial settlement was proposed at $1.3 billion, the Supreme Court ultimately rejected the settlement in 1997, stating that it did not adequately protect the future interests of mesothelioma victims who had not yet developed symptoms. The complexity of the cases led to the creation of asbestos bankruptcy trusts. Many of the companies responsible for asbestos exposure faced so many lawsuits that they filed for bankruptcy. Courts created special trusts funded by the bankrupt companies, which would pay out claims to mesothelioma victims over time. By the 2000s, these trusts had billions of dollars set aside for compensation.[25]

In addition to compensation for the victims, these class action lawsuits played a crucial role in raising public awareness about the dangers of asbestos and pushed for stricter regulation and eventual bans on the substance in many countries. However, asbestos is still not banned in the United States, and legacy asbestos remains in older buildings and products, continuing to pose a risk to workers and residents.

A similar proliferation of lawsuits has recently implicated the weed killer Roundup (glyphosate) for its alleged link to non-Hodgkin lymphoma (a type of blood cell cancer). In 1974, Monsanto introduced Roundup to the agricultural market. It was quickly adopted as a widely used herbicide because of its effectiveness in killing weeds while leaving crops unharmed. Roundup's popularity skyrocketed when Monsanto began selling genetically modified crops in the 1990s that were resistant to glyphosate, allowing farmers to use the herbicide without damaging their fields.

Concerns about glyphosate's safety began to mount as studies emerged suggesting that the chemical might be linked to cancer. In 2015, the World Health Organization classified glyphosate as "probably carcinogenic to humans" due to increased risk of non-Hodgkin lymphoma. A meta-analysis found a 41% increased risk of lymphoma in people with high exposure to Roundup.[26] Monsanto strongly denied these findings, arguing that other studies, including those conducted by regulatory agencies like the US Environmental Protection Agency (EPA), found no conclusive evidence that glyphosate was carcinogenic. Despite these assurances, public skepticism grew, especially among individuals who had used Roundup for years and were now suffering from non-Hodgkin lymphoma.

The first Roundup lawsuits were filed in the mid-2010s, claiming that Monsanto had failed to adequately warn consumers of the potential health risks associated with Roundup and had engaged in deceptive marketing practices by promoting the herbicide as safe. In the lawsuit *Dewayne Johnson v. Monsanto Company*, Johnson, a school groundskeeper from California, had been diagnosed with non-Hodgkin lymphoma after using Roundup for years as part of his job. His case went to trial in 2018, and the jury awarded him $289 million in damages, concluding that Roundup was a substantial factor in causing his cancer and that Monsanto had acted with "malice" by failing to warn consumers about the risks. Although the award was later reduced to $78 million, this case set a precedent for thousands of other lawsuits.[27] Following the success of Johnson's case, thousands of individuals filed similar lawsuits, leading to one of the largest mass tort (wrongful act) actions in US history. By 2020, more than 100,000 individual claims had been filed, alleging that Roundup caused cancer and that Monsanto had engaged in negligence and fraud.

In 2020, German pharmaceutical corporation Bayer, which had purchased Monsanto, announced that it had agreed to settle the bulk of the Roundup lawsuits, committing more than $10 billion to resolve approximately 100,000 claims.[28] The settlement covered both existing lawsuits and future claims related to Roundup exposure. This deal, one of the largest legal settlements in history, was seen as a way for Bayer to manage the growing legal liabilities associated with Roundup without continuing to fight each case in court. In response to mounting legal and regulatory pressure, Bayer announced in 2021 that it would stop selling glyphosate-based products for residential use in the US by 2023, although it would continue to sell Roundup for agricultural and industrial purposes.

While critics have complained that these billion-dollar class actions lawsuits stifle industry and increase costs for consumers, they've also allowed thousands of cancer patients to be compensated for their suffering and in our backward health care system, sometimes even pay off their medical debts. The balance of consumer and worker protections versus the free market continues to be contentious to this day, especially when it comes to less objectively quantifiable dangers to the public good, like pollution and toxic waste.

TOXIC WASTE

The story of DuPont and the Teflon cover-up regarding cancer risk is a troubling example of corporate negligence, environmental pollution, and the dangers of chemical exposure. Striving to make a profit from Teflon, a chemical essential for nonstick cookware and waterproof clothing, manufacturer DuPont covered up the massive spillage of nondegradable, carcinogenic byproducts, exposing their workers and the local water supply.[29]

Teflon was accidentally discovered in 1938 by a DuPont scientist named Roy Plunkett. It was a breakthrough material—nonstick, chemically resistant, and able to withstand high temperatures. DuPont quickly realized its potential for a wide range of applications, from nonstick cookware to military products and industrial uses. By the 1950s, Teflon-coated pans were a household staple, and DuPont's profits soared. However, a critical ingredient in the production of Teflon was PFOA (perfluorooctanoic acid) a synthetic chemical that doesn't break down easily in the environment or in human bodies, making it the first compound to be nicknamed the "forever chemical."[30]

From the 1950s onward, DuPont scientists began noticing troubling signs about PFOA. Early studies showed that it accumulated in the blood of factory workers and laboratory animals. By the 1960s, DuPont had evidence that PFOA could cause health problems, including potential liver damage. Despite these concerns, the company did not publicly disclose the risks and continued using PFOA in Teflon manufacturing. Throughout the 1970s and 1980s, internal documents revealed that DuPont knew PFOA was not only persistent in the environment but also toxic. Studies commissioned by DuPont itself found that PFOA caused numerous types of cancer in lab animals. Yet, the company allegedly continued to downplay the dangers and took no meaningful steps to stop using the chemical or warn the public.[31]

In the 1980s, DuPont discovered that PFOA was contaminating the drinking water near a plant in Parkersburg, West Virginia. Local farmers, whose livestock were dying from unknown causes, began to suspect that chemical runoff from DuPont's facility was to blame. One farmer, Wilbur Tennant, noticed unusual illnesses and deformities in his cattle, leading him to hire a corporate environmental lawyer, Rob Bilott, to investigate.[32]

Through legal discovery, Bilott uncovered a trove of internal DuPont documents that revealed the company had been aware of PFOA's dangers for decades.[33] The documents showed that DuPont had known since at least the 1960s that PFOA was hazardous to both human health and the environment, but had chosen to conceal the information. Bilott's research linked PFOA exposure to serious health issues, including kidney cancer,[34] testicular cancer, ulcerative colitis, thyroid disease, high cholesterol, and pregnancy-induced hypertension.[35]

In 2001, Bilott filed a class action lawsuit against DuPont on behalf of 70,000 residents of the Parkersburg area whose water had been contaminated with PFOA. The lawsuit led to a landmark settlement in 2004, in which DuPont agreed to pay $70 million for medical monitoring and health studies of affected residents.[36]

The fallout from the DuPont case did not stop at Parkersburg. PFOA and other per- and polyfluoroalkyl substances (PFAS) were found to have contaminated water supplies across the US and around the world. These chemicals, due to their persistence and "bioaccumulative" nature, have been found in the blood of nearly all people around the world.[37] In the years since, high PFAS levels have been associated with dozens of new cancer types, as well as higher risk of severe COVID[38] and in one small study, even lower sperm counts and penis size.[39]

Facing growing public pressure and legal challenges, DuPont stopped manufacturing PFOA in 2013, replacing it with similar, but still potentially harmful, chemicals. However, the legacy of PFOA continues. It is still present in the environment, and lawsuits related to PFOA exposure have not slackened. In 2017, after years of litigation, DuPont and its spin-off company Chemours agreed to a $671 million settlement to resolve over 3,500 personal injury lawsuits related to PFOA exposure. These lawsuits were brought by individuals who had developed cancer or other health problems as a result of drinking water contaminated by DuPont's Washington Works plant.[40]

The DuPont Teflon scandal exposed the dangers of corporate cover-ups and the devastating effects that unregulated chemical use can have on public health and the environment. The case became the basis for the 2019 film *Dark Waters,* which highlighted the efforts of Bilott and brought the issue of PFOA contamination to a wider audience.[41]

While the Teflon scandal is among the worst, it is far from an isolated incident. In Niagara Falls, New York, thousands of tons of hazardous chemicals were buried beneath a residential neighborhood, leading to widespread health problems and cancer. In the early twentieth century, entrepreneur William T. Love planned to build a canal linking the Niagara River to Lake Ontario to generate cheap hydroelectric power. Although the project never reached completion, the partially dug canal remained, becoming an ideal dumping ground for industrial waste in the 1940s and 1950s. The Hooker Chemical Company took advantage of the site, using the abandoned canal to dispose of approximately 21,000 tons of chemical waste, including benzene, dioxins, and other highly toxic and carcinogenic substances. Hooker buried the waste in metal drums and covered the canal with clay, considering it a safe method of disposal at the time. The company even purchased the land around the canal, using it as a legal buffer to avoid responsibility.[42]

In the 1950s, despite knowing the land was contaminated, Hooker Chemical sold the site to the Niagara Falls School Board for $1. The deed included a warning about the buried chemicals, but the company did little to prevent development. Over the next few decades, the area around Love Canal transformed into a bustling suburban neighborhood. A school was built directly on top of the canal, and hundreds of homes were constructed nearby. By the 1960s and 1970s, families were raising their children in the community, unaware that beneath their feet lay a ticking time bomb of toxic waste. Over time, the chemicals buried underground began to leach into the soil, groundwater, and basements of homes. The neighborhood became a toxic zone, with residents experiencing severe health problems as a result of prolonged exposure to the hazardous chemicals.[43]

Residents of Love Canal began noticing strange phenomena. Foul-smelling, oily liquids seeped into their basements, and strange residues formed in puddles after rain. Gardens wouldn't grow, and children suffered from chemical burns after playing in the dirt. But these early signs paled in comparison to the mounting health problems that would soon emerge. By the mid-1970s, residents started reporting unusually high rates of miscarriages, birth defects, and childhood illnesses. Families began to see disturbing patterns of disease, including leukemia and liver, bladder, and kidney (the organs responsible for filtering toxins out of the blood) cancers. Community members noticed that many children born in the neighborhood had severe congenital disabilities, such as developmental delays and skeletal malformations.[44]

One of the most notable early activists, Lois Gibbs, a mother of two children who lived in the neighborhood, became concerned when her young son developed severe health issues, including epilepsy, asthma, and urinary tract infections. In 1978, after years of complaints and grassroots organizing by residents, Gibbs and other community leaders brought attention to the crisis at Love Canal. They demanded that the government take action to address the growing health concerns and investigate the cause of the illnesses. Public pressure mounted as media outlets began covering the story, and Love Canal became a national symbol of environmental disaster.[45]

That year, New York State health officials conducted studies and confirmed what residents had long feared: the chemicals buried in Love Canal were indeed seeping into the homes and affecting the health of the community. The studies showed elevated levels of carcinogens and toxic chemicals in the soil and groundwater, as well as a sharp increase in illnesses among residents. The findings were devastating, with hundreds of families living on top of the toxic waste dump facing serious health risks, including cancer.[46]

In response, President Jimmy Carter declared a state of emergency, marking the first time the federal government had taken such an action for a non-natural disaster. The government began evacuating over 200 families from the most severely affected areas, moving them to temporary housing while more investigations were conducted. Lois Gibbs and her fellow activists continued to pressure the government, insisting that all residents of the Love Canal area be evacuated, not just those living directly on top of the former dump site. Gibbs famously held EPA officials hostage in a local office to demand that her community be relocated. Her tenacity paid off, and in 1980, President Carter authorized the complete evacuation of more than 800 families from the Love Canal neighborhood.[47]

The Love Canal disaster became a catalyst for national environmental reform. In 1980, Congress passed a bill for a program known as Superfund, which gave the federal government the power and resources to identify and clean up toxic waste sites across the country and hold companies accountable for environmental damages. Love Canal was designated as one of the first Superfund sites.[48]

The psychological toll on the displaced families was profound. Many faced financial hardship, losing their homes and livelihoods in the process. The neighborhood was eventually declared safe after an extensive cleanup and remediation effort, but by then, the damage had been done. Love Canal remained a symbol of the failure to prioritize public health and the environment over corporate profits.[49]

The Love Canal disaster was a watershed moment in American environmental history. It galvanized the environmental justice movement, drawing attention to the disproportionate impact of industrial pollution on working-class and minority communities. It also highlighted the need for stronger regulations on chemical disposal and corporate responsibility. The Love Canal tragedy also led to broader awareness of the dangers posed by hazardous waste sites across the country. Superfund has since identified and cleaned up thousands of toxic waste sites, though the program has faced funding challenges and political setbacks over the years.[50]

Blunders like Teflon and Love Canal may seem alien to many of us, because these kinds of toxic exposures predominantly happen in poor communities, which have fewer resources to legally protect themselves or move away. On February 3, 2023, a train derailment occurred in East Palestine, Ohio, with a Norfolk Southern freight train carrying hazardous chemicals. The derailment led to a fire and the release of dangerous chemicals into the air, soil, and water, raising serious health and environmental concerns. One of the most alarming potential long-term impacts is the increased risk of cancer among residents due to exposure to vinyl chloride and other toxic substances.[51]

Faced with the risk of a larger explosion, authorities conducted a controlled burn of the vinyl chloride, releasing chemicals such as phosgene and hydrogen chloride into the air. Phosgene is a highly toxic gas used as a chemical weapon in World War I, and hydrogen chloride can irritate the respiratory system and skin. The controlled burn aimed to prevent an uncontrolled explosion, but it led to a massive toxic cloud over the region.[52]

The vinyl chloride released in the derailment is associated with a 45-fold increased risk of hepatic angiosarcoma, a rare and aggressive form of liver cancer. Long-term exposure has also been linked to other types of liver disease, lung cancer, brain cancer, lymphoma, and leukemia.[53] Occupational exposure, where individuals are in regular contact with vinyl chloride, has historically led to higher rates of these cancers, but even lower levels of exposure can carry significant health risks. In the immediate aftermath of the derailment, residents reported a range of health problems, including respiratory issues, headaches, skin rashes, eye irritation, and other symptoms consistent with exposure to toxic chemicals. The black smoke that billowed from the controlled burn likely contained a mix of carcinogens and other harmful chemicals that can have both short- and long-term health effects.[54]

While short-term exposure to chemicals like vinyl chloride can cause acute symptoms, such as dizziness, headaches, and respiratory irritation, the long-term effects, especially the potential for cancer, are more concerning and may not become evident for years or even decades. The EPA and local health authorities began monitoring air and water quality in the area, but concerns remained about the adequacy of testing and the potential for lingering contamination.[55]

Reports surfaced that fish in local streams had died, indicating the presence of toxins in the water. Additionally, there were concerns that private wells and municipal water sources could become contaminated, leading to long-term exposure for local residents. In the months following the derailment, state and federal agencies continued to monitor air, water, and soil quality to assess the extent of contamination. After conducting initial tests, the EPA and local health departments have reassured residents that the air and water are safe, but skepticism among residents remains. The long-term health risks, particularly the cancer risks from prolonged exposure to low levels of vinyl chloride and other chemicals, are difficult to quantify in the immediate aftermath of the incident.

The East Palestine train derailment has sparked a broader conversation about rail safety, the transportation of hazardous materials, and corporate accountability. Norfolk Southern, the company operating the train, faced criticism for its role in the derailment and its response to the disaster. Residents have filed lawsuits, seeking compensation for health issues and property damage,[56] and the incident has prompted calls for stricter regulations on railroads transporting dangerous chemicals.

The derailment has also drawn attention to the environmental and health impacts of industrial pollution in rural and underserved communities. East Palestine is a small town, and many residents feel that their health and safety were put at risk in the pursuit of economic efficiency and corporate profit. The disaster has become a rallying point for environmental justice advocates who argue that the risks posed by hazardous materials are often disproportionately borne by poorer, rural, and urban communities.

That said, US citizens still have more protection against the dumping of toxic waste and pollution than people living in many developing nations. Between 1964 and 1992, Texaco drilled for oil in Ecuador, allegedly dumping over 16 billion gallons of toxic waste into rivers, forests, and soil, leading to widespread environmental damage and severe health problems for local communities, including increased cancer rates. Indigenous groups sued the company over pollution and health impacts. In 2011, an Ecuadorian court ordered Chevron, which had merged with Texaco in 2001, to pay $9.5 billion in damages. However, Chevron refused, claiming the judgment was fraudulent and corrupt, and the case remains unresolved, marked by international legal battles and accusations of corporate irresponsibility.[57]

POLLUTION

Beyond egregious spillage of toxic waste and byproducts, air and water pollution affects our cancer risk on a daily basis. Fine particulate matter (PM), known as PM2.5, in air pollution is particularly associated with a risk of lung cancer and other cancers.

These fine particles are typically released in car exhaust and during manufacturing, and are thus most prevalent in urban and industrial areas. High exposure to PM2.5 is associated with an 8.5% increase in overall cancer incidence, with specific risks for lung, breast, and prostate cancers.[58] Larger air particles, known as PM10, have been shown to increase lung cancer to a lesser degree, probably because the secretions in our respiratory tract have an easier time catching and swallowing the particles before they can do any damage.

Pollutants such as arsenic and benzene in the air have been associated with an increased risk of bladder cancer, skin cancer, and nasopharyngeal cancer—cancer of the tissues that come into regular contact with the outside world or its byproducts. Interestingly, another air pollutant called nitric oxide, which produces high-energy reactive nitrogen species that damage DNA (much like the reactive oxygen species produced by our metabolism), specifically increases the risk of hormone-sensitive cancers like endometrial (the lining of the uterus) and ovarian cancer by about 40%.[59] The mechanism remains unknown, but it is believed to involve hormonal cell signaling and inflammation.[60]

Most of these particles come from car exhaust (particularly diesel) and factories. Cities around the world have been successful in reducing air particulate exposure by reorganizing highways to divert car traffic from dense residential areas, and in turn provide more green spaces with trees that absorb these pollutants. Besides urban planning, there's plenty we can do as individuals to mitigate our exposure. In many parts of Asia, denizens of dense cities routinely don face masks, which can filter out larger air particulates. At home, we can avoid artificial air fresheners, bottles, and plug-ins, which have been shown to contain many of the same cancer-causing airborne particulates.[61] Instead, we can use live plants and air filters to help absorb odors as well as clean the air of toxic chemicals.

Pollution can also affect the water we drink. Most of us remember the fiasco in Flint, Michigan, the financially struggling city that switched its water source from Lake Huron (via Detroit's water system) to the Flint River as a cost-saving measure. The untreated water corroded the city's aging lead pipes, causing lead to leach into the drinking water. It also caused an outbreak of Legionnaires' disease, a severe form of pneumonia caused by bacteria in contaminated water. At least 12 people died, and thousands of children suffered lead poisoning.[62]

The chlorinating agents that many cities use to disinfect their water have actually been associated with an increased risk of bladder cancer. One study estimated that approximately 8,000 of the 79,000 annual bladder cancer cases in the US could be attributed to chlorine byproducts (called THM) in drinking water systems,[63] with the majority of these cases linked to surface water systems serving large populations. The risk is cumulative and relatively mild; one study estimated an 8% increased risk in those with high exposure.[64] It's important to note that it's *chlorine* for disinfecting water, not *fluoride*, which is added to water to prevent cavities, that has been tied to cancer risk. Efforts to eliminate fluoride in drinking water have no basis in science.

While drinking bottled spring water may seem like a safer option, many bottling companies simply use chlorinated water sources from towns that are fed by natural springs, so there is no evidence that bottled water actually contains fewer of these byproducts. Moreover, plastic leaches cancer-causing particles into water (as we'll soon discuss), especially when stored at high temperatures, making plastic water bottles far from ideal. Thankfully, cities around the country are slowly shifting away from chlorination to safer modes of water disinfection. Moreover, activated carbon filters (Brita or any other brand) are particularly effective at removing THMs. These filters work by adsorbing organic compounds, including THMs, from the water. Studies have shown that activated carbon filtration can reduce THM levels by up to 99% under optimal conditions.[65]

PLASTICS BIG AND SMALL

Our modern-day way of life exposes us to toxic waste, water and air pollution, and an inordinate amount of plastic. Unfortunately, our plastic reliance has led to widespread contamination of the environment with tiny plastic particles, known as microplastics. They have been found in oceans, rivers, soil, air, food, water, and people, posing a risk to human health. A recent study found microplastics in the blood of over 90% of people analyzed around the world;[66] in the developed world, essentially all of us are contaminated with plastic.[67]

Microplastics can enter the human body through breathing, drinking contaminated water, or consuming food, especially seafood (as ocean fish and filter-feeders consume an enormous amount of microplastics). Plastic is primarily derived from fossil fuels, such as crude oil and natural gas, through a chemical process called polymerization. The final product is so stable that it could last millions of years, longer than the dinosaurs it came from, and probably outlast the human race. Plastic will leave an indelible footprint on our planet, and on our DNA. Studies suggest that microplastics can cause inflammation, oxidative stress, and damage to cells, which could contribute to long-term health problems. Since microplastics have just recently been identified, and nearly everyone is exposed, establishing their true cancer risk has proven difficult. However, certain chemicals in microplastics, like bisphenol A (BPA) and phthalates, are known hormone disruptors and have been associated with an increased risk of cancers, such as breast, prostate, and testicular cancer.[68] While companies have phased out BPA due to backlash, they have often replaced it with bisphenol S (BPS), which we are now finding has similar cancer risks.[69] Another risk with hormone disruption by microplastics is infertility; a meta-analysis of animal studies suggested an over 20% reduction in sperm viability with high plastic exposure,[70] while observational studies have linked PFAS with a 40% reduction in fertility in women.[71] In a recently published analysis of over 3,000 studies, scientists concluded it was very likely that microplastics increase the risk of infertility (and possibly small penis size[72]), lung and colon cancer, and probably many other forms of cancer. We are actively, shamelessly poisoning ourselves, one bottle, one sip of water at a time.[73] If humanity drives itself to extinction through plastic, it will be an ironic and depressing end to our saga.

The microplastic crisis highlights the urgent need for reducing plastic use, improving waste management, and conducting more research on the health effects of these pervasive pollutants. While microplastics may seem ubiquitous, small changes can greatly reduce individual consumption; for instance, chewing gum, disposable plastic water bottles, tea bags, and plastic cutting boards and utensils have all been shown to increase microplastic consumption. On a grander scale, reducing microplastic release into our water supply can occur on the individual and societal level. While banning disposable plastic bags in grocery stores around the world was met with initial resistance, it's proven highly effective at reducing plastic waste, and quite easy to adapt to (I now find tote bags in the pocket of nearly every jacket). Some sources of plastic are less obvious. Seventy percent of clothes today are made of synthetic, plastic-like fibers (like nylon, acrylic, or polyester), which bleed microplastics into the water supply when washed. Clothes account for around 35% of all global microplastics![74] However, small changes like washing on cold, air drying, or attaching a microfiber filter to your washing machine can significantly reduce microplastic emission. Beyond reducing new production, we must find a way to deal with the giant amount of microplastics already in our water. Novel approaches, like releasing plastic-consuming bacteria into the ocean, are currently being studied, but they have a long way to go until they can match our enormous levels of plastic waste. As with carbon capture technologies for carbon dioxide emissions (mainly from burning coal, oil, and natural gas), these approaches recognize humanity's dependence on our comfortable way of life, but offer harm reduction mechanisms to mitigate the damage while we wean ourselves off our plastic addiction. Like suboxone or methadone for those addicted to opioids, or nicotine patches for smokers, a slow taper will always be more successful than quitting cold turkey. Quitting is possible and necessary.

Of all exposures to manmade toxins around us, the most direct and dangerous source is the food and drink we ingest. Herein, plastics pose a closer danger beyond the ever-present shadow of microplastic pollution. Plastic containers or bottles, especially when heated, have been shown to leach toxic chemicals like BPA into our food and water. Many of these chemicals have been associated with an increased cancer risk, at least in cells and animals. Take those black spatulas most of us use for cooking. One study, which screened more than 200 black plastic products, found high levels of flame retardants, such as polybrominated diphenyl ethers (PBDE), associated with hormonal and development impacts. One variety in the tested items, de-caBDE, was linked to cancer.[75] Similar findings have been shown for the Teflon-covered pots and pans first invented by DuPont (these are usually black and cheaper, as compared to copper or ceramic pans, which don't carry the same risk but are more expensive). Of course, there have not been large human studies to show that people who use Teflon pans or black spatulas have increased cancer risk, because the findings would take decades. In addition, quite frankly, most of us are widely exposed to these plastics, if not in our own kitchens, then in foods prepared by others. Aside from cost and time, such a trial would be impossible because there'd be no true comparison group. Everyone in the developed world is exposed to tons of plastic. Comparing our cancer risk to those in developing nations would also be fraught with error, because there'd be so many other confounding variables (other reasons why their risk would be lower or higher than ours). All this is to say, we aren't likely to prove anytime soon just how bad plastic is for cancer risk. But we can say that heated plastics leach chemicals into food. The safest options are to avoid microwaving food in plastic containers, substitute metal or glass for plastic water bottles, and choose metal, ceramic, glass, or wooden alternatives in your kitchen.

CLIMATE CHANGE AND WILDFIRES

Our environmental damage goes far beyond plastic, and when it comes to cancer risk, we're also shooting ourselves in the foot with carbon emissions. As previously discussed, air pollution from cars, homes, and factories is the second leading cause of lung cancer, after smoking. But these are merely the direct health effects. The carbon dioxide that doesn't make its way into our lungs makes its way into the atmosphere, forming a greenhouse effect, and indisputably heating our planet. While the Earth has certainly seen periods of heating and cooling, never before has it happened this quickly. And in meteorology as in biology, rapid swings can have drastic effects; nowhere is this more evident than the scorched earth surrounding Los Angeles. I flew into LAX airport in February of 2025 to attend a conference on, of all things, lung cancer. I couldn't help but appreciate the irony. From the plane, we saw the swaths of land where buildings and people once stood. But what I couldn't see were the long-term health implications that the catastrophe had borne.

Wildfires are on the rise. From 2018–2022, the average person experienced six more days of intense fire risk compared to 2003–2007, and this is expected to grow to nine days by 2050. And that's a conservative estimate. In the worst-case scenario, where emissions continue to accelerate, global warming leads to collapse of Antarctica's massive glaciers, and Miami finds itself drowning; the wildfire risk could more than double during our lifetimes.[76]

Fire and water, elemental opposites, both affect air, and in turn, our lungs. Coastal flooding due to climate change causes mold, increasing the risk of lung infections and inflammation. Wildfires emit huge amounts of particulate matter, accounting for 25% of emissions in the US (the remaining 75% is from cars, electricity from fossil fuels, and industry). Each year, 44 million people in the US are exposed to unhealthy air due to fires.[77]

In the summer of 2023, I biked to the hospital in a mask and glasses, and I could barely see the road ahead. During the COVID-19 era, I became accustomed to the mask, but I had never seen my clothes turn ashy from a few minutes outside. I was victim of a vicious cycle happening on scales unimaginable.

Carbon dioxide from the cars passing by had overloaded the atmosphere. Summer heat and an unprecedented dry spell had lit Canada ablaze. The soot from as away as British Columbia had made its way thousands of miles to the East Coast. And there I was, in Philadelphia, in an emergency room full of people with worsened asthma and injuries from car accidents. One study found that hospital admissions in New York City for asthma and chronic obstructive lung disease had increased 40%.[78] Another study found that wildfires caused over 4,000 premature deaths.[79] And while we know these particles cause lung cancer, it will take decades for us to truly appreciate the increase in risk. There are skeptics who believe our pollution does not affect climate change or our health. But as Galileo apocryphally replied to a Church that insisted the Earth doesn't move: "And yet it does."[80]

In the short 150 years since we've industrialized, we've polluted shamelessly, leaving no corner of our planet, and no person, free of microplastics or toxic byproducts. Never before has a species done so much damage in so little time. Perhaps we will end up a failed branch on Earth's evolutionary tree, innovative enough to conquer the world, but not wise enough to treasure it. Or perhaps we will cause the end of *all* life on Earth (barring those plastic-eating bacteria, who will be left with a feast). We can't know the future, but we do control the present.

In *Slaughterhouse-Five*, Vonnegut "asked [himself] about the present: how wide it was, how deep it was, how much was mine to keep."[81] The present fiasco of pollution, toxic waste, and plastic stretches wide, and our prioritization of profit over employee and consumer protection comes from deep in our history and our psyche. It will not be easy, nor fast, to change our priorities as a society. But it's ultimately our choice as to how much of our natural world, our health, and our cancer-free survival is ours to keep.

In summary:

- Four percent of global cancers are caused by exposures on the job.

- Asbestos is the only known cause of mesothelioma and a leading cause of other lung cancer among construction workers, plumbers, electricians, and others.

- Hair stylists beware: Hair dye increases bladder cancer risk.

- Pesticides such as Roundup probably increase the risk of lymphoma, and victims can get compensation through class-action lawsuits.

- Toxic waste from manufacturers, such as in Love Canal, New York, or Parkersburg, West Virginia, can significantly increase cancer risk, and disproportionally affects the poor.

- Air and water pollution in urban, industrial, and car-dependent areas, as well as wildfires due to climate change, all significantly increase cancer risk, although air and water filters can help.

- Plastic exposure through food and microplastics (found in all water sources) decreases fertility and probably increases cancer risk; wash clothes in cold water, avoid Teflon, plastic food containers, and plastic water bottles, and minimize plastic waste.

CHAPTER 6

Infinite Reproduction

Sex and Cancer

Don't be a fool, cover your tool.
—Unknown

Science is like sex: Sometimes something useful comes out,
but that's not the reason we're doing it.
—Richard Feynman

Sex is how life has survived on this planet for billions of years. By mixing our genes with a partner's (as opposed to just splitting into carbon copies like bacteria do), multicellular organisms are able create a diversity of colors, shapes, and abilities. The diversity enabled by sex has allowed life to weather Earth's changing conditions and evolve beauty, speed, and intelligence (among other mind-boggling adaptations). Consequently, for the survival of any species, evolution has selected for animals to pursue and enjoy sex. Even humanity's earliest preserved writings are littered with sex. In the Epic of Gilgamesh from Mesopotamia, the oldest (over 4,000 years old) surviving story, Gilgamesh covets the goddess Ishtar, a deity of love, fertility, and sex. In Egyptian mythology, the god Atum creates the universe through an act of masturbation. Early Chinese Taoist texts describe sexual practices designed to preserve health, energy, and vitality.

A lot has changed since, but humanity's desire for sex hasn't. Nevertheless, we are living through a tumultuous time in society's relation to sex. In many countries, the pendulum has swung back and forth between a conservative, often religious, emphasis on chastity and a liberal counterculture focused on sexual liberation, diversity of sexual orientations, and reproductive rights. These issues are politically and morally charged and have often overshadowed the discussion of public health and prevention around sex.

Regardless of your political or religious beliefs, people will engage in sex. Today, more than ever, there is a growing diversity of sexual orientations, practices, kinks, and philosophies, all of which have implications for public health. In certain countries, sexually transmitted infections remain a leading cause of cancer and death, and in most of these nations, contraception is desperately needed, yet often controversial. But even in our daily lives in the developed world, our sexual practices affect our cancer risk and need for cancer screening.

SEXUAL BEHAVIORS AND CANCER RISK

Believe it or not, sex can actually have a protective effect against cancer, in more ways than one. For people with prostates, more frequent ejaculation has been associated with lower risk of prostate cancer. The prostate produces and stores fluids that help sperm survive in the vagina, and it expels its secretions when a person ejaculates. Frequent ejaculation means that secretions spend less time "growing stale" and irritating the prostatic ducts. One study found that people with prostates who reported more than 21 ejaculations per month had a 20% lower risk of prostate cancer than those with under 7 a month.[1] It even seems that more sex for males at earlier ages may protect them against prostate cancer decades later, though the mechanism is still being worked out.[2] Some have suggested that more frequent sex leads to earlier detection of breast lumps in women, but large retrospective trials haven't yet borne this out. All we can say is that, at least for people with prostates, sex reduces the risk of prostate cancer.

For people with uteruses, pregnancy, especially later in life, seems to have a protective effect against ovarian, breast, and endometrial cancers. These cancers are often related to exposure to excess estrogen and progesterone, sex hormones that stimulate hormone-sensitive tissue, like the breasts and ovaries, to replicate. Too much signaling can sometimes lead to too much replication, which increases the risk of mutations and unchecked cell division, resulting in cancer. Pregnancy, however, suppresses the oscillations in the blood levels of these hormones for the duration of the pregnancy and many months after (maintaining high levels of progesterone and low levels of estrogen), which is why many breast-feeding women don't menstruate for months after giving birth. The lack of hormonal cycling also suppresses ovulation, the process by which an egg leaves the ovary to move toward the uterus. The ovulatory cycle is believed to promote ovarian cancer, so reducing the number of ovulations (by getting pregnant, for instance) reduces ovarian cancer risk. In other words, hormonal suppression has a beneficial effect on preventing cancer risk. Similarly, women with late menarche (first menstruation) or early menopause are at lower risk of ovarian cancer.

Ovarian cancer has a particularly poor prognosis because it often does not get diagnosed until it has already spread to the peritoneum (the lining of the abdomen) or elsewhere in the body. There is no approved screening test, and given the anatomy, many people do not feel any pain or symptoms from cancer growth. When it comes to ovarian cancer, the best proven means of prevention is actually pregnancy! A woman's first and second pregnancy decrease her risk by about 25% each, and then the risk reduction levels off with subsequent pregnancies.[3] Similarly, pregnancy appears to decrease the risk of endometrial cancer by about 41% compared to the risk of those who never get pregnant.[4] Whereas older studies suggested that first pregnancy at a young age (under 22) is associated with the lowest ovarian and endometrial cancer risk,[5] these newer studies found the cancer risk reduction benefit of pregnancy was similar at any age. On the flip side, teenagers who get diagnosed with ovarian cancer while pregnant actually had worse survival compared to older pregnant women who had ovarian cancer diagnoses.[6] Bizarrely, when it comes to breast cancer, cancer risk actually increases slightly, shortly after giving birth, but then decreases in the decades that follow.[7] This seemingly counterintuitive pattern makes some biological sense: While estrogen and progesterone initially spike during pregnancy, they remain depressed for months afterward (which is why women often don't have menstrual cycles when they are lactating).

Oral contraceptives (OCs, also known as birth control pills), which similarly suppress the menstrual cycle, are also associated with a significant reduction in the risk of ovarian and endometrial cancers. Women who had ever used OCs had a 28% reduced risk of ovarian cancer and a 32% reduced risk of endometrial cancer compared to never-users, with the protective effect persisting up to 35 years after discontinuation.[8] However, with breast cancer, OCs may actually increase risk. Breast cancer risk increased by 55% for the first three years after women stopped taking their OC but seemed to have normalized five years after stopping OCs.[9] OCs may also increase the lifetime risk of cervical cancer (cancer of the cervix, which is the outer end of the uterus) by twofold (though it's hard to say how much of the effect is because women who used OCs had more sex, thereby increasing their HPV risk and thus their cervical cancer risk).[10] Lastly, for some bizarre reason, OC use also seems to decrease the lifetime risk of colorectal cancer by about 20%.[11] It's important to remember that OCs have other negative health consequences; importantly, OCs increase a woman's risk of blood clots (but not as much as pregnancy does!).

Of course, today there are many means of contraception besides OCs that modulate hormones. Progesterone-containing intrauterine devices (IUDs) provide long-term contraception but have recently been shown to increase breast cancer risk by about 20% with short-term use, about the same amount of increased risk as with OCs.[12] We do not yet have the data to know what the effect with long-term use would be, and whether the increased risk dissipates (as it does with OCs) after the IUD is removed. There are even newer generations of progesterone-secreting contraception such as the Nexplanon implantable rod, but the effects of these on cancer risk remain unstudied. It would seem that for people with uteruses, both pregnancy and hormonal contraception are options to reduce gynecological cancer risk (but increase breast cancer risk), though I doubt that anyone is getting pregnant, or taking OCs, with that motivation in mind.

Ovarian and endometrial cancer metastases commonly leave cancer cells all over the lining of the abdomen and pelvis, sometimes strangling the intestines. Once ovarian cancer has spread, the disease is no longer curable. For these peritoneal metastases, the most aggressive treatment involves hyperthermic intraperitoneal chemotherapy. During this surgery, the abdomen is opened up, the surgeons attempt to remove as much cancer as possible, and then they infuse heated chemotherapy into the abdomen to kill the remaining cancer cells. I remember being a medical student, doing a work rotation in the operating room, and assisting with this procedure, which could take over 10 hours total. Although as a student I was certainly not making any incisions, my bizarre role was to jiggle the patient's warm, protuberant abdomen (so large that it appeared pregnant) full of chemotherapy medication to help keep the chemo solution moving. We were instructed to wear multiple layers of special gloves to prevent hurting our skin with the chemo, so I can only imagine how the patients must have felt, waking up after their abdomens had been surgically manipulated and then soaked in toxins.

Of all the surgeries I observed, the cervical, endometrial, and ovarian cancer procedures were the bloodiest and most impactful. These cancers, if not detected early, are devastating and deadly. No unusual abdominal pain, bloating, or postmenopausal bleeding in women should go ignored. I've heard many physicians (female and male) dismiss these nonspecific complaints, attributing them to women's menstrual cycles. But patients know their own bodies best. If a woman reports that her abdomen or pelvis feels different, it is essential to do the testing. No amount of bleeding or spotting is normal after menopause, and patients should inform their primary care doctors or gynecologists immediately. And while I've seen (but obviously never felt) the discomfort of Pap smears and uterine biopsies, I imagine those pale in comparison to the pain of undergoing extensive pelvic surgery for advanced gynecological cancer.

SEXUAL ORIENTATION

Other aspects of human sexuality seem to have unpredictable effects on cancer risk as well. For instance, women in same-sex relationships have been observed to have a higher risk of breast cancer compared to heterosexual women.[13] Whether this effect is confounded by greater use of OCs in straight women or other lifestyle factors (homosexual women are more likely to be overweight, smoke, drink alcohol, or live under the poverty line) remains uncertain.[14] Homosexual men have a 73% overall increased risk of cancer compared to heterosexual men, mostly because of HIV-associated cancers and HPV-related anal cancer,[15] which we will discuss next. As an important sidenote, gay men also have a 1.7-fold increased risk of skin cancer, likely because of a 3-fold greater use of tanning beds compared to straight men.[16] Either way, sexual orientation and elevated cancer risk are not a matter of direct causation, but rather confounding variables associated with lifestyle choices.

Transgender individuals are also at increased cancer risk. Transgender women (assigned male at birth but identifying as female) who use estrogen for gender-affirming hormone therapy have a risk of breast cancer 20–40 times as great as that of men,[17] although the risk remains lower than that of cisgender women (women who are not transgender). On the flip side, hormone use is associated with a three to five times lower risk of prostate cancer in transgender women.[18] Doctors should remember that most transgender women have a prostate, and not neglect appropriate prostate cancer screening (particularly for people who are at high risk, like those who are Black or have a family history of prostate cancer).[19]

Meanwhile, transgender men (assigned female at birth but identifying as male) who use testosterone may have a slightly increased risk of ovarian or uterine cancer,[20] though this risk is not fully understood. Transgender individuals often face challenges accessing gender-affirming care, leading to lower rates of cancer screenings (for example, Pap smears for transgender men, prostate exams for transgender women).

While sexual activities have some protective effects against cancer, sex can also increase cancer risk, largely through sexually transmitted infections.

SEXUALLY TRANSMITTED INFECTIONS

As soon as we learn about sex in health class, we learn about sexually transmitted infections (STIs). STIs are the nightmare of every sexually active teenager, and every pediatrician (for good reason). The US is suffering from an STI epidemic, with 2.5 million cases of chlamydia, gonorrhea, and syphilis diagnosed annually. Syphilis in particular is at a record high, up over 70% in the past five years.[21] While easily treated if detected early, syphilis can be particularly harmful for fetuses, leading to life-long disabilities. Unfortunately, rates of congenital syphilis (passed to the fetus during pregnancy) have almost tripled over the past five years.[22] While all these STIs carry numerous health risks, especially if left untreated, the most dangerous among them is long-term cancer risk.

Human papillomavirus (HPV) is the most well-documented STI linked to cancer. HPV is actually a family of viruses. There are over 100 types (strains) of HPV, with most just causing warts. When HPV infects skin or mucous membranes (such as in the mouth or vagina), it triggers abnormal, rapid growth in the outer layer of skin, leading to wart formation. Warts can appear on the hands, feet, or genitals, depending on where the virus enters the body. Warts are typically harmless and noncancerous, and often go away on their own. The immune system can recognize and clear most HPV infections that cause warts, and therefore these HPV strains are called "low risk." But a few "high risk" strains integrate their viral replication genes into our DNA, pushing the cells that the virus infects into overdrive, and ultimately causing cancer. In high-risk infections, the virus acts to inhibit tumor suppressor genes. These genes normally control cell growth and prevent mutations, acting as the built-in safeguards against infinite replication and cancer. One of the tumor suppressors turned off by the HPV virus is p53, a master cell-cycle regulator that is mutated in most types of solid tumors.[23] In fact, the high-risk HPV strains, namely strains 16, 18, 31, and 33, are the leading cause of cervical, anal, and head and neck cancers.[24] The presence of high-risk HPV increases the risk for invasive cervical cancer anywhere from 30-fold to 300-fold, compared to people without HPV.[25] In fact, many doctors these days are replacing Pap smears with cervical HPV tests, because the risk of getting cervical cancer without HPV is exceedingly low.

These high-risk HPV strains can infect any mucous membrane they come into contact with, usually through sex. Besides cervical cancer, high-risk HPV increases the risk of anal cancer about 5-fold,[26] and increases the risk of head and neck cancer over 10-fold, compared to those without HPV.[27] As one would expect, penetrative anal sex is a significant risk factor for anal cancer caused by HPV. Interestingly, oral sex performed on a vagina carries a higher risk of HPV transmission and subsequent head and neck cancer than oral sex performed on a penis.[28] HPV also increases the risk of penile cancer, which is very rare in the developed world.

HPV is the reason that sexually active women require regular Pap smears and/or HPV tests until at least the age of 65 for early detection of cervical cancer,[29] and all adults should be getting their mouth examined for cancers by their dentist. But the landscape of HPV-related cancers has undergone a massive shift with the development of one of the most effective, lifesaving breakthroughs in prevention: HPV vaccination.

Since the time of Jenner and the smallpox vaccine, dozens of vaccines have been approved against some of the world's deadliest viruses and bacteria, culminating in hundreds of millions of lives saved. They all work on the same simple principle: exposing your immune system to a fragment of the virus so that it can better recognize and fend off the true invader. There are no microchips, and as of this writing, only the COVID-19 vaccines utilize mRNA technology (which is harmless but has gotten a bad rap in the media). Most importantly, all the vaccines offered in the US are highly safe and effective. The HPV vaccine, which now covers nine of the most high-risk strains of HPV, has an effectiveness of over 99% if administered during the recommended age range.[30] On top of preventing infection, these vaccinations are showing remarkable effects in preventing cancer. The older four-strain HPV vaccine has been shown to reduce cervical cancer risk by over 90%[31] and reduce anal[32] and head and neck cancers[33] by around 80% (and we suspect the new HPV vaccine will be even more effective). While most of my patients appreciate that HPV vaccination facilitates cervical cancer prevention in women, few realize the huge benefits for men. HPV can spread to the penis, anus, and even to the throat via oral sex. Whether or not they engage in these behaviors, men are *more* likely than women to develop HPV-related anal and head and neck cancer. Thankfully, the vaccine reduces the risk of these cancers about five-fold.[34,35]

Importantly, the HPV vaccine seems to have maximal effectiveness when given earlier, because that's when the immune system is most robust. The official recommendation today is to give the first of the two shots at 9 years old and give the second one 6–12 months later.[36] At the latest, both shots should be given before age 15.[37] I recall that on my pediatrics rotation, many parents were hesitant (I know mine were) to give their pre-adolescent children vaccines for a sexually transmitted infection. Some expressed fears that HPV vaccines were "sending the wrong message," giving their children permission to become sexually active too early. What I found most effective was sharing data on cancer risk, and separating medicine from morality. It is not my place, as a doctor, to tell parents or children when or when not to have sex. But I can tell you that because of how our immune system works (and not because I expect your child to start having sex), 11–12 is the optimal age to receive the HPV vaccine. Even if the child waits until marriage, or until 30 years of age, to start having sex, it would still be more protective to have received the vaccine at 11 rather than later in life. Most parents, I've found, were amenable to vaccination after my explanation. Some still refused. Once, I saw a 12-year-old boy beg his mom to let him get the vaccine, because he had learned about it in school and wanted to avoid cancer. When the mom still refused him, I was heartbroken, but there was nothing I could do. Thankfully, if teens do not get this vaccine, "catch up" vaccination is recommended until age 26 for women and 21 for men.[38] After those ages, the data on effectiveness is limited.

While we're talking about vaccines, let me say definitively that there is **no** evidence they cause autism. Yes, we've seen a rise in autism diagnoses over the past decades, but that is mostly because we've been screening and diagnosing children more. In centuries past, autistic people like me were just the town recluses, living out in the woods, out of public perception. Any fairy tale will assure you they existed. Today, we're forced to constantly interact, so autism stands out more. Perhaps growing up with technology has also dampened some of our social skills and made behaviors like maintaining eye contact feel less comfortable and natural. But I can assure you that autism has *nothing* to do with vaccines.

Many other vaccine horror stories you may hear are either cherry-picked manipulations of the data, or flat-out lies. The most common side effects from vaccines are arm pain and harmless injection site reactions (I'm writing this while "recovering" from a joint flu/COVID-19 jab). There have been rare, life-threatening side effects like myocarditis (inflammation of the heart lining) or Guillain-Barré (a paralysis syndrome) reported with COVID or flu shots (and all other vaccines), but it's important to note that these complications are actually *even more common* with COVID-19 or the flu, so the vaccine actually decreases your risk. Vaccines have been modern medicine's most miraculous tool, allowing us to eradicate smallpox, a virus that had killed millions, and nearly eradicate polio, which caused the paralysis of tens of thousands of people each year and the deaths of thousands of children in the US during the early and mid-twentieth century.

While HPV is the worst STI when it comes to cancer risk, it's certainly far from the only one. Chlamydia and gonorrhea, while typically thought of as "curable," have been shown to increase ovarian cancer risk later in life by about twofold.[39] Trichomonas, a parasite, leads to yellow-green discharge and cervical inflammation described as "strawberry cervix" (what is it with bizarre medical descriptors and foods?). It has also been shown to increase cervical cancer risk.[40] As for people with penises, studies have found that a history of gonorrhea, HPV, or any STI significantly increases the risk of prostate cancer later in life.[41] In addition, sexual activity can spread viral hepatitis, which infects the liver and can cause liver cancer.

Safe-sex practices are essential in reducing the rates of STIs and associated cancers. While the HPV vaccine is the single most effective cancer-reducing tool, condoms, dental dams, and other barrier contraceptives have been shown to reduce the risk of STI transmission. Consistent condom use decreases the risk of HIV transmission by 71%–80% in heterosexual relationships and by 70%–91% in men who have sex with men.[42] While providing teens with condoms and safe-sex education in schools remains controversial in some parts of the US, the data for such initiatives is overwhelmingly positive and shows that sex education does *not* lead to an increase in sexual activity.

Of course, the most dangerous and deadly of the STIs is HIV. HIV infects T cells, critical immune cells that police others to detect and destroy infections or cancer. Advanced HIV, particularly AIDS (when nearly all of your T cells have "died"), is associated with increased risk of dozens of cancers. Certain rare cancers, like Kaposi sarcoma, have only really been seen in patients with AIDS. HIV and HPV co-infection, in particular, lead to the highest risk of anal and throat cancers. Thankfully, with advances in highly active antiretroviral therapy (HAART) like the medication Biktarvy, these AIDS-related cancers have become much rarer. Modern HIV therapies (HAART) attack the HIV virus on multiple fronts at once, which makes them over 99.9% effective in suppressing the virus and preventing transmission to others (when the medicines are taken as instructed). Nonetheless, many feel that the research and public health initiatives against HIV were far "too little, too late," largely because of HIV's original association with homosexuality, which led to a lot of missed opportunities for prevention, education, and scientific studies during the AIDS epidemic of the 1980s.

HIV AND THE LEGACY OF HOMOPHOBIA

In the early 1980s, when the first cases of a mysterious illness began surfacing in the gay communities of major cities like San

Francisco and New York, few could have foreseen the devastation that would follow. The epidemic—soon to be known as AIDS—was quietly taking root in the lives of men who loved men, but most of the rest of the world chose to ignore thousands of deaths rather than provide desperately needed health care for people who developed this mysterious disease.

By the end of 1981, more than 100 men in the US had died from a strange condition that doctors unfortunately labeled Gay-Related Immune Deficiency (GRID).[43] It wasn't long before the disease spread beyond just the gay community, but the stigma remained. "It's only affecting gays," people would say. "It's a punishment for their lifestyle." The media barely reported on it. Politicians, eager to maintain their distance from an issue tainted by homophobia, chose silence. Ronald Reagan's administration, deeply conservative and heavily influenced by the religious right, refused to even acknowledge the crisis publicly. It would take four years—until 1985—before Reagan mentioned AIDS in a speech, by which time tens of thousands of people had already died.[44]

Gay men would find themselves falling ill with a flu that often would pass. But soon they would notice white patches of fungus in their mouth, or dark lesions growing on their skin, which doctors would later identify as Kaposi sarcoma, one of the hallmark signs of AIDS. Doctors didn't have answers. The hospitals were overcrowded with men with unknown illnesses, and the lack of federal recognition and funding meant little research was being done to find out why.

News channels avoided talking about the epidemic directly, instead talking around the issue and passing moral judgments. Pundits referred to the disease as a "gay plague." Rush Limbaugh, the conservative radio host, hosted a weekly "AIDS update" in which he mocked gay people who had died of the disease.[45] Hatred of homosexuality wasn't just a sentiment; it was policy.

Lawmakers refused to fund early research, claiming that AIDS was confined to "degenerates," not worth diverting public health dollars for. The government, under pressure from religious conservatives who saw the illness as divine retribution, resisted helping the dying men who flooded the hospitals.

As the government turned a blind eye, grassroots efforts rose from the ashes of grief. The Gay Men's Health Crisis (GMHC) and the AIDS Coalition to Unleash Power (ACT UP) were born out of necessity. These were not just activist groups—they were lifelines, distributing pamphlets about safe sex, visiting the sick, and fighting the pervasive misinformation that allowed the epidemic to grow unchecked.[46]

By the time Rock Hudson, the Hollywood heartthrob, died of AIDS in 1985, the disease could no longer be ignored. Hudson's death shocked the public; a famous, "straight" man had fallen victim to a disease people thought to affect only gay men.[47] In 1984, Ryan White, a 13-year-old boy with hemophilia, was diagnosed with AIDS due to a contaminated blood transfusion.[48] It was clear that anyone could contract HIV and AIDS. For a brief moment, the veil was lifted. But the damage of years of government neglect was done. Tens of thousands of people were dead, and tens of thousands more were infected.

Only after sustained pressure from activists did the government start to take action. ACT UP members staged die-ins at the headquarters of pharmaceutical companies and in front of the White House. They chained themselves to government buildings, forcing the world to look at the bodies they were ignoring. "Silence = Death" became their rallying cry. Through it all, the gay community became its own source of resilience. While the government faltered, they took care of each other. Lesbian women, often overlooked in conversations about the epidemic, were some of the fiercest caregivers, organizing support networks and blood drives, and standing by their brothers in arms.

By 1985, AZT or zidovudine, the first antiretroviral medication for HIV to be discovered, was finally showing promise in early studies, and it became a leading candidate for human trials. Interestingly, AZT had originally been synthesized as an anticancer drug in the 1960s, but proved ineffective, and was shelved for over 20 years until some interested scientists found a new purpose for it. The first human trial concluded in 1986, showing reduction in infection and death, and the drug was approved 20 months later—a record turnaround for the FDA.[49] Unfortunately, the original doses were far too high, leading to severe side effects, and the drug was first priced at over $10,000, making it inaccessible to many marginalized groups, such as people living in poverty and people of color. Moreover, HIV, like cancer, was capable of evolving, and soon AZT was becoming less and less effective. By the early 1990s, researchers began combining different antiretroviral drugs to prevent HIV from mutating and becoming resistant (much like we use combination therapies in oncology). It wasn't until 1996 that scientists first started using HAART, a combination of three drugs that we still use today. With the use of HAART, HIV deaths in the US fell by over 40% in a year.[50] Finally, the suffering of the gay community was being heard and addressed—but 15 years too late.

The story of sex and cancer is one that is often repressed or ignored because of society's prejudices. Children are deprived of early HPV vaccination, and LGBTQI+ (short for lesbian, gay, bisexual, transgender, queer, intersex, and others) individuals are denied access to appropriate health care, because of morality judgments around sex. Sex is a personal decision, and in many cultures, a familial or religious decision. But it certainly should not be a policy decision. We as doctors should not have any say in when, or how, someone decides to have sex (although many exasperated ER docs will advise a flared base if you're putting anything up your butt). Neither should the government. It should not be up to members of one religion, or one family, to tell another how to vaccinate their kids, to dictate legislation on abortions, or to tell a school how they should teach about safe sex. Furthermore, in medicine we value the life of a child above the beliefs of their parents. Parents are not allowed to refuse lifesaving medicine for their children. By the same token, some would argue that parents should not have the right to refuse vaccinations or education for children that have been shown to prolong life and reduce risk of cancer. The debate on autonomy and public health, especially when it comes to minors, is controversial but necessary.

Everyone seems to have an opinion about sex: doctors, parents, politicians, religions, ancient and contemporary societies, and last and often listened to least, sexually active individuals. But to best serve public health, we must all set our judgments aside and approach the medical aspects of sex like we would any other behavior. Sex has risks and benefits to health, and there are many evidence-based means of easing the risks. Applying your religious or moral views to other people, or sticking your head in the sand, won't stop other people from sticking other things in other places.

In summary:

- Oral contraceptives reduce risk of ovarian and endometrial cancer, but may increase risk of breast cancer (in the short term); hormonal IUDs may do the same.

- Frequent ejaculation decreases men's risk of prostate cancer.

- LGBTQI+ patients are at higher risk of cancer due to hormone therapy and less access to health care.
- HPV is the leading cause of cervical and head and neck cancer, but childhood vaccination can reduce cancer risk by more than 90%.
- HIV increases the risk for dozens of cancers, and thousands senselessly lost their lives due to bigotry and ignorance during the AIDS epidemic.

CHAPTER 7

Virtue and Vice

Smoking, Vaping, Alcohol, and Other Drugs

Every virtue carried to the extreme is a vice.
—Aristotle

Three be the things I shall never attain:
Envy, content, and sufficient champagne.
—Dorothy Parker

Beer is civilization's oldest beverage. Residue of beer has been found on pottery as old as 13,000 years. As soon as people learned to harvest grain, they began to drink beer. After all, alcohol is naturally antiseptic. Before clean drinking water was available, beer was the healthier alternative.[1]

As agriculture expanded, so did the many types of alcohol produced. Nearly any starch could be fermented. Alcohol became humanity's salvation, keeping people content enough to labor in the harshest conditions. It was an opium of the masses before opium had made its way around the world.[2]

Then in the fourteenth century, Christopher Columbus's plunder of the Caribbean and its people, paid for by the Spanish crown, brought tobacco to Europe. French ambassador Jean Nicot, after whom nicotine is named, introduced the leaves as snuff to French royalty, and soon the stimulant was all the rage. As beer had fueled the agricultural revolution, tobacco would now fuel the industrial revolution. With the African slave trade at its peak and farming transforming the New World, tobacco became the lifeblood of factory workers in Europe, who had to somehow stay awake for 16-hour shifts in grueling factories.[3]

Alcohol and tobacco are intertwined with the history of our civilization. These so-called vices have perhaps enabled some of humanity's virtues. But there's no free lunch. Tobacco, and to a lesser degree alcohol, have become the leading causes of cancer around the world.

Nearly everyone today knows that smoking causes lung cancer. But how we got to this realization, and everything that's happened since, is a story of greed, persistence, and public health legislation in action. As industrialization brings tobacco smoking to more countries around the world, and alcohol and drug use surge as public health crises, humanity must rethink its love-hate relationship with these addictive substances.

TOBACCO AND CANCER

Smoking tobacco causes cancer through the inhalation of multiple carcinogens produced from combusting tobacco leaves at high temperatures. Some carcinogens, like polycyclic aromatic hydrocarbons, arise from burning any organic compounds, while others, like N-nitrosamines, are unique to burning tobacco.[4] These substances induce DNA damage, leading to mutations in critical genes such as KRAS and p53, which are essential for cell cycle regulation and cell death. When these genes are damaged, cancer cells can replicate rapidly, unperturbed by the body's built-in tumor suppression mechanisms. Even nicotine, the addictive substance in tobacco, while not a direct carcinogen, promotes tumor growth and metastasis by activating nicotinic acetylcholine receptors. These in turn stimulate various signaling pathways involved in cell proliferation and survival.[5] The same pathway that provides our brains with some extra energy also fuels a cancer's growth.

It's not surprising then that the lungs, which are exposed to all of the inhaled smoke, are the primary source of tobacco-caused cancer. In fact, some 85% of all lung cancer cases are tobacco related.[6] But this is far from the only consequence of using tobacco. The compounds in tobacco smoke cause cancer in every tissue they touch. The mouth, throat, esophagus, and even stomach are at heightened risk of cancer due to tobacco exposure. The carcinogens poison our blood and accumulate in the kidneys and bladder, whose job it is to filter and excrete toxins. Smoking is even associated with cervical, pancreatic, colorectal, and liver cancers, as well as leukemia, through various, often ill-defined mechanisms.[7] Tobacco also increases the risk of heart attacks and strokes. There seems to be nearly no tissue that smoking does not harm. Chewing tobacco likewise increases the risk of primarily oral cancer, but is also associated with gastrointestinal cancers.

And yet, tobacco use is still growing at a rapid pace around the world. While only 11.5% of Americans smoke (down from 42% in 1960),[8] 22% of adults across the globe now smoke, and this percentage is quickly increasing in Southeast Asia, Africa, and the Middle East.[9] As countries become industrialized and adopt the "western" way of life, they also adopt many of our worst habits. It seems that tobacco, as a powerful and affordable stimulant, may help people cope with the grueling conditions of industrialization. To add insult to injury, nicotine is among the most addictive substances known. On average, it takes smokers 11 attempts before they are able to successfully quit.[10]

Although we've used tobacco for centuries, much of the research on its harms has only been published in the last few decades. The data on tobacco's dangers had been actively suppressed by a select few, who continue to profit from their deception to this day.

THE SMOKE SCREEN: HOW BIG TOBACCO LIED

In the early twentieth century, smoking was seen as glamorous. Celebrities lit up on the silver screen, soldiers were given cigarettes in their rations, and ads declared that a smoke would calm your nerves or help you stay slim. The dangers of smoking weren't widely known—at least, not to the general public. But behind closed doors, the tobacco industry knew more than they let on.

By the 1940s and 1950s, millions of people around the world were hooked on cigarettes. Tobacco companies made fortunes as smoking became a cultural norm. But even as sales of cigarettes filled their bank accounts, something sinister was happening. Early scientific studies began linking smoking to lung cancer,[11] heart disease,[12] and a range of other health problems. Doctors, at first, didn't know the full extent. Some thought that the rise in lung cancer cases might be due to pollution or even genetics. But as more research came in, the evidence became harder to ignore: Smoking was dangerous, and it was killing people.

"Big Tobacco" knew the tide was turning, so they hatched a plan to fight back. Instead of acknowledging the health risks, they tried to sow doubt. In 1954, several of the largest tobacco companies banded together to form the Tobacco Industry Research Committee. On the surface, this group seemed to support research into smoking's effects. But in reality, its main goal was to confuse the public and delay any potential regulations.[13]

The tobacco companies hired scientists who would challenge the studies linking smoking to cancer. They funded research designed to cast doubt on the dangers of smoking. Their message was simple: There's no solid proof. The science isn't settled.

While behind the scenes they worked to manipulate the science, Big Tobacco ramped up its advertising. They paid movie stars and athletes to endorse their products. They claimed that certain cigarette brands were safer than others or even "recommended by doctors." Cigarettes were promoted as part of a healthy lifestyle—despite the fact that, by the 1960s, even the US government had acknowledged the harms of tobacco.[14] One of the most telling moments came in 1969, when a tobacco executive wrote a now-infamous memo stating: "Doubt is our product."[15] The strategy was clear. As long as the public was uncertain about the risks of smoking, people would continue buying cigarettes, and regulators would pause on passing stricter laws.

This tactic worked for decades. The tobacco industry spent millions on public relations campaigns, lobbying efforts, and "scientific" studies meant to keep people in the dark. It wasn't until the 1990s that lawsuits brought by states, patients, and antismoking advocates began to peel back the curtain. Internal tobacco industry documents were made public, revealing how much the companies had known about smoking's dangers—and how hard they'd worked to suppress that information. Some of the most shocking evidence showed that Big Tobacco had not only known about the deadly effects of smoking but had also actively worked to increase nicotine levels in cigarettes to keep people addicted.

Finally, in 1998, the tobacco industry agreed to a historic settlement. As part of the Master Settlement Agreement, the major US tobacco companies paid billions of dollars in damages and agreed to major restrictions on advertising.[16] They were also required to make many of their internal documents public, exposing just how deeply the industry had deceived the world.

Even today, the story of how Big Tobacco hid the truth about smoking serves as a reminder of the power of corporate influence. For decades, millions of people suffered and died because a few companies put their profits first. It was only through persistent efforts by scientists, doctors, journalists, and activists that the full truth finally came to light.

Unfortunately, despite hefty legal fees and taxes on tobacco, profits have only accelerated. In the late twentieth century, several large tobacco companies began merging with other companies to counteract the losses from declining cigarette use. Philip Morris merged with Kraft foods in 1988 and then rebranded as Altria, and Nabisco (creator of Oreos, Chips Ahoy, etc.) was acquired by tobacco giant R. J. Reynolds and then by Kohlberg Kravis Roberts & Co.[17] Millions of people will never get their loved ones back from cancer, but tobacco companies recovered their profits very quickly by replacing one carcinogenic product with another.

VAPING, NICOTINE, AND MARIJUANA

Vaping, or the use of electronic cigarettes (e-cigarettes), has been marketed as a "safer" alternative to smoking traditional cigarettes. While safer because they avoid high temperature combustion, vaping products are still associated with cancer risk. E-cigarette aerosols contain harmful substances such as formaldehyde, acetaldehyde, and other volatile organic compounds that are suspected to cause cancer. Studies have shown that heating the liquid in e-cigarettes can produce harmful byproducts, including substances that damage DNA and increase cancer risk.[18] Early research has shown that vaping damages DNA in lung cells and hinders DNA repair.[19] E-cigarettes have not been around long enough for scientists to be able to estimate the long-term cancer risk.

While marijuana smoke contains fewer chemicals than tobacco smoke, it still contains carcinogens, including polycyclic aromatic hydrocarbons and benzene, both of which are known cancer-causing substances. Research on the link between marijuana smoking and lung cancer has produced mixed results. A large study found no definitive link between moderate marijuana use and lung cancer, although there were concerns about potential risks with heavy, long-term use. The study noted that marijuana smokers tend to inhale more deeply and hold smoke in their lungs longer than tobacco smokers do, which could increase exposure to harmful carcinogens.[20] In addition, increasing evidence links marijuana use to testicular cancer. A 2012 study reported a doubled risk of these cancers among frequent marijuana users, though the reasons for this association remain unclear.[21]

WOODSTOVES AND CAMPFIRES

In many developing countries, stoves that burn wood (along with other solid fuels like charcoal, crop residues, and dung) are commonly used for cooking and heating. This practice exposes households to high levels of indoor air pollution, which has been linked to serious health problems, including an increased risk of cancer. Wood-burning stoves produce smoke that contains a complex mixture of harmful pollutants, including: particulate matter, polycyclic aromatic hydrocarbons (same as in tobacco), carbon monoxide, formaldehyde, and more. Studies have consistently shown that prolonged exposure to indoor air pollution from wood-burning stoves increases the risk of lung cancer by about 1½ to 2½ times. The risk is particularly high for women in rural areas who are responsible for cooking and spend long hours near the stove.[22] Indoor stoves, especially gas ones, have also been associated with cancer of the bladder and of the respiratory (breathing) and digestive tracts. The International Agency for Research on Cancer, part of the World Health Organization, classified indoor emissions from household combustion of wood as Group 1 carcinogens (carcinogenic to humans).[23]

Campfires produce all the same carcinogenic compounds, but given that exposure is outdoors and tends to be less frequent, the cancer risk remains unclear. Studies of outdoor workers and frequent campers have noted an increased risk of respiratory problems, and possibly lung cancer, over time.[24] Exposure to wildfires, and particularly burning plastics and inorganic compounds (like the first responders during 9/11 experienced), has been associated with a number of cancers, including lung, prostate, and blood cancers.[25]

ALCOHOL

Research has shown that drinking alcohol increases the risk of several types of cancer. This link is well established, and even moderate drinking can raise cancer risks over time. When we consume alcohol, the body breaks it down into acetaldehyde, a toxic chemical. Acetaldehyde can damage DNA and prevent cells from repairing this damage, leading to cancer. Alcohol, like the metabolism of fatty foods, also generates reactive oxygen species that damage cells, promotes hormone (such as estrogen) imbalances, and makes it easier for harmful chemicals to enter the body.

The evidence shows that several types of cancer are linked to alcohol consumption. Alcohol irritates and damages the cells lining our throat, especially in people (and for some reason, especially in women) who drink heavily and smoke. Just one drink a day has been shown to increase head and neck cancer risk by 38%.[26] Breast cancer risk is notably increased even with light to moderate alcohol use. For women, consuming just one serving of alcohol per day is associated with a 13% increased risk of alcohol-related cancers, primarily driven by breast cancer.[27] Colorectal cancer risk also rises with alcohol intake; moderate drinking (two to four drinks per day) and heavy drinking (equal to or greater than four drinks per day) are associated with a 21% and 52% increased risk, respectively.[28]

Most people know that long-term drinking is associated with degeneration of the liver, known as cirrhosis. Cirrhosis is a truly terrible condition, leading to bleeding in the esophagus, bleeding and clotting all over the body, confusion, weakness, kidney failure, and early death. But cirrhosis also significantly increases the risk of primary liver cancer. All patients with cirrhosis have about a 3% risk of developing liver cancer each year,[29] about 10 times higher than the average person.[30] Heavy drinking, even without cirrhosis, is associated with a twofold increased risk of liver cancer.[31] Other cancers associated with alcohol include pancreatic, lung, and endometrial.

With every alcoholic drink, you are imbibing a cancer-causing toxin; the more you drink, the higher your risk. There is no "safe" level of drinking when it comes to cancer. For example, heavy drinkers (more than three to four drinks per day) have a three to four times higher risk of cancers, compared to people who do not drink. Even moderate drinking—defined as up to one drink per day for women and two for men—has been shown to increase the risk of breast, esophageal, and other cancers.

A lot of countries, including the US, struggle with a problematic drinking culture. Alcohol is deeply embedded in American culture; it's often associated with college, celebrations, sporting events, and simply recreation on weekends. Heavy drinking is normalized in many settings, leading to an acceptance of behaviors like binge drinking and excessive alcohol use. Defined as consuming enough alcohol to bring blood alcohol concentration to 0.08% or higher, binge drinking is common, particularly among young adults and college students. Binge drinking in particular contributes to accidents, injuries, and alcohol poisoning, and it has the strongest association with developing liver cirrhosis and its many complications. Excessive drinking contributes to around 140,000 deaths annually in the US, along with $250 billion in costs from health care, lost productivity, and accidents.[32] It also plays a role in crime and domestic violence incidents.

The question of why we drink is one that philosophers have grappled with for millennia. In my opinion, drinking, or any psycho-modulating substance for that matter, is a means of coping with stress, anxiety, and depression. Even in the most common circumstances, people use substances to "loosen up" and escape the ever-looming burden of social anxiety. Unfortunately, the more we rely on alcohol to allow us to relax and enjoy others, the more we become unable to make the same connections or have the same experiences without alcohol, leading to dependency and addiction. Fanning the flames is the alcohol industry's heavy marketing of its products in ways that glamorize and normalize drinking (unlike tobacco companies, alcohol companies are allowed to have much more liberal advertising). Ads frequently target young adults and associate alcohol with social success, relaxation, and adventure.

Learning to enjoy experiences and the company of others without substances is a skill to work on like any other, and it requires going against decades of conditioning. I recognize that I myself too often rely on a drink or two to deal with the stress of life, and I empathize with my patients who struggle more than I do. Of course, the health risks of an occasional drink, or cigarette, or edible marijuana are negligible. As with dieting or exercise, it's unrealistic to aim for perfection, and most of us aren't keen to give up all earthly pleasures. Occasional inebriation can also have positive effects, such as dampening inescapable stressors, enhancing creativity, and suppressing fear. But it is important to recognize when we rely on these substances as a crutch or band-aid for other problems, and try to intervene upon dependency before it becomes an addiction. When life is too stressful to handle sober, that is precisely the *wrong* time to drink. Instead, those are the times to seek help from our loved ones or mental health professionals, to take a much-needed vacation, or to go on a run or participate in whatever hobby brings us joy. These are approaches I've seen patients use to turn their lives around, and lessons I've relied upon during my share of rainy days.

Alcohol, tobacco, and other addictions are more a symptom than a root cause of psychological and societal ills. These addictions arise and prosper due to unfulfilled human needs, due to facets of modern-day life that are maladaptive and incongruous with how our primate brains were wired to work. Unfulfilling desk jobs leave many turning to alcohol for thrill and human connection during their limited time off, while the never-ending judgment of social media has exacerbated social anxiety. The biggest root cause of addiction, and most other preventable medical diseases, is poverty. It comes as no surprise that the communities hit worst by opioid, tobacco, and alcohol addiction are low-income rural and urban communities, where economic opportunities are sparse, and fulfilling recreation and connection are difficult to come by. While educating children on the dangers of alcohol and drugs and promoting rehabilitation programs are certainly meaningful endeavors, the most successful reforms to address the root causes of addiction would be safety net and job programs like those used by our government during the Great Depression. Investing in people before they become ill is the solution we ignore far too often.

VICTIM BLAMING

Lung cancer patients often report feeling judged, shamed, or dismissed due to the perception that they "caused" their cancer by smoking. This stigma can lead to depression, isolation, and feelings of guilt, making it harder for patients to cope with their diagnosis and treatment. Stigma may also hinder someone from seeing a doctor due to the fear of being blamed for their symptoms. This delay can lead to later-stage diagnoses, when lung cancer is harder to treat. Lung cancer research is underfunded compared to research on other cancers, partly due to the perception that lung cancer is self-inflicted, reducing public sympathy and support for funding. Breast cancer receives significantly more research funding and public awareness, despite lung cancer being a leading cause of cancer deaths.

ADDICTION AND AUTONOMY

We doctors are guilty of imbuing our recommendations with our own biases. I once worked with a cardiologist who was a muscular Israeli American former military man. I would some-times see him aggressively riding his bike, weaving through center-city Philadelphia traffic. He counseled his heart failure patients with the same aggressive focus on exercise. Perhaps he was right to push his patients, perhaps not. I try to be vigilant about my own complicated history with diet and body image when I give advice. My wife will be the first to say I like to get on my soapbox, so I try not to offer unsolicited advice. With pa-tients who've definitively said they have no interest in quitting smoking, I don't push the issue.

Medicine is no longer the "wild west," where doctors exper-iment on patients or push them into treatments without their consent. As the son of Soviet refugees, I value bodily autonomy more than most. Sometimes, patients fail to recognize their own autonomy. I once had a patient who was hesitant to get the shin-gles vaccine, but upon further discussion, reluctantly agreed to do it. I stepped out to grab the nurse, and when I returned to the room, he was gone. He had fled without checking out. Perhaps he was a people pleaser who couldn't say no, or got cold feet while waiting. Either way, I have learned to always doublecheck and triple check that a patient actually wants what I'm offering them, even if I know it's what's best for them medically.

A problem arises when we're not certain that a patient un-derstands their situation enough to make an informed decision; in medical lingo this is called "capacity." I once had an elderly gentleman come in with severe, life-threatening anemia, or low blood count, due to gastrointestinal bleeding. When we came to offer him a blood transfusion, we were surprised to find him adamantly refuse. It's not unusual to meet people, namely Jehovah's Witnesses, with religious beliefs that preclude them from receiving blood products. But this patient wasn't a Jeho-vah's Witness. When asked why he was refusing, he would offer rambling, inconsistent answers. At one point, he claimed his religion, Islam, did not allow him to accept blood, which neither I nor my Muslim colleagues had ever heard before. Most importantly, he could not articulate the risks (in this case, death) of refusing blood. When we called his family, they likewise did not understand his apprehensions, and asked that we give him the blood. Upon exhaustive discussion with the patient and his family, we decided to give him blood against his wishes, deeming that he did not have the "capacity" at this time to make this decision. The next day, after we had treated his bleeding, he was a completely different person, and actually thanked us for giving him the blood. Stories like these highlight the balancing act of the art of medicine—knowing when to blindly respect a person's wishes, and when to probe deeper.

When it comes to addiction, whether alcohol or opioid, the picture gets even muddier. One of the hospitals where I've worked is the safety net hospital for West Philadelphia, and we have borne the brunt of the fentanyl, and now xylazine, epidemics. Over half the patients I see there are hospitalized with drug-related diseases, whether it be skin infection and bacterial growths in the heart from injectable drug use, or life-threatening withdrawal symptoms. These cases are particularly frustrating because, despite our best efforts, many of these patients decide to leave against medical advice prior to completing therapy, and are often then brought back days, weeks, or months later in even worse condition.

In the spirit of harm reduction, this hospital has started an addiction medicine service that provides opioid-dependent patients with long-acting opioids like methadone or suboxone, or just plain oxycodone, to help stave off withdrawal symptoms and keep them in the hospital long enough to treat their medical issues and help facilitate transfer to substance rehabilitation.

Unfortunately, oftentimes even sky-high doses of opioids are not enough, or the patients are not yet ready to give up the addiction, and they end up leaving to use again on the streets. I've even had patients in police custody, with officers stationed outside their room, manage to escape. Addiction is a powerful motivator.

I remember one young woman who came in with life-threatening vegetations (clumps of bacteria) growing in her heart, who had been stabilized and was pending transfer to substance use rehab with long-term intravenous (IV) antibiotics. Every day, she was pleasant, thankful, and committed to changing her life. Her pain was well controlled, and she claimed she had no desire to go back to using. Then suddenly, the day prior to her transfer to rehab, she was adamant that she had to leave. We pleaded with her to stay, then tried to set up some last-minute, long-acting IV antibiotics, but it was all for naught. As soon as she signed the papers, she was out the door. I was disappointed, but I hoped for the best for her. Then I overheard, about a week later, that she was back, this time in the ICU. The bacterial growths in her heart, left untreated, had led to a massive stroke. She passed away a few days later.

I found myself in tears, and then I felt angry. All our hard work was for nothing. If only we could *make* people stay, we could save them from killing themselves. I've worked with so many cancer patients who fight tooth and nail for an extra few months of life, only to see young, otherwise healthy people throw away decades.

As much as I've wanted to force people to stay, to have their medical issues and addiction treated, I remember the horror stories my parents share of practicing medicine in the Soviet Union, where alcoholics would be locked up, shaved, and dumped in freezing water as the standard of care for withdrawal.

My father told me the story of one man who had saved up for years to get a hair transplant in Turkey, came back home to celebrate with his friends, got a little too drunk, and then woke up in a hospital to find his million-ruble hair shaved off. And these were the "reformed" times. In the decades prior, recurrent alcoholics would be sent to gulags (prison camps) in Siberia along with murderers and political prisoners. As Alexander Solzhenitsyn, the Nobel-winning author of *The Gulag Archipelago* who spent eight years in Siberia among alcoholics and criminals for critiquing Stalin in a private letter put it, "We didn't love freedom enough."[33] Freedom means accepting that people have the right to use drugs, to become addicted, and even to lose their lives. As long as people are able to understand the risks of their choices, it is not our place to stop them, or even to judge them. Heaven knows they get plenty of judgment as it is.

When I first heard that my former patient had died, I felt sad and furious. But after treating a few more patients like her, I'm afraid to say I grew used to it. Now it's just the norm. The same tragedy is playing out all across the country. Addiction is a public health epidemic. Around 17% of Americans have a substance use disorder, and another 10% suffer from alcohol use disorder[34] (while this is considered the less-stigmatizing terminology, I've met plenty of patients who prefer to be called "alcoholics"). Prior to COVID-19, the US life expectancy had actually been declining, partly due to drug overdoses, and it's only gotten worse with all the new synthetic opioids that have hit the streets. Many are laced with all sorts of toxic additives, and the medical field is playing catch-up trying to deal with the consequences.[35]

For instance, I've seen hundreds of people with wounds all over their bodies due to xylazine, an additive to fentanyl that causes the high to wear off faster and also damages the skin where it is injected. The chemical chokes off blood vessels, causing blackened, dead, gangrenous tissue. Some patients even develop these wounds in places on their body where they haven't yet injected, and as of this writing, we haven't figured out why. The wounds are at risk of getting so badly infected that patients must have their limbs amputated to save their lives. The surgeries and amputations to deal with the wounds result in more pain and more opioid dependence, fueling a vicious cycle that has only one escape: death. I've seen a lucky few break the cycle and get their health back, but I've seen many more lives lost to the greed of drug dealers and the feebleness of our social safety net. Whether you see it in your community or not, this is the America we live in today. Relatively few opioid deaths are cancer related, barring the occasional cancer cases that get diagnosed late and go untreated; this can happen when patients who have substance use disorder neglect to get screened for cancer and are too ill to tolerate chemotherapy. Nonetheless, addictive substances like alcohol, opioids, and tobacco continue to pose an existential danger to our marginalized groups, to our health care system, and to our society at large.

As a society, we are addicted to many things: coffee, alcohol, accolades, narcotics, money, sex, popularity, or weed, just to name a few. Each one fuels the others. Tobacco and alcohol arose as tools of greed and productivity, and have since become accomplices to popularity, sex, and success. To prevent cancer, we absolutely must invest in public health initiatives and education to curtail alcohol and tobacco use. Moreso, we must address the cruel social circumstances that lead people to addiction. But we should also take a deeper look within ourselves, and consider why we've chosen to rely on substances and external gratification to find happiness. Addiction will only ever be truly solved when society can provide for all, and people learn to find happiness from within.

In summary:

- Tobacco is the leading cause of cancer—lung, bladder, head and neck, and more—and its use is rising worldwide.

- Tobacco companies operated a "smoke screen" to conceal the dangers of tobacco for decades, and after public backlash, have changed their names and merged with processed food companies, growing their profits.

- Alcohol consumption increases the risk of liver, breast, and esophageal cancer; the more you drink, the higher your risk, but no amount is totally "safe."

- Vaping produces fewer dangerous particles than tobacco smoke, but likely also carries cancer risk, which may take decades to appreciate.

- Addiction is an epidemic fueled by social and economic conditions, and addressing the root causes, like poverty, is actually cheaper than dealing with the consequences.

CHAPTER 8

All the Rays We Cannot See

UV Light and Radiation

I'm not afraid of God. I'm afraid of man.
—Svetlana Alexievich, *Voices from Chernobyl*

Nothing in life is to be feared, it is only to be understood.
Now is the time to understand more, so that we may fear less.
—Marie Curie

Her bone marrow had stopped making blood cells (known medically as "aplastic anemia"). Without red blood cells, she could not deliver oxygen from her lungs to the rest of her body. Without platelets she could not stop bleeding, and without white blood cells, she could not fight infections. By the time Marie Curie died of radiation poisoning at the age of 66, she was nearly blind from cataracts and chronically ill. Her daughter and son-in-law, who would continue her research, also died of radiation-induced disease. To this day, Curie's notebooks are kept behind lead because they remain dangerously radioactive.[1]

Marie Curie and her husband Pierre were awarded Nobel Prizes for transforming our understanding of radiation with the discovery of radium and polonium. After Pierre died in a tragic carriage accident, Marie went on to apply her discoveries to create the world's first x-ray imaging, used in the battlefields of World War I. Others built upon her work to advance radiation therapy, first used against cancer of the throat in 1902 and still relied on to this day.[2] Marie had unlocked a Pandora's box for medicine and society, for decades handling her discoveries with bare, inflamed hands. Little did she realize that the high-energy, invisible rays from her newly discovered elements were depositing that energy in her cells, causing the DNA sequences that her cells relied upon to grow and duplicate to mutate. These mutations accumulate, causing either cellular aging and death, resulting in organ dysfunction, or a disabling of the pauses in cellular replication, resulting in uncontrolled cell division and cancer. In both ways, radiation kills.

Today we know much more about radiation, and how to mitigate its inherent danger, thanks to the sacrifices of pioneers like Marie Curie. Nonetheless, every day we are exposed to radiation from the sun, from the Earth, and from ourselves.

UV RADIATION AND SKIN CANCER

I once saw an elderly patient in the hospital, admitted for heart failure and kidney disease, who was now complaining of a huge, irritated lesion on his back. It was around eight centimeters in diameter, oozing, and excruciatingly painful. Nurses and doctors, of around a dozen different specialties, all looked at it in passing and brushed it off as a bed sore. "Just move him around in bed and apply gauze and ointment," went the mantra. The only problem was, it didn't get better. When a dermatologist took a closer look, and decided to look at a sample under the microscope, we learned that it was actually a huge basal cell carcinoma, the most common type of skin cancer. We had been ignoring it for weeks as it slowly dug its way deeper and deeper into his back.

This patient had been a farmer, and had spent decades with his back exposed to the grueling sun. Never having looked at his back, he had no idea what must have been growing there for years. Evidently, whoever looked him over when he first got to the hospital, before the cancer got inflamed from him lying in bed all day, never took a good look, either. Thankfully, basal cell has the best survival rate of all skin cancers, and this patient was able to get the cancer removed and recover fully. Not all skin cancer patients are so lucky.

Skin cancer is the fourth most commonly diagnosed cancer in the world. One in five Americans will develop skin cancer at some point in their life, and around 10,000 Americans are diagnosed with this cancer every day.[3] There are about 3 million new cases each year of basal cell, squamous cell, and Merkel cell carcinoma,[4] and another 325,000 new cases of melanoma (as of 2020 estimates).[5] The nations with the highest rates are Australia and New Zealand, which have about twice as many cases as North America (though North America still exceeds the world average by six times!).[6] The vast majority of all these cases boil down to one major risk factor: UV light.

The sun emits copious ultraviolet (UV-A and UV-B) photons that hit our skin. Tanning beds produce UV-A, UV-B, and additionally, UV-C. Much like the high-energy rays of radioactivity that we previously discussed, UV-C light has the most direct impact on our DNA, greater than UV-A and UV-B. Remember that DNA is the code that allows our cells to function and consists entirely of four bases: A (adenine), T (thymine), G (guanine), and C (cytosine). In a chemical reaction, the energy causes two adjacent pyrimidine bases (the As and Ts) to stick together, creating bulky "pyrimidine dimers" that our DNA machinery doesn't know how to handle. An estimated 10,000 of these reactions occur in every skin cell every day, due to sun exposure.[7] UV-B causes an estimated 1,000 times more mutations per photon, and is thus responsible for most sunburns, but UV-A exposure in sunlight is 20–40 times greater than UV-B, based on the season, latitude, and altitude.[8]

UV light should not be taken lightly. When skin gets exposed to excessive UV, a bad sunburn, where the damaged cells just die and flake off, is the best-case scenario. At worst, one of the molecularly damaged cells deep in the skin's basal layer survives and becomes deranged. It starts making replicas of itself and accumulating new mutations to avoid the body's immune system and cellular checkpoints. It grows uncontrollably, ulcerating or darkening the skin. In other words, it becomes skin cancer.

If this scenario makes you paranoid, it might (or might not) reassure you to learn that the cells in your body will accumulate quadrillions of new injuries to your DNA every day.[9] This damage occurs primarily from UV light, metabolism (the breakdown of food), and inflammation. Thankfully, the body has evolved an intricate array of safeguards that recognize and repair DNA when damaged and destroy the cells deemed irreparable before they can become cancer. In health care, we use the "Swiss cheese model" to describe how a medical error happens when failures in all the safeguards line up just right. Cancer is much the same. Millions of cells in your body, each day, start on their path to become cancer. 99.999999999% of them get stopped in their tracks, recognized by the immune system or by the inherent safeguards in DNA replication or cell division. The average cancer cell accumulates over 10,000 mutations,[10] of which 1 to 10 may be considered "driver mutations," essential to tumor survival against all the safeguards.[11] In other words, the constellation of mutations that a cancer evolves over years must be "just right" to fool the constellation of safeguards our cells have evolved over billions of years to protect us.

If numbers on this scale are too confusing to follow, suffice it to say that more mutations means greater cancer risk. Our bodies evolved to avoid DNA damage and mutations. One such evolution against skin cancer is melanin, the pigment that gives skin its color. Melanin absorbs the high-energy rays of UV light (just like dark surfaces get hotter in the sun than light ones do), and is also known to be an antioxidant and radical scavenger, which means it interferes with the high-energy molecules that cause DNA damage. As you would expect, individuals with darker skin, and more melanin, are thus at lower risk of skin cancer. Of note, the melanin also prevents UV light's destruction of a vitamin called folate (or folic acid, found in all prenatal supplements), which is essential to the development of baby brains and spinal cords. One team of researchers has hypothesized that melanin could have evolved more to prevent the destruction of folate than to prevent skin cancer.[12]

The original *Homo sapiens* who left Africa around 60,000 years ago, and from whom all non-African people today descend, were most likely Black. However, as they encountered climates with less UV light, they faced a new challenge; UV light is required to produce 90% of vitamin D3, which is essential for bone strength and immune function. Our ancestors in northern climates like Europe thus had to lose their melanin (which, as you recall, absorbed UV rays) and develop lighter skin to produce enough vitamin D3 with less direct sunlight.[13] Of note, although very visible, these changes happened relatively recently in the story of human evolution; this means there is actually *more* genetic variation among different groups in Africa than among Africans, Europeans, and Asians.[14] In other words, skin color doesn't mean all that much in genetic terms.

When we look at skin cancer today, we see that it occurs most commonly in individuals with paler skin living in climates like Australia, New Zealand, and parts of North America, where inhabitants get much more UV exposure than their ancestors would have. As we live longer, and get more UV light than our skin can handle, our cancer risk increases exponentially.

Another contributor to the *more than doubling* of skin cancer cases over the past three decades is the depletion of the ozone layer. The ozone layer within the stratosphere of the atmosphere acts as a natural filter, reducing the amount of UV-B that reaches our skin. The destruction of the ozone layer has occurred with the dumping of chlorofluorocarbons and halons into the atmosphere, which are released in industrial production, aerosols, and refrigeration. Climate change due to the accumulation of carbon dioxide in the atmosphere, released from the burning of fossil fuels, may be exacerbating the issue. Studies suggest that the risk of UV-induced skin cancer increases with every one-degree rise in temperature, although the mechanism is still not fully understood. Particularly in Australia and New Zealand, which are closest to the ozone hole over the South Pole, skin cancer has become a significant public health hazard.[15]

Thankfully, with the Montreal Protocol, implemented in 1987, which has limited ozone-depleting gases, the ozone hole has begun to repair itself. As of 2022, the hole is about 15% smaller than it was at its largest, in 2006. But over the same time period, emissions of carbon dioxide contributing to climate change have continued to worsen.[16] The Montreal Protocol was an impressively successful public health intervention, and certainly not the only one. Australia has led the way in raising awareness and implementing regular hat and sunscreen use, which will likely change the skin cancer risk in that country for generations.

Public health initiatives have a median return on investment of around 14, at least according to a 2017 meta-analysis of 3,000 campaigns from around the world. In other words, for every $1 invested, $14 are saved in future health care costs and improved social productivity. Every day we can keep someone out of the hospital or chemo infusion suite gives society back thousands of dollars and an extra day of work.[17] And yet, our proportion of spending on public health has consistently decreased over the past decade. When it comes to skin cancer, we may well be burning ourselves.

In 1988, the State of Victoria in Australia started the Sun-Smart program, which used television advertising to stress the use of hats and sunscreen. A subsequent study found that the rate of sunburns had been more than halved by 2002, with those who viewed more of the advertisements more likely to use skin protection. Of course, even with copious advertising, there were still holdouts. While adults are often stuck in their ways, youth tend to be more impressionable, and thus the best candidates for educational interventions. An extension of the SunSmart program created a school accreditation that required hat wearing, shade seeking, and positive sun-protective behavior role modeling for grade-school students, including providing sunscreen for those who did not have it. After 20 years of implementation, the proportion of schools in Victoria, public and private, that had policies in place to meet these requirements increased from 17% in 1993 to 89% in 2013.[18] With initiatives like this one across its states, Australia's rate of melanoma, the deadliest skin cancer, peaked in 2005. In the US, our peak is not expected until 2022–2026.[19]

The US EPA adopted a narrower program, called SunWise, that also provided education to schoolchildren on skin protection. From 2000 to 2015, SunWise is estimated to have prevented 11,000 cases of skin cancer and 50 deaths from skin cancer, saving $2–$4 in health care spending for every $1 invested.[20] It seems that investment in sun protection education is a no-brainer. And yet, a study of 828 US schools found that only about 15% provided sunscreen, scheduled activities around sun intensity, or reminded parents to apply sunscreen.[21] While public health is often kept in the shadows, our children, unfortunately, are not.

PREVENTING SKIN CANCER

While the chambers of our legislature slowly mull over funding these well-established public health initiatives, what can we, as individuals, do to alleviate our skin cancer risk?

Sunscreen and hats are the best-established protection against UV light when outside. Fewer than 40% of Americans report practicing adequate skin protection, and less than 20% apply sunscreen to all exposed skin surfaces.[22] In order to fully protect oneself, the American Dermatology Association recommends a broad-spectrum sunscreen (meaning it blocks both UV-A and UV-B rays) of at least 30 SPF is a mathematical ratio of how long it would take the average skin to redden with and without sunscreen. So, an SPF of 30 means that, with proper application, skin with that sunscreen on would take 30 times longer to burn than skin without it. As you may recall, sunburn is predominantly a consequence of UV-B, so SPF is really a measure of how much UV-B gets blocked. SPF 15 sunscreen blocks around 93% of UV-B light, while SPF 30 blocks around 97%. After SPF 30, you get diminishing marginal returns, with SPF 50 blocking 98% and SPF 100 blocking 99%.[23] Some experts suggest that consumers with SPF above 50 feel emboldened to stay out in the sun longer, even though the difference in protection they get is insignificant, actually resulting in a higher chance of getting sunburn. To ensure your sunscreen also blocks UV-A light, associated with DNA damage and resulting in skin aging and cancer, look for broad-spectrum sunscreens with at least 3% avobenzone or 15% zinc oxide.[24]

Optimal use of sunscreen means applying it 30 minutes before you go out on all exposed skin and reapplying it every 2 hours when out and about. Likewise, most sunscreens get washed off and degrade in water, so reapplying upon exiting the water is necessary.[25] Unfortunately, many commercial sunscreens contain chemicals that may harm marine life like algae, corals, fish, and even dolphins, though these studies of marine life have largely been laboratory-based as opposed to real-world studies. Looking for sunscreens specifically made to avoid these chemicals, and wearing ultraviolet protective factor (UPF) swimwear instead, can help preserve the very environments we want to safely explore.[26]

Unlike SPF, UPF is measured as the denominator in the fraction of how much UV light passes through the clothing to reach your skin. For example, a UPF of 50 means only 1/50, or about 2%, of UV rays reach your skin, and 98% are blocked. Clothing with higher UPF includes darker colors (it absorbs the rays, thus heating up in the sun) made of unbleached cotton, shiny polyester, and satiny silk, preferably loose fitting, so the sun-blocking fabrics don't get stretched out.[27] Avoiding outdoor activity in the sun at peak hours of overhead sun, around 10 a.m.–2 p.m., dependent on season and latitude, is also a great way to protect your skin. In addition, high altitudes as well as snow reflection can cause sunburn quickly, so wear sunscreen when hiking in the mountains and while on ski slopes.

The sun is not the only source of UV exposure. An estimated 7.8 million women and 1.9 million men use tanning beds annually, despite the International Agency for Research on Cancer identifying tanning bed radiation as a carcinogen due to levels of UV exposure higher than that from daily sun (for most latitudes). As expected, more time spent tanning is associated with greater cancer risk, with the greatest risk for people who have tanned for decades, beginning at an early age. In fact, a 2020 study estimated that stopping indoor tanning among people under 35 years old would prevent around 450,000 cases of melanoma, the most dangerous form of skin cancer.[28] In fact, 97% of women who develop melanoma before age 30 have an extensive tanning history. A single session increases one's lifetime risk of basal cell skin cancer by 67% and squamous cell skin cancer by 29%. Fortunately, tanning is falling out of favor among US high school students, with the proportion who tan decreasing from 15.6% in 2009 to 7.3% in 2015. White, non-Hispanic women continue to be the group with the highest usage. Although often frowned upon in social media, sunless (spray) tanners are the only fully safe way to achieve a tan.[29] Another, nonmedical consideration is how much tan is too much, especially in a society with an evolving appreciation of our inherent colorism. Celebrities and models with naturally pale skin have been accused of racial insensitivity as social "beauty standards" have driven them to emulate darker, historically undesirable skin tones. While the social and medical aspects of tanning are two very different beasts, it is medically well established that the influence of social media on beauty standards, which includes but is not limited to skin tone and weight, has a detrimental effect on mental health, especially among girls and young women.[30]

Although by far the largest, UV light is not the only contributor to skin cancer. Immunosuppression from disease (such as HIV) or medications is also associated with an increase in skin cancer.[31] UV light has been shown to suppress the immune cells in the skin, known as Langerhans cells, that are responsible for monitoring against cancer development.[32] On the flip side, many cases of melanoma and squamous cell carcinoma are being successfully treated with immune-stimulating antibodies known as checkpoint inhibitors (currently approved for skin cancers are brand names Keytruda, Opdivo, and Libtayo). These drugs, approved for dozens of types of cancer, take the brakes off the T cells, encouraging them to recognize and destroy cancer cells. Treatment for immunosuppressive diseases like HIV or leukemia can improve skin cancer risk, although patients with this history or those taking immunosuppressive drugs (such as steroids) long term should be more vigilant about skin protection and examination.[33]

While the US Preventive Services Task Force *does not* recommend skin examinations for all adults, it does recommend it for anyone with a family history of skin cancer, genetic predisposition, immunosuppression, history of intensive sun exposure, or paler skin.[34] Many studies have found a benefit to regular skin examination, although one suggested that lesion-directed examination, where patients identify lesions and show them to their doctors, was six times faster and equally effective as whole-body exams by the doctor.[35] In other words, when done correctly, whole body self-examination with mirrors or friends/family can improve skin cancer detection.[36]

What to look for on your skin is a whole science unto itself. Moles are technically precursors to melanoma, so the more moles a person has, the greater their risk of eventually developing melanoma. The risk of any single mole transforming into melanoma is, of course, rather slim, ranging from 0.0005% in those under 40 years old to 0.003% in those over 60 years old. Another study found that people with greater than 100 moles have a sevenfold increased risk of melanoma.[37] When it comes to melanoma, all moles are not created equal. The ABCDE criteria, used to identify high-risk moles, stands for Asymmetry,

Border irregularity, Color variation, Diameter greater than 6 mm, and Evolution (or change). Any mole that meets any of these criteria is best taken off and observed under a microscope to find out whether it is cancerous.[38]

Moles, however, are but the tip of the iceberg when it comes to precancerous skin lesions. For instance, an actinic keratosis is a scaly, rough patch of skin that develops after years of sun exposure, often on the scalp, face, arms, or hands. It is also a direct precursor to squamous cell skin cancer. Related to actinic keratosis is actinic cheilitis, a similarly scaly lesion that usually forms on the lower lip (which is exposed to more UV light than the upper lip).[39] Bowen disease is another precancerous lesion associated with sunlight, and it can be scaly, flat, raised, itchy, red, or brown (in other words, it can show up in various ways). All of these lesions have a significant risk of transforming into cancer, and for this reason, all of them ought to be cut out and evaluated with a microscope.[40]

There are other types of skin cancer, particularly melanoma, which is much more likely to metastasize early (often to the brain or lungs) and thus has a poorer survival rate than other skin cancers. Around 10% of melanoma patients have a family history of the disease, suggesting a hereditary component. Mutations passed on from parents to children, such as those in the CDKN2A gene, disable one of the many cellular safeguards against cancer. Children who have this mutation have a higher risk of one of their melanocytes, or melanin-producing cells, accumulating the critical load of other carcinogenic mutations (either from UV light, metabolic damage, or just random chance) to become melanoma.[41] Similarly, people born with a faulty repair mechanism for UV-induced DNA damage, a condition known as xeroderma pigmentosum, have a 20,000-fold increased risk of getting any skin cancer.[42] Children born with dysplastic nevus syndrome have hundreds, if not thousands, of high-risk moles, any of which can transform into cancer.[43] Once inherited, there is not much we can do about these conditions, except watch the skin vigilantly and cut out anything suspicious. Advances in genetic testing are finally allowing parents to test themselves, a fetus, or even an embryo to identify these conditions early, as we will discuss later.

Besides avoiding UV light, we are now learning that other lifestyle changes may lower skin cancer risk. Some, but not all, studies have suggested that being overweight increases one's risk of melanoma.[44] Fat cells are notorious for producing inflammatory cytokines, or signaling molecules, that increase one's risk of a whole host of cancers. Metabolism, or the breakdown of food into energy by our cells, creates high-energy particles, much like UV light, that damage our DNA. Those who eat more, metabolize more, contributing to the cancer risk of obesity.[45]

On the other hand, some skin cancers are not inherited nor caused by our choices, at least as far as we know today. Acral melanoma often occurs on the palms, soles, and nailbeds, which get minimal sun exposure. It is particularly common in people with darker skin, who are otherwise at *lower risk* of skin cancer.[46] Uveal melanoma is melanoma of the colored part of the eye, and it has a very poor prognosis, with over half of patients diagnosed with late-stage disease. Unlike other melanomas, uveal melanoma has *not* been associated with UV light, and may even be prevented with more UV light. Vitamin D3, which is synthesized by UV light, seems to have a protective effect.[47]

As I've heard many times throughout my training, *cancer doesn't read the textbook.* For all the many cases of skin cancer that are predictable and preventable, there will always be the few that we are unable to explain, at least with our current understanding. Further research will shine light on the development of skin cancer.

In terms of sheer numbers of cancerous lesions, UV light is by far the deadliest form of radiation. But many other invisible cancerous rays, known as ionizing radiation, lurk right next door, above our heads, or beneath our feet.

RADIATION FROM THE GROUND

Radiation is the rare foe we cannot see, hear, smell, or feel. The majority of lung cancer patients I've seen in the clinic were smokers. They had, for decades, inhaled toxic particles produced by high-temperature combustion—particles that they could smell and taste, but whether through ignorance or misinformation, judged to be worth inhaling. A select few were nonsmokers who had the misfortune of developing a random mutation like EGFR or ALK that changed the cells in their lungs. Then there were a few miners. They were all elderly gentlemen, some of whom had smoked, some of whom hadn't. In my area of the country, they were a dying breed, bygones of a time when men toiled in the darkness year in and year out. Around the country, some 140,000 people still work in mining.[48] Most work with coal or precious minerals. An exceedingly rare few mine uranium. I've never seen a uranium miner in the clinic, but I have learned that about an hour north of Philadelphia, back in the '60s, '70s, and '80s, active uranium mines existed.[49] Like coal miners, uranium miners are also at a far greater risk of lung cancer, but through a completely different and invisible mechanism.

Uranium naturally releases alpha radiation and degrades into the element thorium and then into the element radium. These are the elements that Marie Curie tirelessly studied, sacrificing her health, and possibly her sanity, in her pursuit of knowledge. They are elements crucial to countless industries today, from x-ray machines (which we will discuss later) to energy production. These elements are found in small amounts all over the Earth, but most people outside these industries have little exposure to their radioactivity. However, these elements are also the precursors of radon gas.

Radon is produced when uranium or radium, found in the soil in small amounts, naturally degrades. Unlike its precursors, radon is a gas, which means it can spread far and wide. It can also penetrate through almost any material, and itself degrade into radioactive "radon daughters," producing more and more alpha radiation throughout the process. These radon daughters stick to dust in the air, get breathed in, and get trapped somewhere along the respiratory tract, emitting small amounts of radiation, potentially for years. The nearby cells soak up the radiation, accumulate the damage, and ultimately transform into cancer. As you'll see over and over, it is the cells, whether they be in the skin, the gut, the bladder, or the lungs, exposed to our environment and our consumption of food and drink, that account for almost all cancers.[50]

Eight times denser than air, radon sinks and accumulates in low, confined spaces, like basements. Radon levels vary geographically, with North Dakota and Iowa having the highest levels, and certain areas in most states being designated as "radon zones." Historically, areas naturally high in radon in the US and Europe were advertised as "radon spas." People would bathe and soak in these spas, hoping the radon would treat chronic pain and improve mood. This practice may have indeed worked for a select few, like people with rheumatoid arthritis, in whom the radiation would have suppressed the immune system, decreasing their painful autoimmune flares. Today, we know radon spas are dangerous, although they remain open in several countries.[51] Even if a spa is shut down, that doesn't address the natural levels of radon in certain places. In Armenia, for instance, radon accounts for about 30% of all lung cancer cases. In fact, radon is so prevalent that it is considered the second leading cause of lung cancer in the US and around the world, after smoking. An estimated 21,000 deaths due to lung cancer each year can be attributed to radon, making it the deadliest source of radiation worldwide.[52]

Radon cannot be sensed by humans, but it can be measured. The EPA recommends that all homeowners measure their radon levels, particularly in the basement. All over the country, millions of people live in high-risk zones, areas where uranium deposits occur naturally and used to be mined. Approximately seven million homes in the US are estimated to have radon above safe levels.[53]

Anyone with a radon level above the baseline level that is found outside, about 0.4 pCi/L (picacuries per liter of air), should hire a professional to help ventilate the radioactive gas from the home. The most common method is called soil suction, which involves pumping out the air from the basement or confined space up and outside the home, where it can be diluted by the outside air. Other methods to dilute radon include sealing cracks in basement walls to slow its diffusion and improving airflow with windows or vents, but without some form of pump, these methods are considered insufficient. It is estimated that if all homes across the country followed these recommendations, we could decrease lung cancer deaths by about 4%.[54]

For many families, radon testing and mitigation may simply be unaffordable. The average soil suction system costs around $1,000, though it may run to over $3,000, depending on the size and complexity of the home. For over 30 years, the EPA has sponsored the State Indoor Radon Grants program, which helps share the cost with states, territories, and tribes to install radon elimination systems or sponsor the construction of radon-proof buildings.[55] This program is not available to individuals. People with low income are left to cover the cost on their own, or not at all, exacerbating the already striking racial and income disparities in lung cancer risk.

It would cost the federal government around $1,000 to eliminate radon in a home, or about $400 per individual (the average US home has 2.5 residents). In contrast, the immunotherapy medication Keytruda, which is now one of the treatments recommended for nearly every case of metastatic lung cancer, costs around $185,000 per year.[56] Economic analyses suggest that eliminating radon in high-risk homes would easily pay for itself.[57]

DAILY RADIATION

Setting radon aside, we are bombarded with many other forms of radiation every day. Trying to avoid each and every one of them would drive anyone crazy. Avoiding medical scanners or cellphone towers and sporting a tinfoil hat isn't likely to make you significantly safer, from a cancer-risk perspective.

The greatest source of your daily "radiation intake" is actually cosmic radiation, fast-moving particles from our sun and the rest of outer space that bombard the Earth every day. Thankfully, our atmosphere and natural magnetic fields intercept most of them (which is, incidentally, responsible for the beautiful light show of the aurora borealis in the polar skies).[58] Given that all of us inhabit the same planet, it is impossible to study how much these cosmic rays contribute to cancer risk, because we have no control group that is not exposed to these rays. Some studies suggest that airplane pilots, who spend more time higher up in the atmosphere and are exposed to more cosmic radiation, have a higher rate of skin cancer, but these are just observations, and other lifestyle elements are difficult to control for. Consider this: If your job allowed you to travel to the world's beaches and golf courses (like a pilot does), would you always responsibly wear sunscreen? Also, pilots as a group tend to be white and male, the two groups at highest risk of skin cancer.[59] While cosmic radiation is an important consideration for our astronauts on a space station, here on Earth, it's not something we can significantly change, and thus not something for most of us to worry about. However, some people on Earth fly "closer to the sun" than others. For instance, airline attendants may have higher rates of breast cancer, per one meta-analysis.[60]

When it comes to the cancer risk of additional ionizing radiation, on top of the baseline level of radiation we get from the Earth and the sky, most of our data comes from the victims of the atomic bombs dropped on Hiroshima and Nagasaki, Japan. The laws of physics make it fairly straightforward to calculate the level of radiation exposure for those living many miles from the blast, and enough time had passed that scientists could observe and quantify their cancer risk relative to the rest of Japan at the time. The flaw in this method is that all that radiation was delivered at the same time, while our exposure from flying or x-rays happens gradually, stretched out over many years. One large exposure gives the cellular machinery much less opportunity to repair the DNA damage, compared to a slow, steady exposure. Nonetheless, based on the studies of the survivors, scientists have designated 100 millisieverts (mSv) as the annual level of radiation above which cancer risk begins to increase (by about 0.2%).[61]

The accepted level of 100 mSv, as an upper limit, can help put some of our daily exposures into perspective. Flying in a commercial plane adds about 0.003 mSv per hour.[62] Doing the math, you would have to fly 33,000 hours a year to exceed that level, which is impossible, as there are only 8,760 hours in a year. Another common source of radiation is actually food. Plants and animals, by virtue of the soil they grow in and water they use, accumulate naturally occurring radioactive isotopes. For instance, Brazil nuts are known to be up to 1,000 times more radioactive than other foods. Other "radioactive foods" include red meat, carrots, and lima beans, though none of them compare with Brazil nuts. Nonetheless, when you calculate the actual level of radiation, you find that you would have to eat 400 nuts a day, every day, to exceed the annual level of 100 mSv.[63] Moreover, Brazil nuts are among the best dietary sources of selenium, a deficiency of which, although rare in the US, is medically more dangerous than the amount of radiation in the nuts.

The greatest contributor to our increased radiation exposure over the past decades has been medical imaging. The proportion of total daily radiation that comes from health care has grown from 15% in 1980 to 50% today, with computed tomography (CT) scans accounting for 24% of that. But even with a whole-body CT scan, one of the most radioactive medical imaging tests, it would take about five scans a year to exceed the threshold. In comparison, it would take 1,000 chest x-rays to exceed the 100 mSv threshold. One study looking at the risk of cancer in patients 22 years after they got CT scans found an elevated cancer risk of 0.7%, but the risk was skewed by those who had gotten 5 CT scans or more over the 22-year period. Among those patients, the cancer risk may have been as much as 12% higher. Of note, CT scanners have gotten safer and "less radioactive" over the past decades.[64]

Ionizing radiation is particularly harmful to children, both because their longer life expectancy gives cancer greater opportunity to arise, but also because their growing bodies have more dividing cells that are susceptible to DNA damage. However, parents should not hesitate to take children on vacation or get an x-ray for a fracture. The radiation from food, airplane travel, and even x-rays is negligible; only the exposure from repeated, frequent CT scans may actually be enough to tip the scales.[65]

When CT scans are recommended, patients can ask their doctors if they would be good candidates for "low-dose" CTs, ultrasound, or magnetic resonance imaging (MRI), the latter two having no radiation whatsoever. Children and people who are exposed to a lot of radiation should be particularly wary of receiving CT scans, however, sometimes medical necessity outweighs the risks. Certain acute, life-and-death conditions, like a brain bleed or appendicitis, cannot be quickly diagnosed without a CT scan. Modern medicine is a blessing, but we must remain vigilant and conservative in its applications. It will take decades for us to fully observe the long-term risks of relatively recent innovations like the CT scan. Our world is inherently radioactive, now more than ever, but at least we are finally learning to measure, mitigate, and even wield this mighty force. Yet sometimes, with overconfidence, we attempt to control forces of nature that are far more powerful than we are.

RADIOACTIVE CATASTROPHES

Dnipro is an old industrial city in Eastern Ukraine. With a population roughly that of Fort Worth, Texas (at least before the current war), it was also home to one of the highest percentages of Soviet Jews. Jews from all over the Russian Empire were made to leave their homes beginning in 1791 and forced to live in a designated region of Ukraine named the "Pale of Settlement," where they were constantly terrorized by officially sanctioned attacks known as pogroms.[66] Dnipro and its surrounding towns and villages are where my grandparents hail from and where my parents grew up. It is also less than 300 miles from Chernobyl.

My grandfather, the last devout member of my family, died just days before my bar mitzvah, of multiple myeloma, a cancer of immune cells housed in our bones. My grandmother, who was my cheerleader for all things academic, died of a rare lymphoma transformed to leukemia just days before my valedictorian speech. While I'd found my way into the world of medicine as their translator and advocate, after they passed, I found myself wanting to stay. Their early deaths got me involved in laboratory cancer research in high school and set me on the path that has brought me here. Their deaths may also have been preventable.

In the middle of the night on April 26, 1986, the number 4 reactor at the Chernobyl nuclear power plant suffered a catastrophic meltdown rated a 7 (the maximum) on the International Nuclear Event (INE) Scale. (The only other such nuclear accident was the Fukushima nuclear power plant disaster in Japan in 2011.) In a safety test gone wrong, the leakage of the coolant and loss of power resulted in an explosion, destroying the building and rupturing the reactor core. A fire ensued for over eight days, which released airborne radioactive contaminants all over the Soviet Union and the whole of Europe.

It took over three days to evacuate the residents of the neighboring city of Pripyat. On May 1, while the fire was still raging, my mother recalls being forced to march for International

Workers' Day, a major communist holiday, blissfully unaware of the radioactive contaminants raining down on her. The Soviet Union was not known for its transparency. The disaster may never have been announced to the public had scientists at the nuclear plant in Forsmark,[67] Sweden, not picked up the signals of radioactivity two days after the explosion.

My father was a conscripted fireman at the time, stationed in Kiev, not far from Chernobyl. All of his superiors were summoned, in secret, to help put out the fire, with no warning of what they were to face. Most of them never came back. Many of the engineers and firemen at Chernobyl suffered a similar fate to Marie Curie, but much more acutely. Decades before they could develop cancer, the rapidly dividing cells in their skin, intestines, and bone marrow accumulated an unsustainable number of mutations, causing them to die and slough off. In a situation such as this, the only chance at survival is supportive and bone marrow transplant to replace the vital blood cell progenitors that have been lost.[68]

Those who do survive a disaster like this are still at risk of cancer, particularly blood and thyroid cancer. The thyroid is especially at risk of cancer from radiation because it takes up and stores iodine to make thyroid hormone, and iodine itself can become radioactive. Patients exposed to radioactive fallout are often treated with a form of iodine to help replace the radioactive iodine in their thyroid and prevent cancer development. This is the only prophylactic, or preventative, treatment available for radiation exposure.[69] Thankfully, being a fledgling recruit fireman, my father was not called upon; if he had been, I probably would not be here. While this book emphasizes all the deaths we fail to prevent, it is important to appreciate all the lives that are saved, by intervention or by chance.

My family will never know exactly why both my grandparents developed relatively rare blood cancers, at the same age, despite no family history or established risk factors. It is tempting to blame Chernobyl, which, according to the World Health Organization, is estimated to have resulted in over 10,000 early cancer deaths (although the "official" Soviet death toll was 30).[70]

I once met a patient who had been diagnosed with metastatic lung cancer, and a year later, aggressive lymphoma. Her misfortune seemed astronomically unlikely and unlucky. But it turned out that present-day luck had nothing to do with it. Her fate had been sealed decades ago. She had lived in the Ukrainian town of Pripyat, adjacent to Chernobyl, when the nuclear reactor suffered its infamous meltdown. She was among the clueless masses who were kept in the dark, both literally and metaphorically, following the tragedy. It took two days of cover-up and bureaucratic stalling before officials finally decided to evacuate. Unlike the police, civilians were told nothing and provided with no protection or masks. (Could a mask have prevented her lung cancer? We'll never know.) Our bodies are resilient and have built-in redundancies. We carry two copies of all tumor suppressor genes, both of which must be shut off for cancer to take hold. Chernobyl's radiation delivered a "hit" to this patient's DNA, causing the first mutation in a master cell regulator gene called TP53, leaving her with only one functional copy to spare. After decades of life, she randomly developed another mutation, and then the cancers took off.

Those precious hours after the explosion, wasted by a politburo with a wanton disregard for human life, had sealed this woman's fate some 40 years ago. She reminded me of my grandparents; we cried and reminisced about the "old world" and all its bygone ways. As she left the hospital, I wished her well, leaving her with my coy "I hope to never see you back here again."

Months later, I came across her chart. To my dismay, she had actually "beaten" her lung cancer, only to then die of the lymphoma months later. Two hits to her genes, two days, two cancers, one death.

*   *   *

But Chernobyl was only the tip of the iceberg. Public safety was never a priority in the USSR. My grandfather worked his whole life in a steel factory with no precautions, and he recalled many of his colleagues and superiors taking "early retirement." Extensive uranium mining in the area and dumping of radioactive residue from the nearby Prydniprovsky chemical plant are suspected to contribute to the unusually high number of thyroid cancers in the area,[71] though large studies have never been undertaken. My parents recall, as children, smashing mercury thermometers and playing with the indicator beads, which they did not know were dangerous. They, too, now fear for their cancer risk. My mother was recently diagnosed with an extraordinarily rare leukemia that, while indolent (that is, unlikely to rapidly progress), still keeps her up at night. Even I may carry the legacy of radioactivity, mutations that my parents may have accumulated from radiation, somewhere in my genes. For people who cared so much about our genes being Jewish, they cared very little about the genetic mutations they may have wrought.

Without a doubt, the corner-cutting, cover-up culture of the Soviet Union contributed to the nuclear meltdown and radioactive fallout. But we mustn't delude ourselves into thinking that we're immune from such a catastrophe. Seven years before Chernobyl, and less than 100 miles from my home in Philadelphia, the Three Mile Island nuclear power plant suffered a partial meltdown, rated 5 out of 7 on that INE scale.[72] Similar failures in design and cost-saving measures possibly contributed to that accident. Similarly, the administrators of the plant tried to cover up the full extent of the leakage. Radioactive gases spilled into nearby cities, people were evacuated (albeit also after some delay), and even the Hershey chocolate company paused production due to fears of contaminated milk.[73] Luckily, the limited spill of radioactivity has not been found to have contributed to excess cancer,[74] although locals have unsuccessfully sued for what they call an unusually high burden of health problems. It was by sheer chance that this accident did not result in a full meltdown, a steam-fueled explosion, and a fire, as in Chernobyl. While the last functioning nuclear reactor at Three Mile Island was shut down in 2019, it will take till 2079 to fully dispose of all the radioactive material. The consequences of radiation last for generations, while accidents can happen in mere seconds.

The greatest death toll from manmade radiation was in Hiroshima and Nagasaki, where the atomic bombs dropped by the US resulted in approximately 166,000 and 80,000 immediate deaths, respectively.[75] Over the decades since, some 800 to 3,000[76,77] excess cases of cancer have been attributed to the radioactive fallout. It may come as no surprise that when Robert Oppenheimer, the father of the Manhattan Project, saw the first nuclear detonation, he recited from the sacred Hindu text *Bhagavad Gita,* "Now I am become death, destroyer of worlds."[78]

THE FUTURE OF RADIATION

Radiation is the story of what we can see and what we cannot, and the gaping chasm between the two. Marie Curie could see the vast potential of her life's work, but she couldn't see it slowly eating away at her. My mother saw a beaming parade dedicated to her homeland, championing equality for the masses. She couldn't see the radioactivity raining down on her because the masses were anything but equal. As a child, I saw my grandparents as constant. Every day after school, I expected to see my grandfather standing there to take me home. When I got older, I expected them to be at home waiting for me, with snacks prepared, ready to go to the park or work on the garden. I saw them, their love, their comfort. I couldn't see the damage they carried within their genes, the molecular clock ticking away at their mortality, the frailty of their existence. I couldn't see them gone from my life, until I did.

The danger of radiation is that it goes unseen. We can see the sun's light and feel its heat, but the UV rays seem like a figment of science fiction—that is, until we get burned. It's tempting to imagine that the air in Chernobyl somehow felt heavier or smelled strange during the fallout, that there was some sign of the impending death lurking, but we know full well there wasn't. Everything felt totally normal, until it didn't. The firemen sent to their deaths in Chernobyl had no sense of the irreparable damage that was accumulating in their cells. Eventually, after a few minutes of exposure, they would get tired, or nauseated, or start coughing up blood, but at that point it was too late. Their future could not be changed. The damage from UV light and radon is on a scale so infinitesimally small it cannot be perceived, and yet that doesn't make it any less real. The cancer that gets diagnosed decades later feels so temporally distant from the cause, and yet they are inextricably linked.

Radiation is the story of having to take steps to avoid risks we cannot see. It takes a great level of discipline to apply sunscreen every day, even when we feel it doesn't make any sort of difference. It takes sacrifice to spend your last dollars testing for a gas you could blissfully ignore for decades. Public health initiatives are much the same. They require significant investment, and decades of patience, to produce results. They require putting aside judgment and envy ("Why should my tax dollars pay for his radon test when I already paid for my own?") for the public good. They require lawmakers to think beyond the scope of the next election cycle, and doctors to think beyond just treatment. Like radiation, cancer prevention requires us to know what we cannot see.

Yet sometimes the effects of radiation, or scientific advancement in general, are all too visible. The power of the atom is a blessing and a curse. The energy allows us to rely less on fossil fuels, which poison our atmosphere and our lungs (resulting in *far* more deaths than the risk of radioactivity from nuclear power plants). But in the hands of the most violent species on the planet, atomic weapons may prove fatal. It would feel almost ironic, if it weren't so bleak, that the same land where my family suffered at the hands of radioactive fallout may now be the catalyst for atomic war. Was Marie Curie correct in saying that understanding will always mitigate fear? Only time will tell.

In summary:

- UV radiation from the sun and tanning beds increases the risk for all types of skin cancer, particularly melanoma—a leading cause of cancer deaths.

- Programs encouraging the wearing of hats and sunscreen (any SPF of 30 or higher) have significantly reduced rates of skin cancer.

- Radon exposure in basements across the US is the second most common cause of lung cancer; get your basement tested, and if the level is high, invest in a radon reduction system.

- Airplane travel, CT scans, and even Brazil nuts are common sources of radiation, but they are unlikely to significantly contribute to cancer risk for the average consumer.

- If implemented safely, nuclear power may actually *prevent* cancer by decreasing fossil fuel pollution; when implemented poorly, nuclear power can be catastrophic.

CHAPTER 9

In Their Genes

Hereditary Cancer Risk

The sins of the father are to be laid upon the children.
—SHAKESPEARE, *THE MERCHANT OF VENICE*

An individual doesn't get cancer; a family does.
—TERRY WILLIAMS

I was the kind of kid who met many of their friends at "cancer camp." More precisely, I was fortunate to be accepted to an outreach program for high school students that allowed me to spend my summers working in a cancer research laboratory and attending lectures with other likeminded high schoolers. But as a kid, I felt cheeky calling it "cancer camp."

I met a girl there who was fiercely obsessed with cancer genetics. As a high schooler, Jennifer knew the genes, the pathways, like the back of her hand. She also had about her a maturity that I had seldom met. Jen had her whole life planned out: how many kids she wanted, when she wanted them, when her career had to be at its peak. As a fellow type A neurotic, we got along well, and began to get to know each other. Then, casually over lunch one day, she dropped a bombshell: Her mom had died a decade ago of ovarian cancer, and had left her daughter carrying a BRCA1 mutation. Jen had become a cancer genetics expert by necessity. She was planning her reproductive and professional life because she was, quite literally, running out of time.

Looking back today, I recognize a lost innocence. As a kid, Jen had wanted to play soccer and make art. I suspect she had no inkling of cancer genetics until she suddenly lost her mom to a disordered gene. She was now cursed with a constant reminder of her childhood trauma, and her own perilous mortality. At the time, as I got to know her better, I began to feel an awkward hesitancy. I liked her, as a high school boy likes a girl, but I also felt a glimpse of the enormous burden she shouldered. She told me she needed to find a husband, have kids (genetically tested, of course), and get her ovaries, fallopian tubes, and breasts removed as soon as possible. Every year she delayed, she increased her chances of early death. She had accepted that she would die young, like her mom, and she wanted to find a husband who could raise her kids as a single dad. It was an admirable yet precocious maturity. No child should have to plan out their whole life and stare down their own mortality.

Eventually we drifted apart and lost touch. Years later, I found her on Facebook and saw that she was happily married, likely pursuing her plan to have kids via pre-implantation genetic diagnosis, and then undergo extensive surgery, as soon as possible. I'd always wished her the best, but I've also worried about the wisdom of having children when you know you may leave them earlier than most parents do. After falling in love with my now wife, who has also lost her mother, to a sudden and, we hope, uninheritable rhabdomyosarcoma (cancer of soft tissue), I've changed my views. Cancer is unpredictable, striking without rhyme or reason, and it is a fool's errand to live in fear of it. When an individual gets diagnosed with cancer, a family suffers, both from the loss of their loved one, but also from the fear that the curse lurks within them, too. The increasing diagnosis of hereditary cancers has opened countless ethical and psychological Pandora's boxes, all revolving around our most basic need: protecting ourselves and our children.

CANCER FAMILIES

In the early 1900s, Scott Warthin, a dedicated pathologist in Michigan, found himself captivated by an unusual case. He encountered a family with an alarming history: generations plagued by colorectal cancer and other malignancies. Intrigued, Warthin began to delve deeper, interviewing family members and meticulously charting their medical histories.

As he pieced together their stories, a pattern emerged; multiple relatives had battled cancer, often at a young age. This familial link sparked Warthin's curiosity about hereditary factors influencing cancer risk. With each conversation, the weight of their struggles became clearer, revealing not just statistics but real lives affected by this silent menace. Warthin meticulously documented his findings, hypothesizing that this family was suffering from a genetic syndrome. In 1913, he published his groundbreaking work, highlighting the connection between genetics and cancer, coining the term "hereditary nonpolyposis colorectal cancer," which would later be recognized as Lynch syndrome after Henry T. Lynch, an American geneticist who would build upon Warthin's findings 60 years later.[1]

We now know Lynch syndrome occurs because of inherited (that is, carried in eggs or sperm cells) mutations in mismatch repair proteins, which are responsible for repairing damaged portions of DNA where the two strands no longer "match up." Without this repair process, mutations accumulate, culminating in deranged cells without a blueprint or genomic guardrails—cancer. Lynch syndrome, now called hereditary nonpolyposis colorectal cancer, accounts for approximately 2%–3% of colorectal cancer cases. This genetic condition carries a high lifetime risk of colorectal cancer, ranging from 30% to 74% for carriers of the most common mutations.[2] Lynch syndrome also significantly increases the risk of other malignancies (cancers), including endometrial, stomach, small intestine, pancreatic, biliary tract, ovarian, urinary tract, and brain cancers.[3] Despite being the most common genetic cancer syndrome, Lynch is underdiagnosed, which underscores the importance of genetic evaluation for anyone with colon or endometrial cancer, or a family history of other cancers. Interestingly, diagnosing Lynch syndrome has implications beyond familial risk. Colon, endometrial, and other cancers that are mismatch repair deficient, as in Lynch syndrome, respond better to immunotherapies because the cells are so disturbed that it's easier for the immune system to recognize them.[4] Also, colon cancer grows much faster in patients with Lynch syndrome, so they should be getting colonoscopies every 1–2 years as opposed to the usual 10 years. Therefore, finding out whether a person has Lynch syndrome is essential for treatment selection as well.

Warthin had inadvertently stumbled upon the first "cancer family." His research laid the groundwork for understanding inherited cancer risks and led to the discovery of numerous other hereditary cancer syndromes.

The most infamous of the inherited cancer syndromes is BRCA1/2, commonly known for causing breast cancer. BRCA, which stands for breast cancer, made headlines when actress Angelina Jolie learned she carried the gene and decided to undergo a double mastectomy (surgical removal of both breasts) to reduce her risk. But the story of BRCA begins decades prior.

In the late 1980s, the world of genetics was buzzing with promise and possibility. Researchers were eager to follow in the footsteps of Dr. Lynch and uncover the secrets of hereditary cancers that plagued families for generations. Among them was Mary-Claire King, a determined scientist at the University of California, Berkeley. She began investigating families with a striking pattern of breast and ovarian cancer.

In the days before genetic sequencing (finding out the order of the C, T, A, and G nucleotide bases in DNA), this meant relying on rudimentary techniques to look at normal cells and cancer cells of people with these strong family histories to identify a pattern. Techniques included karyotyping, where cells are frozen at a certain time in their cell cycle and the chromosomes (bodies of DNA) are examined under a microscope. Karyotyping is how the "Philadelphia chromosome," a fatal, erroneous exchange between the arms of chromosomes 9 and 22, which leads to chronic myeloid leukemia, was first discovered. Going a step further, scientists then learned to label certain locations on the chromosomes with fluorescent probes, and painstakingly examine whether a certain gene or chunk of a chromosome was missing or mutated.

In 1990, the dedication of King and her team paid off when she successfully identified the BRCA1 gene on chromosome 17, fittingly, after 17 years of work.[5] This groundbreaking discovery linked the gene to hereditary breast cancer, igniting excitement in the scientific community. A few years later, a team led by Mark Skolnick, a student of King's, unveiled BRCA2 on chromosome 13, revealing yet another critical piece of the puzzle. Per a 1994 *New York Times* article, "No one is more surprised and gratified than Dr. Mark H. Skolnick of the University of Utah, whose team plucked the gene from a crowded stretch of chromosome 13 and out of the grasp of 12 other teams that had thrown hats and hopes into the ring."[6] Both discoveries were monumental, confirming that mutations in these genes significantly increased the risk of breast and ovarian cancer.

Women with both BRCA1 and 2 have a 60%–80% lifetime risk of breast cancer (about 10 times the average risk) and a 15%–45% lifetime risk of ovarian cancer (with BRCA1 worse, at 44%, and BRCA2 better, at 17%).[7] Interestingly, BRCA1 increases the risk of male breast cancer by about fourfold, and BRCA2 by a whopping 44-fold.[8] But breast and ovarian cancers are far from the only risks. BRCA1 and 2 also increase pancreatic,[9] prostate, bladder, and stomach cancer risk by 200% to 600% (relative risk),[10] with BRCA2 more likely to cause these non-breast cancers. While the relative risk of different cancers is actually rather similar, the absolute (lifetime) risk varies dramatically. Since prostate cancer is much more common to begin with (the most common cancer in males), men with BRCA2 have a whopping 27% lifetime risk of developing prostate cancer, compared to 2.5% for pancreatic, and 0.4% risk for breast cancers.[11]

Lynch syndrome and BRCA are the most common cancer syndromes. Lynch occurs in about 1 out of 440 people,[12] and BRCA in around 1 out of 400 people.[13] However, certain ethnicities are more likely to carry the mutation. For instance, 1 out of about 40 (10 times the average rate) Ashkenazi Jews, like my family, carry the BRCA mutation.[14] This "amplification" of genetic syndromes in small populations like Ashkenazi Jews occurs due to the "founder effect," when a small group of individuals from a larger population establishes a new population, carrying only a limited gene pool. With reduced genetic diversity, natural selection is unable to get rid of unfavorable mutations like BRCA (moreover, evolution doesn't care if you die *after* you have kids). The founders' genetic makeup heavily influences future generations, making them more susceptible to specific inherited conditions. This phenomenon is often observed in isolated communities or in cases where a small group migrates to a new area, illustrating how historical events can shape genetic variation.

In the case of Ashkenazi Jews, the original population was around 350 people.[15] They were isolated in the Pale of Settlement by the Tsar's decree and rarely started families outside their towns and villages. Due to pogroms and genocide, they then underwent numerous waves of "population contraction." Consequently, Ashkenazi Jews suffer from numerous genetic conditions, the most common being BRCA, Tay-Sachs, and Gaucher (diseases of cellular waste disposal, which affect all organs, including the brain and liver, and the blood).[16]

GENETICS AND THE HUMAN GENOME

The landscape of inherited cancers was completely turned on its head with the mapping of the human genome, completed in 2003, the culmination of centuries of work in genetics. The foundation of genetics began with Gregor Mendel in the nineteenth century. His experiments with pea plants in the 1860s established the principles of inheritance, though his work went largely unrecognized until the early twentieth century. Mendel discovered that traits are passed from parents to offspring through discrete units, which later came to be known as genes.

Mendel, a monk and self-trained botanist, got lucky that he chose to experiment with peas. Peas are simple—all genes are either dominant or recessive. When he cross-pollinated two yellow peas, the offspring would always turn out yellow. Human genetics are far more complicated, especially when it comes to cancer. Certain genetic diseases, like Huntington's, have strong penetrance, which means inheriting the gene *guarantees* the disease. For one gene to cause so much suffering, the gene must be essential, and the mutation itself must destroy the function of the gene. Cancer genes are different. Even the aforementioned BRCA or Lynch mutations, which greatly increase cancer risk, do not guarantee cancer. Cancer develops with a group of mutations, each of which slowly chips away at a cell's normal function. BRCA may be the catalyst, the so-called "driver mutation," but it must first recruit many passengers to reach its destination. Even in patients with the BRCA mutation, lifestyle and environment still influence cancer risk. The complex interplay of genetic and environmental factors has only come to light over the past few decades.

In the 1950s, James Watson, Francis Crick, Rosalind Franklin, and Maurice Wilkins made a groundbreaking discovery—the double-helix structure of DNA. After the structure of DNA was discovered, scientists began to focus on understanding the sequence of nucleotides (the building blocks of DNA) that make up genes. Over the next few decades, technologies to sequence DNA improved rapidly. By the late 1970s, the first complete DNA sequence of a virus was achieved using methods developed by Frederick Sanger, a pioneering scientist in this field.

The human genome consists of about three billion base pairs of DNA, so sequencing it was a daunting challenge, to say the least. If you wrote out all three billion letters of the human genome end to end, they would stretch about 250 million inches—almost 4,000 miles. It would take a group of visionary scientists decades to complete the arduous task of sequencing all our DNA.

In 1990, the Human Genome Project (HGP) was formally launched as an international effort, with the initial target for completion being 15 years, but advances in technology sped up the process. While the HGP was making steady progress, in

1998, a private company called Celera Genomics, founded by scientist Craig Venter, entered the race to sequence the human genome. Celera aimed to sequence the genome much faster and more cheaply using a technique called shotgun sequencing. This involved breaking the genome into random small pieces, sequencing them, and then using computational methods to piece them together. The competition spurred rapid advances in sequencing technology and methodology.

On April 14, 2003, the HGP was declared complete—two years ahead of schedule and under budget. The final version of the human genome covered over 99% of the gene-containing regions, with an accuracy greater than 99.99%. This marked the beginning of a new era in genomics, with the sequence providing a foundation for further understanding the role of genes in health, disease, and human biology.

The discovery of the full human genome sequence opened new frontiers in science. Researchers began exploring how variations in the genome contribute to disease, leading to the development of personalized medicine, where treatments can be tailored to an individual's genetic makeup. It has enabled the targeted and gene therapies that have revolutionized cancer care and other medical disciplines. It's also allowed us to discover the genetic underpinnings—thousands and thousands of them—that increase cancer risk.

In order to understand and act upon these findings, researchers have collected The Cancer Genome Atlas (TCGA, a clever use of the first letters of the four nucleotide types in DNA), an encyclopedia of all mutations associated with cancers, in the hopes of identifying new targets to attack with cancer therapies.[17] However, in human genetics, things are never that simple. The heterogeneity and sheer number of different cancer mutations across individuals, tumors, and even cells within a tumor have made it difficult to identify the few mutations that are the "drivers" (those that fuel the cancer and can be targeted) among the thousands that are mere "passengers." Researchers are left trying to separate the wheat from the chaff, or more accurately, trying to find the needle in the haystack. The struggle to make sense of all this information has fallen upon doctors and patients, creating countless opportunities and challenges.

GENETIC TESTING

Everyone's genome is about three billion letters long, and only 1% of those code for valuable proteins (that we know of). Instead, most consumer DNA testing services scour your genes for single nucleotide polymorphisms (SNPs),[18] one letter variations among people that often correspond to mutations that lead to certain conditions. Different services look for different SNPs, and most don't report the vast majority of the results they find.

For instance, the company called 23andMe sequences about a quarter of all known SNPs, which is more than most other services but less than Ancestry.com does. Of these results, it offers ancestry reports (like ethnicity and Neanderthal DNA) and various health reports, with BRCA1/2 recently included in their panel. 23andMe also offers a number of wellness reports and over 40 carrier-status reports.[19] Most of the conditions tested are relatively rare, but could be valuable for those planning on starting a family, especially if you and your spouse belong to a historically small population like Ashkenazi Jews or French Canadians.

Ancestry.com tests the most SNPs of all consumer services,[20] almost half of all the known ones. However, it does not use this data to offer information about your health or disease risk. Instead, Ancestry offers more comprehensive ethnicity results, with a "DNA story" that may trace the migrations of your ancestors. In addition, it gives more detail on ethnicities—in my case, "Northeast Poland, Lithuania, Latvia & West Belarus" instead of just "Baltic" (from 23andMe).

Both 23andMe and Ancestry offer a feature to connect to relatives, which may also be used to track you down[21] if you or a relative happen to be a killer who leaves DNA at the scene of the crime. More recently, 23andMe has filed for bankruptcy, leading to a lawsuit by 27 states to prohibit the sale of the genetic information of millions of consumers.[22]

The most comprehensive way to utilize consumer genetic testing is through a little-known online application called Promethease, used by scientists and enthusiasts looking to dive deeper into their genetic results. For only a few dollars, you can upload your 23andMe or Ancestry data to Promethease,[23] which connects your results to the SNPedia,[24] a database of all known SNPs and their possible clinical significance. In turn, Promethease provides a long list (with thousands of entries) of all the possible disease risks, pharmacogenetic variations, and other tidbits that your raw data from 23andMe or Ancestry revealed but which those services did not report. Remember that neither company tests all the SNPs in your genome, so depending on which you try, you may receive different results.

The trouble comes in finding what's meaningful amid the noise. Promethease offers a "magnitude" rating to help individuals determine whether the particular result is reliable and important. Generally, magnitudes under 3 are usually not worth worrying about.[25] Promethease also has a search function that allows you to search for certain conditions or locations in your genome. So, for any risk reported on the 23andMe health report (and many more), you could find out which SNPs they used (each has an rs [reference SNP] number), and search for them on Promethease.

For instance, if you're worried about BRCA1/2 mutations (but got only the 23andMe ancestry test), you can find the rs numbers that correspond to them and search them. Promethease also offers an odds ratio, which suggests how much greater risk you have, compared to the average person. Keep in mind that for a rare disease that occurs in 0.1% of people, even if your odds ratio is 10 times the normal rate, your risk is only 1%. Promethease is a blessing wrapped in a curse. It has all the information one could want and way, *way* more, so for people willing to take the time to learn and sort things out, it could offer valuable insights.

Finally, numerous medical-grade germline genetic tests are used to evaluate DNA for hereditary cancer syndromes, either in people with a family history of a cancer or who are diagnosed with a given cancer. These tests use technologies that are more expensive but more reliable than the consumer tests, and they require a doctor to order them and health insurance to cover them. Even women whose breast cancer, for example, is found to have a BRCA mutation are still told to get a "germline" BRCA test, to determine whether they inherited the faulty BRCA gene or just spontaneously developed the mutation (known as a "somatic" mutation) in their breast cancer. Other groups at high risk, like Ashkenazi Jews, women with a family history of breast, ovarian, pancreatic, and prostate cancer (when at least two first-degree relatives, meaning siblings, parents, or children, have that cancer) or *anyone* diagnosed with pancreatic cancer, is currently recommended for germline genetic testing for BRCA. Likewise, doctors recommend that anyone with a family history of colorectal or endometrial cancer gets Lynch syndrome testing. BRCA and Lynch syndrome are the most common but far from the only inheritable cancer syndromes. Other rare cancers like pheochromocytoma (cancer of the adrenal glands), medullary thyroid, retinoblastoma (a cancer of the eyes), and certain blood cancers are all associated with germline mutations and warrant genetic testing.

Many of my patients have worried that findings revealed on genetic testing may lead to discrimination by their health insurer or employer. Thankfully, the Genetic Information Nondiscrimination Act (GINA) was enacted in 2008 to protect individuals from discrimination based on their genetic information.[26] Its primary goal is to encourage people to take advantage of genetic testing and medical advances without fear of misuse of their genetic data. Per the law, health insurers are prohibited from using genetic information to determine eligibility, premium rates, or coverage terms. Insurers cannot request or require individuals to undergo genetic testing. Employers also cannot use genetic information in hiring, firing, promotion, job assignments, or other employment decisions. It is illegal for employers to request, require, or purchase genetic information about an employee or their family members. Unfortunately, GINA does not have provisions covering life insurance. Furthermore, while genetic information is currently protected, as soon as a condition manifests itself in a patient, such as an early-stage cancer, it is considered a pre-existing condition. Considering that people with hereditary cancer risk get screened more frequently, they are more likely to be diagnosed with conditions that are found incidentally (like random lung nodules and colon polyps). Thankfully, under the Affordable Care Act, insurers are currently prohibited from discriminating against patients with pre-existing conditions, but the fate of these protections has been put in jeopardy by recently proposed health care policy changes.

While genetic risk can help motivate patients to change their lifestyle and receive appropriate cancer screening, it's a double-edged sword. Patients may fear their genetic information being used against them or their families in the uncertain future of US health care. Moreover, for patients predisposed to catastrophizing, I've found that knowing their increased risk of cancer can sometimes be counterproductive and just cause more anxiety and depression. All this is to say that genetic testing ought to be a patient-driven decision, and genetic counselors are very helpful in explaining and discussing risks and benefits for a patient and their family.

SECONDARY PREVENTION

As we've previously discussed, primary prevention refers to avoiding the underlying causes of cancer. In patients with inherited conditions, this is unfortunately impossible. But there are still significant benefits from secondary prevention—medical screenings, surgeries, and treatments to mitigate the risk conferred by their inherited mutation.

For patients with BRCA mutations, the American Society of Clinical Oncology recommends annual mammography and breast MRI starting at age 25–30 for BRCA1/2 mutation carriers. This combined approach has shown a sensitivity of 94% for detecting early-stage breast cancer when it is surgically removable and may not require chemotherapy.[27] For male BRCA2 mutation carriers, the National Comprehensive Cancer Network (NCCN) recommends annual prostate-specific antigen screening starting at age 40, due to the significantly elevated risk of aggressive prostate cancer.[28]

But prevention can take forms much more aggressive than just screening. Many women, like Angelina Jolie, opt for risk-reducing mastectomy, which can decrease the risk of breast cancer by 90%–95% in BRCA1/2 carriers.[29] The NCCN also recommends considering risk-reducing removal of ovaries and fallopian tubes from ages 35 to 40 years for BRCA1 carriers and from ages 40 to 45 years for BRCA2 carriers; this surgery also reduces breast cancer risk by approximately 50% in BRCA2 carriers (since much of breast cancer is hormonally driven).[30] Of course, these procedures come with surgical complications and the risks associated with early menopause, like cardiovascular disease and low bone density (osteoporosis) that can lead to fractures.

Additionally, hormone treatments like tamoxifen are options for chemoprevention in BRCA2 mutation carriers, though their effectiveness for BRCA1 carriers is less clear.[31] The use of oral contraceptives has been shown to reduce the risk of ovarian cancer in BRCA1/2 carriers, but their impact on breast cancer risk is still debated.[32]

For people who have Lynch syndrome, the American Gastroenterological Association recommends surveillance colonoscopy every 1–2 years starting at age 20–25, or 2–5 years before the youngest age of colorectal cancer diagnosis in the family.[33] Lynch syndrome colon cancers grow much faster than the average colon cancer, so the usual 10 years is not frequent enough to catch them early. Having a colonoscopy every 1–2 years has been shown to significantly reduce colorectal cancer incidence and mortality for patients who have Lynch syndrome. For women with Lynch syndrome, many doctors recommend risk-reducing removal of the uterus, ovaries, and fallopian tubes after childbearing is complete, to prevent endometrial and ovarian cancers.[34] Interestingly, aspirin has been studied extensively for its role in chemoprevention. The CAPP2 trial demonstrated that daily aspirin use can reduce the incidence of colon cancer in people who have Lynch syndrome, although the optimal dose (81 mg vs 325 mg) and duration are still under investigation.[35]

Lastly, when it comes to family planning for people with inherited conditions, recent innovations are providing previously unheard-of opportunities. First and foremost, all people with known genetic conditions who are planning to have kids should speak to a genetic counselor, who can walk them through the complexities surrounding testing, risks, and choices.

Some of my patients with mutations like BRCA have been choosing to undergo preimplantation genetic diagnosis (PGD), wherein in-vitro fertilization (IVF) embryos are screened for mutations, and the healthiest embryo (without BRCA, for instance) is implanted into the mother.[36] Mutations like BRCA are autosomal (not on the sex chromosome) dominant, meaning there's a 50% chance that an affected woman's embryo would have the mutations. PGD eliminates the risk.

Of course, PGD has not been without its critics. While curing deadly, congenital diseases is one thing, the possibility of modifying our children to our liking raises many ethical questions. Where to draw the line has become a matter of fierce debate. For instance, Iceland's campaign to eliminate Down syndrome (via abortion) has received criticism from many on the political right, with critics comparing it to eugenics and calling it "the death of humanity."[37] On the other hand, some deaf parents have increased their odds of having a deaf child,[38] and some dwarf parents have aimed to ensure having dwarf children.[39] While some see this as promoting a disability, others consider that stance an example of ableism.

In the midst of this ongoing controversy, a US company called Genomic Prediction has developed a PGD test for low intelligence.[40] While intelligence is based on a myriad of genes, the company believes they have identified a "risk score" that can predict whether an embryo is at a high risk of having an IQ below 75,[41] which counts as "intellectual disability." Parents could screen for, and thus eliminate, embryos with this increased risk of lower intelligence. The company has stressed that test results will not be used to help parents pick embryos with high IQs, only to eliminate low-IQ embryos. The test is likely to be approved and offered in the US, which has lax laws for PGD, relative to European nations. IVF clinics in the US are allowed to offer sex selection of embryos, which many have argued is also unethical (especially with the ongoing infanticide of female babies in some countries).[42]

Technologies for genetic selection and recent approvals of genetic editing for conditions like sickle cell anemia and hemophilia are ushering in a new era of gene-informed medicine. But permanently messing with our biologic code is not without risk. Continued debate on the ethics and implications of genetics in medicine is paramount, lest we repeat one of the worst chapters of our history.

EUGENICS

The legacy of genetics will be forever tainted by eugenics, a pseudoscience that culminated in the mass murder of millions. The eugenics movement began in the late nineteenth century, inspired by Charles Darwin's theory of natural selection. Francis Galton, Darwin's cousin, coined the term "eugenics" in 1883, promoting the idea of improving the human race by encouraging reproduction among people with "desirable" traits and discouraging or preventing reproduction among those with "undesirable" traits. Early eugenicists believed that traits like intelligence, criminality, and mental illness were inherited and that selective breeding could prevent social problems. This idea spread across Europe and the US (where it was applied against Black people) in the early twentieth century, gaining widespread support among intellectuals, politicians, and scientists.[43]

In Germany, eugenics found fertile ground, especially after World War I, when the country was reeling from economic hardship and political instability. The eugenics movement merged with rising nationalism and anti-Semitism, influencing political groups like the Nazis, who sought to restore the nation's perceived racial purity. Adolf Hitler was a firm believer in eugenics and "racial hygiene." His views were shaped by the belief that the "Aryan" race was superior, while Jews, disabled individuals, Romani people, and others deemed "genetically defective" threatened the purity and strength of the German nation.[44]

When Hitler came to power in 1933, he quickly implemented eugenic policies. The Nazi regime passed the Law for the Prevention of Hereditarily Diseased Offspring, which led to the forced sterilization of around 400,000 people—those with disabilities, mental illness, or certain physical conditions—deemed genetically unfit.[45] The Nazis also promoted marriage loans and rewards for "racially pure" Aryan families with many children, encouraging the expansion of the "master race." Meanwhile, Nazi propaganda portrayed Jews, Romani, and other marginalized groups as biologically degenerate and dangerous to society, dehumanizing them and laying the groundwork for more extreme policies.

The Nazi obsession with racial purity and eugenics escalated into what became known as the T4 Program, the systematic murder of those deemed "unworthy of life." Beginning in 1939, under the guise of euthanasia, the T4 Program targeted disabled and mentally ill Germans, resulting in the deaths of approximately 70,000 people.[46] The techniques developed during this program, such as gas chambers and mass shootings, would later be used in the larger-scale genocide of the Holocaust.

The Holocaust was the culmination of Nazi racial ideology, which combined eugenic theories with deep-seated anti-Semitism and other forms of racism. When all other solutions, like deporting all Jews to Madagascar, had failed,[47] and other countries had turned their backs on the displaced Jews, the Nazis resorted to what they called the Final Solution: the extermination of all of Europe's Jews. Between 1941 and 1945, approximately six million Jews were systematically murdered in concentration and extermination camps like Auschwitz, Treblinka, and Sobibor. The Nazis also targeted millions of Romani, Poles, Soviet prisoners of war, disabled individuals, homosexuals, and others deemed racially or genetically inferior. The Holocaust represents the horrifying end result of eugenic thinking taken to its extreme, where the goal of creating a "perfect" race justifies the wholesale extermination of human beings, like my great-grandparents.

My grandmother and grandfather grew up on the run, in hiding in Kazakhstan as the Nazi war machine tore through the Soviet countryside. When they were able to return to Ukraine, they found their villages, language, and culture decimated. They were forcibly integrated into the rest of Soviet society, losing the last vestiges of their Jewish identity. What started off as a twisted initiative to purify Germany's genetics deprived families like mine of our genetic heritage.

Genetics holds the key to the future of medicine and cancer prevention. It has provided opportunities to identify those at increased risk and even intervene with screening, treatment, and surgery to decrease their risk. Our innovations have even paved the way to prevent future generations from inheriting our flawed genes, and possibly fixing the genes when they do. But they've also brought about a slippery slope, raising concerns about abuse of our innovations against marginalized groups or people with disabilities. In countries like China and India, a legacy of preference for male children has led to widespread murdering of female babies. Genetics is a double-edged sword, and one we must use carefully to avoid repeating the fatal mistakes of the past.

In summary:

- Patients with a family history of cancer should get tested for genetic syndromes like Lynch or BRCA; early detection and intervention can reduce the risk of death from cancer.

- The Genetic Information Nondiscrimination Act prevents discrimination by employers or insurance companies based on genetic results (but does *not* apply to life insurance).

- People who have Lynch syndrome should have a colonoscopy every 1–2 years, while patients with BRCA may benefit from surgery to remove the breasts, ovaries, and fallopian tubes.

- Eugenics, the belief in genetic "superiority," was a key principle used by the Nazis to justify discrimination and genocide.

CHAPTER 10

Burning Questions

Inflammation, the Microbiome, and Cancer

A fire from the ashes shall be woken,
a light from the shadows shall spring . . .
—J. R. R. TOLKIEN

You always said, don't face a problem, burn it.
—RAY BRADBURY, *FAHRENHEIT 451*

The word "inflammation" comes from the concept of fire. Doctors of past centuries, faced with the angry, swollen, vermilion
joints of gout, described them as appearing "burnt," and so "inflammation" was born. Today, we understand the finer details,
the countless signaling molecules and cells involved in the immune response that produces that burnt-like appearance. Our
body, primed to fight invaders, mistakenly attacks itself, heating up healthy cells in its wake. But deep below the swollen
joints or reddened skin of various inflammatory conditions, the
heightened immune response leaves its mark on healthy cells
around the body, damaging their DNA and increasing cancer
risk. Cancer is, at its root, a disease of too little, and too much,
immunity. Blazing the trail to cancer prevention means getting
to the root of inflammation.

INFLAMMATION

Inflammation is your body's natural response to injury, irritation, or infection. It's a defense mechanism that kicks in when your body senses a problem, such as a cut, burn, or any opening through which bacteria may invade. The goal of inflammation is to protect against intruders and clear out debris to facilitate the healing process. Inflamed areas are red, warm, and swollen because your immune system sends more blood to the area, along with immune cells that help fight off germs and initiate tissue repair. The entire process is governed by a cascade of signaling molecules, called cytokines, that tell the immune cells to arrive and the blood vessels to dilate. The key to addressing inflammation is understanding and modulating this signaling cascade.

Inflammation is meant to occur with infection, injury, and toxic irritants. However, in this modern day, where we deal with diminishingly few infections and injuries (compared to millennia ago), inflammation can often occur inappropriately, and hurt the body more than help it. The simplest examples are allergies and asthma. These processes occur when immune cells recognize harmless particles, like cat hair, dandruff, or pollen, as infections, and launch their signaling cascade to "fight them off." An inappropriate inflammatory response ensues, leading to a rash on our skin, or even life-threatening closure of our airways (asthma). A common treatment for all these processes are corticosteroids, which "throw a wet blanket" on the fire, halting our entire immune system in its tracks.

Inflammation doesn't just affect the tissues that the white blood cells target. It also causes the release of the signaling molecules that lead to immune activation all over the body. When the immune system is activated, it can use numerous tools that were designed to fight invaders. T cells identify and "kill" infected cells, while B cells produce antibodies that coat infected cells, labeling them for destruction. Like the burning of Moscow ahead of Napoleon's advance, the immune system achieves a Pyrrhic victory. Its heavy-duty weapons are a powerful tool to fight microbes in the short term, but these weapons cause collateral damage to the host, and can become particularly dangerous when they remain activated in the long term.

When inflammation is chronic, it means your body is in a constant state of "attack and repair." The nonstop battery by overzealous immune cells inflicts damage, killing off most cells, but leaving some "traumatized" survivors. To repair damaged tissue, your body speeds up cell growth. However, when cells are forced to multiply too rapidly, mistakes (mutations) can occur during cell division. If these mutations affect genes that control cell growth, they can lead to cancerous changes. The process of metabolizing energy to power this constant cellular repair also leads to dangerous production of free radicals, which are unstable molecules that can damage DNA. Damaged DNA in cells increases the likelihood of mutations, some of which might make the cell grow uncontrollably—a hallmark of cancer.

During chronic inflammation, immune cells are always present in the inflamed area, constantly releasing chemicals to fight the perceived threat. These chemicals, the cytokines, support the survival and growth of cells with mutations, allowing them to become cancerous. Over time, chronic inflammation creates a "microenvironment" that supports tumor growth. Inflammation may help nourish tumors by promoting the growth of new blood vessels (a process called angiogenesis) or by suppressing the immune system's ability to recognize and destroy abnormal cells.[1] Like the boy who cried wolf, the over-activated immune cells can no longer tell friend from foe, and fail in their duty to keep cancer in check. In the simplest terms, inflammation is an adaptive process our body needs to deal with infection or injury, but when chronic, it inadvertently paves the way for cancer development.

CHRONIC INFLAMMATORY DISEASES

There are numerous chronic autoimmune diseases, which essentially all occur because our body's immune system gets primed to attack itself. The targets may differ, like joints with rheumatoid arthritis or the kidneys with lupus nephritis, but the process is always the same. Consequently, most of these conditions respond to drugs such as steroids that dampen the immune response. Unfortunately, any immunosuppressant medicine carries risks, such as life-threatening infections, if taken long term. Steroids, in particular, act on dozens of processes in the body, causing everything from diabetes to psychosis, and are notoriously terrible for your health if taken for months on end.

Given that these conditions cause the constant release of inflammatory cytokines and continual immune-mediated damage of tissue, over decades they lead to increased cancer risk. For instance, chronic hepatitis, either from a virus that won't go away on its own or from repeated liver damage from drinking alcohol, increases the risk of liver cancer by over 10 times. Chronic inflammatory diseases of the colon, like ulcerative colitis and Crohn's disease, increase the risk of colorectal cancer. After 20 years of ulcerative colitis, the absolute risk of colorectal cancer increases fivefold, to 5%.[2] Given the increased risk, guidelines recommend starting colonoscopy screening 8 years after diagnosis of ulcerative colitis or Crohn's disease, and repeating every 1–3 years (as opposed to every 10 years) due to the heightened risk.[3]

Some autoimmune diseases, like lupus and sarcoidosis, can affect nearly all the tissues in the body. These diseases involve creating antibodies and activating immune cells to recognize friend as foe, and lead to a nonstop, indiscriminate attack fueled by inflammatory mediators. The constant damage and immune activation lead to increased cancer risk, particularly lymphoma, or cancer of our immune cells. The overall risk of cancer for people who have lupus is increased by about 62%. Specifically, non-Hodgkin lymphoma risk increases by 5.4 times, and Hodgkin lymphoma risk increases by 3.3 times.[4] Thankfully, many immunosuppressive drugs have been discovered that quiet the immune response in lupus. Unfortunately, many of them affect cells other than the immune cells and inadvertently increase cancer risk; for instance, cyclophosphamide, used to treat lupus nephritis, increases the risk of bladder cancer.[5]

Even for patients who do not have autoimmune disease, chronic inflammation is believed to be at the root of over half of all cancer cases worldwide. Any process or chemical that damages a certain tissue leads to an immune response, and often that immune response is what ultimately leads to increased cancer risk. The many occupational exposures, like silica or asbestos, that lead to lung cancer, do not in and of themselves cause cancer; instead, cancer occurs because the immune cells in the lungs, faced with a foreign object they can't destroy, get stuck in a chronic inflammatory state that damages the lung tissue. Likewise, fat tissue is by its very nature pro-inflammatory, because it releases numerous cytokines that stimulate our immune cells.[6] This is why excess fat, as in obesity, increases cancer risk throughout the body, and even eating meat with a lot of fat, like beef, is associated with increased cancer risk.[7] While in these cases inflammation is not the root cause of the cancer, it is still the process that drives cancer development.

Chronic inflammation from poor diet and obesity is increasingly being identified as the culprit behind far more than just cancer. Heart failure with preserved ejection fraction (HFpEF), the most common type of heart failure, was for decades believed to be caused exclusively by high blood pressure. But recently, cardiologists have begun to see HFpEF as another facet of "metabolic syndrome," the deadly triad of obesity, diabetes, and blood pressure that causes chronic inflammation and likely underlies most other chronic diseases in modern-day Americans.[8] HFpEF has been associated with all the inflammatory markers of obesity, and is almost exclusively diagnosed in patients who are obese or diabetic.[9] Similarly, fatty liver disease, which is caused by metabolic syndrome, is overtaking alcohol as the leading cause of cirrhosis (or liver failure) in the US. And, as we've previously discussed, obesity is now considered the primary risk factor behind common cancers like colorectal and breast. Add in all the mechanical issues caused by obesity, such as arthritis of the hips, knees, and ankles, and you quickly see how excess weight has become the single leading cause of preventable disease in the US.[10]

With all this in mind, what can be done to decrease the risk of inflammation-induced cancer? For patients with autoimmune disease, chronic lifelong therapy (ideally not with steroids) to keep their disease in check is the first step. Likewise, regular monitoring and appropriate screening, like colonoscopies and mammograms, are key to detecting cancer early, before it spreads, when it's still removable and curable (that is, patients can achieve remission and cure).

Then there's the concept of the anti-inflammatory diet. Certain foods are rich in antioxidants, natural compounds that capture those cancer-causing free oxygen radicals created by inflammation. Foods rich in antioxidants are usually colorful fruits and vegetables, like blueberries, pomegranates, peppers, and more. Many companies, from those who produce supplements to "superfoods" to juices, have jumped on the antioxidant wagon with more concentrated, and more expensive, antioxidants. Data has shown that a higher proportion of antioxidants in one's diet is associated with decreased colorectal, gastric, and endometrial cancer risk.[11] However, these are also the cancers associated with obesity, and we know that people who eat more fruits and vegetables are also less likely to be obese. Therefore, it's difficult to distinguish the benefit of antioxidants specifically from the benefit of a healthy diet overall. Moreover, a study of prostate, lung, colon, and ovarian cancers found that while dietary intake of more antioxidants was associated with lower risk, antioxidant supplements did not seem to affect cancer risk.[12] My recommendation to patients is to skip the supplements and juices (which often have way too much sugar), and instead opt for whole fruits, vegetables, and fiber-rich foods (like whole wheat bread, quinoa, or brown rice)—the specific dietary changes that have been clinically shown to reduce cancer risk. There is no clinical difference between "superfoods" like acai berries, compared to blueberries, pomegranates, or whatever local, seasonal berry is available.

Other common anti-inflammatory nutrients are omega-3s. These are a type of unsaturated fats found in nuts, fish, and flax seeds. While we used to think of all fats as promoting inflammation, modern science has revealed that certain unsaturated fats like omega-3s are actually anti-inflammatory. In fact, omega-3 supplements have been shown to decrease the risk of heart attacks in specific patients by reducing cholesterol and inflammation in the coronary arteries. When it comes to cancer risk, the data is more tepid. Numerous meta-analyses (studies of studies) have found no conclusive reduction in cancer risk with high omega-3 intake.[13] One study did note a 17% risk reduction in digestive cancers,[14] but once again, it's difficult to attribute that to omega-3s specifically (as opposed to a healthy diet overall). As with antioxidants, the best advice is simply to eat a diet rich in nuts, seeds, and fish like salmon or tuna. As we discussed in the chapter on diet, processed foods high in sugar, and processed or smoked meats, contain cancer-causing chemicals and are often pro-inflammatory, so reducing the amount of these in our diet is key. And the complement to diet is exercise. Studies have found that both strengthening and aerobic exercise work on the molecular level to reduce the levels of inflammatory signaling molecules[15] and calm inflammatory cells.[16]

Overall, maintaining a healthy weight to minimize the amount of fat tissue is central to reducing inflammation. Interestingly, location of weight and weight-loss goals can vary by race and sex. For complex reasons, weight carried around the waist is more pro-inflammatory, and worse for heart disease and cancer risk, than weight carried in your hips or butt. Asian people seem to carry and store excess weight differently, and therefore they should aim for a lower BMI (less than 25) than white people (BMI less than 30) to maintain the same diabetes risk; some studies distinguish between South Asians (BMI less than 27) and East Asians (BMI less than 25).[17] Meanwhile, Black people tend to have a higher BMI corresponding to the same percentage of fat, compared to white people.[18] Women, in general, are at higher risk of inflammatory diseases because of pregnancy, female hormones, and having two X chromosomes. Yet women also naturally have a higher healthy proportion of body fat, and are less likely to store the fat around the waist as compared to men. For all these reasons, one's goal body weight or BMI is highly variable, and should be discussed with your primary care doctor. It's not realistic, or even healthy, for everyone to aim for the same BMI. In fact, one recent meta-analysis of 20 studies found that poor cardiac fitness, rather than high BMI, increased the risk of death by two to three times.[19] In other words, people who are overweight, but fit, seemed to live longer than people who were skinny but out of shape.

Inflammation is at the root of most cases of cancer, and diet and exercise are the key to keep this inflammation in check. Unfortunately, new harbingers of inflammation lurk all around us; the latest to strike has been the infamous virus COVID-19.

COVID-19

I would wake up every morning an hour early and bike the desolate, post-apocalyptic streets to work. All my nonmedical friends were working from home, enjoying (or hating) the company of their families. Meanwhile, I was working longer hours than I ever had. Outside the hospital, I'd don my N95 mask, suffocating in the summer, and wait in line to have my temperature taken before entering the building. Many attending physicians were sheltering at home, so we medical students and residents would gown and mask up, head to toe, grab an iPad, and video call our supervising doctors to fumble through a burgeoning list of patients. The hospital, emergency room, and intensive care units were overflowing. Everyone had coronavirus disease (COVID-19), and none of us really knew what to do. The Zoom call would cut out and I, a student, would be left alone and feeling awkward, while a frightened patient sized up my alien attire. Perhaps there was some solidarity between us; we were both stuck in the hospital for weeks on end, the patient separated from all family, me separated from my supervising physicians. We were both equally clueless about what was going on or what the next day would hold. Sometimes, the only thing we could do for a patient dying of COVID-19 was flip them on their stomach to help oxygenate their lungs. To my surprise, that simple fix often did the trick, and they survived. Medical training during the height of the COVID-19 pandemic was a baptism by fire.

All doctors have gained a healthy fear of the intense inflammatory response caused by COVID-19. Often, it's not the virus itself that kills you, but your body's reaction to it. With COVID-19, the most dreaded complication was ARDS—acute respiratory distress syndrome. As you may guess from the name, we weren't really sure how it happened or why, at least at first.

ARDS is a life-threatening lung condition that results in severe inflammation and fluid buildup in the lungs, making it difficult for oxygen to pass into the bloodstream. When the COVID-19 virus entered a person, it preferentially infected the cells of the lungs. The body's immune system would react by sending immune cells to the lungs to attack the virus, but unable to contain or understand it, the immune system would go into overdrive, producing copious amounts of those inflammatory signaling molecules called cytokines. The condition that ensued was labelled a "cytokine storm"; the immune cells would damage the cells lining the lungs and cause small blood clots, causing fluid to leak into the spaces meant to be filled by air.[20] As the cytokine storm raged and the fluid accumulated, COVID-19 patients would literally suffocate while getting 100% oxygen through a breathing tube. The inflammatory response in the lungs was unlike anything doctors had seen before.[21] Even if we got the patients through the acute phase, the lungs would become stiffer, and the oxygen exchange membranes damaged, leading to chronic lung disease for many patients. There were even hypotheses that the intense inflammatory damage may increase long-term cancer risk.

The data remain mixed, and it's far too early to draw conclusions about long-term cancer risk after severe COVID-19 infection. One study found an increased risk of breast, esophageal, colorectal, and stomach cancer after severe COVID-19, but it remains unclear whether this is caused by the virus, or by some unknown genetic factor (probably an immune mediator). This unknown factor may predispose certain people to severe COVID-19 and also make them more susceptible to those cancers.[22] Interestingly, an association with lung cancer, which I'd expect, was not observed. We do know that the immune-system milieu created by COVID-19 contains all the factors that would predispose someone to cancer, and we've seen it play out in the laboratory.[23] Severe COVID infection has also been observed to increase the risk of a cancer of immune cells called multiple myeloma,[24] as well as other rare blood cancers.[25] It may simply be too soon to tell how COVID-19 will affect our cancer risk decades down the line. Keeping all this in mind, it will be especially important for those who have recovered from severe COVID-19 to stay on top of their cancer screenings—colonoscopies, mammograms, endoscopies if a person has chronic reflux, and lung cancer screening if a person has a smoking history. Unfortunately, the COVID-19 pandemic also resulted in many of these screening tests being delayed or forgone; this will result in over 10,000 extra breast and colorectal cancer deaths in the US, and over 200,000 additional deaths from late cancer diagnosis across developed countries over the next decade (extrapolating from a study of Canada).[26] This additional mortality is on top of the seven million global deaths from COVID-19 itself so far.

Some medical mysteries from the COVID-19 epidemic may never be solved. The "Spanish" flu pandemic of 1918–19 resembled COVID-19 in many ways (least of which, they happened nearly 100 years apart). This early-twentieth-century virus was believed to have infected nearly a third of the world population, culminating in over 50 million deaths. A century later, many questions remain. For instance, a mysterious pandemic of sleeping sickness arose around the same time. Over a million people were randomly stricken with weakness, coma, and bizarre Parkinson's disease–like symptoms, resulting in half a million deaths. Some had been sick with flu, others had not. After that the disease, called encephalitis lethargic (EL), simply vanished. Present-day doctors are still flabbergasted. The prevailing hypothesis about EL is that it was an autoimmune reaction to the flu, and certain patients were for some unknown reason predisposed to inflammation of the brain (much like some people are predisposed to inflammation of the lungs from COVID-19). The fact that such medical mysteries persist, despite all our advances, speaks to the complexity of our immune system. The more we learn, the more questions we raise, leaving us chasing the horizon.

THE HYGIENE HYPOTHESIS

We've discussed how the bacteria *Helicobacter pylori* (*H. pylori*) is the chief culprit behind stomach cancer, the third most deadly cancer in the world. Like COVID-19, it causes chronic inflammation in the stomach, and over decades, that cell damage can transform into cancer. However, after decades of eradication efforts, global health experts are now reconsidering their approach toward the stomach bug.

H. pylori has been identified as the cause of up to 90% of non-cardia stomach cancers,[27] the more common of the two sub-types of stomach cancer. The two subtypes are named after their anatomical locations: Cardia occurs toward the top of the stomach, where the heart is (hence the name), while noncardia occurs toward the bottom of the stomach, near the small intestines. Doctors have waged a war against the bacteria, nearly eradicating it from much of the developed world. But then a twist occurred: As noncardia stomach cancer rates fell, the rates of cardia cancer, the other type of stomach cancer, has risen sevenfold.[28] Ironically, it seems that while *H. pylori* promotes inflammation in the noncardia region, it actually decreases inflammation in the cardia region and in the esophagus.[29] Eliminating the bacteria has simply helped trade one stomach cancer for another.

The antibiotic war against *H. pylori* and numerous other bacteria has raised a broader issue: too *much* hygiene. Believe it or not, many doctors now think that our lives being clean and sterilized is actually a bad thing, particularly for immune system development during childhood. Supporters of the "hygiene hypothesis" point to research that shows those raised in hyper-sanitary environments, for example, without siblings or pets, have far greater rates of allergies and autoimmune disorders.[30] Meanwhile, kids exposed to dirt, animals, and other gross stuff early on actually have less of a chance of developing allergies later in life. Other studies have shown that parasitic infections actually decrease your risk of type 1 (autoimmune) diabetes[31] and multiple sclerosis.[32] Our immune systems need microbes to train on, so when they go "understimulated" due to our sanitized way of life, they start getting antsy and attacking normal cells, resulting in autoimmune disease. These autoimmune diseases, as we've discussed, then increase your cancer risk. Obviously, *H. pylori* is still worth treating in many cases, especially if it's causing symptoms. But further research is required on the mysterious interplay among genetics, diet, infection, and inflammation, to explain why some nations, like India, have astronomical rates of *H. pylori* infection but very few cases of stomach cancer.

There's also the brewing crisis of antibiotic resistance. As we treat common bacteria like *H. pylori* with antibiotics, as well as treating all sorts of viral infections and treating most of our livestock with antibiotics, we've noticed the rise of antibiotic-resistant "superbugs" like methicillin-resistant *Staphylococcus aureus*, flesh-eating bacteria, and gonorrhea. Like with cancer, when you treat bacteria with an antibiotic, if even a few cells survive, those cells have probably gained resistance to that antibiotic. Most antibiotics belong to only a few different "classes," so once a bacterial species has developed resistance to all of them, doctors are literally out of options. Last year, 25,000 Europeans died of resistant superbugs, which scientists are calling the next big medical crisis.[33] That's why it's important to take the full course of antibiotics your doctor prescribes, and equally important to not take antibiotics at all if your likelihood of bacterial infection is low.

THE GUT MICROBIOME, STRESS, AND INFLAMMATION

We're now learning that a lot of inflammation, antibiotic resistance, and autoimmune disease can be traced to the gut microbiome. The gut microbiome refers to the trillions of microorganisms (bacteria, fungi, viruses, and other microbes) that live in the digestive tract, mainly in the intestines. These microbes play a crucial role in digestion, immune function, and overall health. Each of us has a unique and balanced ecosystem growing within us that helps regulate various bodily processes. In fact, there are more types of bacterial cells in your microbiome than there are types of "human" cells throughout the rest of your body.

Your microbiome helps regulate nutrition, your immune system, and even your mental health. Gut microbes help break down complex carbohydrates, fiber, and other substances that human enzymes can't fully digest, converting them into nutrients and vitamins (like B vitamins and vitamin K) that the body can absorb. The gut microbiome also communicates with the immune system, helping to distinguish between harmful invaders and harmless substances, reducing the risk of immune overreaction. Just like the hygiene hypothesis we discussed earlier, exposure to many different bacteria in your gut gives your immune system the practice it needs to distinguish friend from foe.[34] Beneficial gut bacteria also ferment dietary fibers to produce short-chain fatty acids (SCFAs) like butyrate, acetate, and propionate. These compounds have anti-inflammatory properties and help maintain the integrity of the intestinal lining. The microbiome also helps maintain the gut barrier, preventing harmful substances from leaking into the bloodstream, which can trigger an immune response and inflammation.

When the microbiome goes awry, it can lead to all sorts of autoimmune dysregulation and disease. Lack of healthy gut bacteria, like after long courses of antibiotics, can weaken the gut barrier, leading to a condition called increased intestinal permeability or "leaky gut." Leaky gut allows harmful substances, like toxins, undigested food particles, and bacteria, to pass through the gut lining into the bloodstream. These foreign substances trigger an immune response, causing inflammation throughout the body.[35] An imbalance in the gut microbiome (dysbiosis) can lead to the overgrowth of harmful bacteria or the loss of beneficial bacteria, which disrupts the immune system's regulation and contributes to inflammation.[36] Dysbiosis has been linked to Crohn's disease, ulcerative colitis, rheumatoid arthritis, and multiple sclerosis. Dysbiosis can also trigger low-grade chronic inflammation, even outside the gut. As we've discussed, chronic inflammation is at the root of nearly all chronic disease, from heart disease to cancer. Chronic inflammation plays a role in atherosclerosis (plaque buildup in arteries), increasing the risk of heart disease, and insulin resistance, a key factor in the development of type 2 diabetes. In fact, doctors are now studying fecal microbiota transplant, literally putting one person's "healthier" gut bacteria into someone else's intestines, as a treatment for a wide array of illnesses. If conventional treatments have failed, fecal transplant is now recommended for people who have Crohn's disease or ulcerative colitis.[37] It is also showing promise for those with type 1 diabetes,[38] lupus, autoimmune liver disease, and Hashimoto's thyroiditis.[39] Basically, with any disease that includes chronic inflammation, fixing the gut microbiome can help.

Dysbiosis of the gut is also linked to cancer risk. Specific microbial species and their metabolites can promote carcinogenesis by inducing DNA damage, activating pro-inflammatory pathways, and altering the immune response. For instance, with periodontal disease, certain bacteria growing in the mouth actually cause inflammation in the colon, increasing the risk of colon cancer about 20%.[40] On the flip side, beneficial gut bacteria produce SCFAs, which, due to their anti-inflammatory properties, also decrease colon cancer risk.[41] In fact, it seems that people who develop colorectal cancer have a different gut microbiome from those who don't,[42] and research is now starting to focus on the microbiome to predict, prevent, or even treat colon cancer.[43] Similarly, doctors have identified differences in the vaginal microbiome in women with gynecological cancers, and differences in the urinary microbiome in people with bladder or prostate cancer.[44] The study of the delicate interplay among bacteria, inflammation, and cancer is in its infancy, but holds transformational promise when it comes to cancer prevention.

The gut microbiome can even affect mental health, stress, and dementia. Emerging evidence suggests that gut microbiome imbalances may influence brain inflammation, contributing to conditions like depression, anxiety, and neurodegenerative diseases (e.g., Alzheimer).[45] The bacteria that live in your gut help your body produce the building blocks of the neurotransmitters used in your brain, and those anti-inflammatory SCFAs may actually help regulate cognitive function and mood.[46] This association is believed to underlie the link between gastrointestinal conditions (such as irritable bowel syndrome) and mental health, and between gastrointestinal problems and pain syndromes like fibromyalgia. All this data isn't yet ready for prime time, but I anticipate that in the years to come, we will see much more about the fascinating mind-gut-cancer axis.

The interplay of stress, mental health, and the gut microbiome may even be linked to cancer risk and survival. Chronic psychological stress has been shown to induce dysbiosis, which can exacerbate cancer progression. For instance, chronic stress reduces the presence of beneficial gut bacteria such as *Lactobacillus johnsonii* and its metabolite protocatechuic acid, leading to increased risk of colorectal cancer progression.[47] Chronic stress activates the sympathetic nervous system (which controls the fight or flight response), resulting in systemic inflammation and immune system dysregulation. This pro-inflammatory state can promote tumors and cancer progression by creating a tumor-supportive microenvironment.[48] Stress truly takes a mental and physical toll on the body, and often presents itself in surprising ways. I had a young veteran in my clinic at the VA who had severe knee and back pain, unaffected by pain medications and physical therapy. But on a routine screening during the visit, I learned he suffered from recurrent nightmares, feelings of guilt, hyperarousal, and anxiety—all hallmarks of PTSD. We started him on antidepressants and psychotherapy, and lo and behold, his back and knee pain resolved. I've seen dozens of similar examples, where treating a patient's underlying mental health issue improved their physical health. Treating depression has been shown to prolong life expectancy in patients with heart disease and cancer.[49] What's more, reducing stress can extend life and may reduce cancer risk for all patients.[50,51]

A Slow Burn

Chronic inflammation is a slow burn. Unlike the angry ankle of gout or a pus-filled skin infection, chronic inflammation is a nefarious, surreptitious process brewing deep in our cells. Even though we don't see it, we may feel its effects all over. Inflammation disrupts our gut bacteria balance, which in turn worsens the inflammation, creating a spiral of chronic disease. Inflammation is associated with autoimmune disease, heart disease, diabetes, dementia, depression, and even cancer risk. There doesn't seem to be a chronic disease process that hasn't been linked to inflammation in some way these days.

Addressing inflammation may be the key to disease prevention, but it's not quite as easy as just taking anti-inflammatory medicines like aspirin or anti-inflammatory supplements. For one thing, inflammation also fights infections, and immunosuppressant drugs actually increase cancer risk. Other anti-inflammatories, like aspirin or ibuprofen, are good to take in the short term, but in the long term, they lead to kidney disease and increased bleeding risk. In the whole market of anti-inflammatory "snake oils," none have been clinically proven to bring about the benefits of reduced inflammation. As with most things, the most effective supplement is the natural one.

Thankfully, there are many ways to promote beneficial gut bacteria and reduce inflammation. Fiber from fruits, vegetables, whole grains, and legumes feeds beneficial gut bacteria and promotes SCFA production (and also reduces colon cancer risk). Fermented foods like yogurt, kefir, sauerkraut, and kimchi contain probiotics (beneficial bacteria) that support gut health. Prebiotic fibers, found in foods like garlic, onions, and bananas, nourish beneficial gut bacteria. On the other hand, high-sugar and high-fat diets (especially those including red and processed meats) can promote the growth of harmful bacteria. Regular physical activity supports gut health and reduces inflammation. And then there's the mind-body axis. While it may sound like woo-woo medicine, the effects of psychological health on physical health are very real. Stress-reduction techniques like meditation, yoga, deep breathing, or whatever works for you personally, can help improve gut health and reduce inflammation.

The gut, the mind, bacteria, and immunity are linked. The study of integrative medicine has found so many ways that lifestyle affects chronic disease, even as researchers are still struggling to explain it all. So next time you're chowing down on a plant-based stir-fry or fruit salad, or taking a break to stretch or enjoy some music, you may actually be reducing inflammation all over your body and reducing your cancer risk. If you trust your body's signals, and take good care of it, you increase your chances of enjoying a good mood and a long, healthy life.

In summary:

- Inflammation causes genetic mutations and immune system dysfunction, increasing cancer risk.

- People with autoimmune diseases like Crohn's, ulcerative colitis, or lupus are at increased risk of cancer.

- Antioxidants have not been shown to reduce cancer risk, but weight loss, probiotics, and foods rich in healthy bacteria (like yogurt) help reduce inflammation.

- COVID-19 has been hypothesized to increase cancer risk, but it's too early to know the answer—although missed screenings due to the lockdowns have led to more than 200,000 early cancer deaths in the US alone.

- Over-sanitation in childhood increases the risk of autoimmune disease like asthma; it's important for children to play in the dirt, and even get sick from time to time.

CHAPTER 11

To Prevent the Recurrence of Misery

Cancer Relapse and Screening

To prevent the recurrence of misery is, alas! beyond
the power of man.
—THOMAS MALTHUS

Even if they do let you go home, you'll be back here pretty quick.
The Crab loves people. Once he's grabbed you with his pincers,
he won't let go till you croak.
—ALEXANDER SOLZHENITSYN, *CANCER WARD*

In his novel *Cancer Ward*, dissident Alexander Solzhenitsyn drew
an extended analogy between the cancer patients around him
and his homeland, plagued by a philosophical cancer: the Soviet regime. He believed that, like a cancer cell, the ideals of
communism had mutated into something nefarious, and me-
tastasized until they had subjugated every human right. He saw
doctors attempt all sorts of "hail Mary" treatments, from surgery to radiation to poison, but the tumors would always come
back. In the book, these treatments were metaphors for the
many failed attempts at social reform, and their side effects were
grueling. "There's something noble about treating oneself with
a strong poison. Poison doesn't pretend to be a harmless medicine," he wrote.[1]

Funnily enough, Solzhenitsyn did successfully cure his testicular cancer, in part with an herbal remedy from mandrake root, which decades later would be developed into the widely used chemotherapy agent etoposide.[2] But Solzhenitsyn's outlook for his country's struggle with communism remained bleak. Could the cancer be cured? It seemed it had been defeated in 1991, when the USSR collapsed, allowing Solzhenitsyn to return and live the rest of his days in his native Russia until 2008. Thankfully, he did not live to see Russia's return to totalitarianism in the years since. Perhaps he was right that some cancers always return.

This book has addressed the many roots of cancer development and the strategies, on an individual and social level, to mitigate them. But what can be done when cancer has already arisen, or the risk factors for it have already been cast? Cancer survival was once the stuff of fantasies. Today, survival is an expectation for many people who have cancer. Over 5,000 years ago, the ancient Egyptians described breast cancer as incurable. Today, the 10-year survival rate is 83%. For breast cancers detected early, the survival rate is 99%. The millions of people who have "defeated" their cancer are, in most cases, at heightened risk of the cancer coming back. Sometimes, even the chemotherapy or radiation we use to fight cancer can lead to new cancers decades later. So, what tools can we use to monitor for cancer recurrence? And can these same tools be applied to everyone to help us catch and cut out cancers early, before they spread and become deadly?

CANCER RECURRENCE

In 2022, about 18 million cancer survivors were living in the US, or approximately 5% of the population. That figure is projected to increase to 26 million in 2040.[3] Cancer recurrence risk varies highly by tumor type, stage, and treatment, but it is safe to say that most of these millions of people are at increased risk of their cancer returning, compared to the general population's risk of developing cancer. Given that many people who have had cancer are immunocompromised or have received potentially cancer-inducing chemotherapy and radiation, they are at an increased risk of secondary cancer (a cancer of the same type, showing up in another location) as well. How we monitor for disease recurrence is a rapidly evolving field, and advances may trickle into new screening technologies for the general population.

The same suggestions for cancer prevention apply to preventing cancer recurrence. The greatest lifestyle factors that affect the success of cancer therapy, and the risk of recurrence, are exactly what you would expect: smoking and alcohol cessation, healthy diet, and physical activity. In fact, a recent clinical trial of colon cancer patients across six countries found that a structured exercise program after surgery and chemotherapy decreased the risk of recurrence or death by a whopping 37% compared to no exercise program.[4] On the flip side, all those supplements and snake oils that lack data on preventing cancer are equally ineffective in preventing recurrence. What patients can do, though, is stay vigilant. The symptoms of recurrence often mirror those of the original cancer. New, unintended weight loss over 5% of a person's weight, lumps or bumps, bruising or bleeding anywhere, or other changes to your health should never be ignored. All cancer survivors should follow up with some doctor regularly, either their primary care provider or an oncologist. Although anecdotal, many of my patients have said they can feel their cancer coming back before the scans show it. On the flip side, though, hindsight is 20/20, and constant anxiety itself has a myriad of health repercussions. I've seen my mom lose sleep for days in anticipation of her regular blood tests. It is a difficult line to toe between vigilance and anxiety, and in my experience, sharing those feelings with family or a therapist is one of the best ways to cope. Seeking help with mental health is never a sign of weakness or failure, and is in fact specifically recommended for people who have or had cancer.

All that aside, testing for recurrence is an evolving medical arena. Imaging and blood tests for recurrence vary highly by tumor type, but as a general rule, they reflect the tests that were originally used to diagnose the disease. Mammograms and MRIs diagnose breast cancer, and are relied upon to monitor for recurrence. It's the same with CT scans for cancers of the lungs or abdomen. Blood tests like prostate-specific antigen (PSA) for prostate cancer or carcinoembryonic antigen for colorectal cancer should be continued after treatment. But most tumors don't have reliable blood tests, and imaging can be costly, inconvenient, and even dangerous, as with the radiation and risk of kidney damage with CT scans. What if there were a way to detect cancer by the shadow it casts, to read its signature without seeing the actual cell? That's where testing for cancer DNA in the blood comes into play.

Since cancers replicate wildly and die, they release copious amounts of DNA or ribonucleic acid (RNA). Testing for these molecules, also known as liquid biopsy, was first invented and approved as a supplement for tissue biopsy. For many cancer types, it is essential to test the cancer for driver mutations that can be targeted with specific therapies, significantly improving survival. In scenarios when a tissue sample cannot be procured, either because of the location of the cancer or the health status of the patient, liquid biopsy could be used instead. The mutations could be determined by isolating cancer DNA in the blood and sequencing it. But on top of mutational testing, the levels of that DNA could also be used to confirm whether the cancer is truly gone or if minimal residual disease (MRD) remains, and also monitor for recurrence.

MRD testing was originally a concept used exclusively for blood cancers, whose cell populations can be easily quantified with blood tests, but the advent of cell-free DNA has allowed us to expand MRD testing to solid tumors as well. For instance, the Signatera cell-free DNA test was shown to successfully predict residual disease, and disease recurrence, in patients who had undergone surgery for colorectal cancer. These findings could be used by doctors to decide who should receive additional chemotherapy, and who was at a low enough risk that they didn't need it. Liquid biopsy is now a $5 billion industry, with over a dozen companies vying for indications for different tumor types.[5] But while the race is on, little reliable data exists on how much, if at all, this early detection and prognostication can translate into improvements in survival. The technology may be the next Google, or it may be the next Google Glass. Whether it catches on will depend on valid clinical trials, designed to minimize the statistical bias inherent in this imperfect science.

SURVIVAL AND BIAS

Any study of cancer survival is subject to statistical bias. Bias is when our approach to answering a scientific question affects our result, leading us away from the truth. In World War II, the US military was deciding how to improve their fighter planes. They noticed that most airplanes recovered after battle had holes in their wings, so they assumed the wings ought to get re-inforced. But when they asked mathematician Abraham Wald, he drew a different conclusion. The planes that sustained damage to the wings survived and returned to be analyzed, while the planes that got hit in the engine were destroyed in battle. This was a classic case of selection bias. The military went on to re-inforce the engine, not the wings, and the rest is history, or so the story goes.[6]

Selection bias is equally at play in medicine. If doctors are comparing two cancer drugs, and they choose healthier patients for the experimental drug, we cannot trust the results, even if those patients live longer. Did the drug cause the difference in survival, or was it selection bias? Even if doctors subconsciously perceive their patients receiving an experimental drug as doing better, they can bias the results. That's why most phase III (large trials across centers comparing a treatment to the current standard of care) clinical trials are double blinded: neither the patient nor the physician knows who is getting which treatment. In the interest of controlling for bias, these clinical trials must be large, held in academic institutions across the country, and stiflingly expensive. The company must offer their medicine for free and pay the doctors and hospitals for all costs incurred. The average cost of a "pivotal" trial, based on which the FDA approves (or does not approve) a new cancer therapy, was around $32 million in 2017.[7] Nonetheless, that value pales in comparison to the total that pharmaceutical companies in the US spend each year on marketing their products to patients and doctors: over $30 billion as of 2019.[8] Clinical trials have also come under fire for being more accessible to men, white people, and those of higher socioeconomic status.

Studies of surveillance techniques can be similarly fraught with bias. Two common biases here are "lead-time" and "length-time." Lead-time bias occurs when survival doesn't actually change, but the time to death appears to get longer because the cancer was detected earlier. If, for example, I found a stage I (small and confined to one area) cancer but the patient didn't do anything about it, that person may live for five more years. If a patient didn't get screened until they developed symptoms, they may be diagnosed with stage IV (spread to other organs) disease four years later and then die after a year. The survival may appear to have increased from one year to five, but the disease course was actually the same; we just found the cancer earlier.

The other bias is length-time. Length-time bias occurs when screening mostly detects the slow-growing tumors, while the aggressive ones do not get caught on screening. As such, it may seem that the group that got screened, versus the one that didn't, had better survival, but actually the screening just found a lot of cancers that probably weren't going to cause death anyway. In short, it is easy to fall into a statistical trap and conclude that screening makes a huge survival difference, when in fact it doesn't. For this reason, trials of screening approaches are conducted rigorously with thousands of patients, and only a few screening protocols have actually passed the test and are regularly recommended for prevention.

In medical lingo, there are many "tiers" of prevention. Primary prevention corresponds with the lay definition of prevention: eliminating the risk factors that lead to disease. This is what the rest of this book has dealt with. Secondary prevention is preventing death or suffering by catching disease earlier, when it is easier to treat and cure.

Catching cancer early is an admirable goal. For most solid tumors (versus blood cell tumors, which do not form solid masses), taking out a localized cancer and any lymph nodes to which it may have spread, with or without chemotherapy (given after surgery), is often curative. Many cancers, especially those of internal organs that do not have nerves and thus cannot feel pain, tend to spread before they become symptomatic. Pancreatic cancer, for instance, is a notorious silent killer. Over half of pancreatic cancer cases are diagnosed after the tumor has spread, at which point the five-year survival is a bleak 3% (while localized disease has a 44% five-year survival rate).[9] Early detection is literally vital. For these reasons, patients at higher cancer risk, such as adults over 50, and people who are overweight, drink alcohol excessively, or smoke, are advised to see their doctor with any new fevers, chills, bleeding, skin yellowing, gastrointestinal changes, or unintended weight loss. A recent study has actually identified two unexpected symptoms that have been shown to be early warning signs of pancreatic cancer: increased thirst and dark urine. While they are certainly not specific to pancreatic cancer (and are far more commonly seen with diabetes and kidney disease), they should at least prompt a discussion with your doctor and initial lab testing. These symptoms may arise a year or more before the cancer would otherwise be diagnosed.[10]

Of course, many tumors can start off with no symptoms. For select cancers, secondary prevention can take the form of screening protocols that are offered to all patients of a certain demographic group (for example, age or sex) in search of tumors common enough to justify the cost. Four cancer screenings are currently recommended by the US Preventive Services Task Force (USPSTF) and American Cancer Society (ACS) for healthy adults with no symptoms (based on age, sex, and smoking history): breast, cervical, colorectal, and lung. These four cancers are common and deadly enough that universal screening has been proven, by thousands of data points, to save years of life and save money for society. Prostate cancer screening was previously recommended for all men above a certain age but has since become more controversial, as its cost- and life-saving value have come into question.[11]

I've encountered many people who express hesitancy about cancer screenings. It can often feel like you go to see a doctor feeling completely healthy, only to learn you've got health issues brewing, or are at risk of life-threatening disease. Some have even accused me of making up illnesses for profit (I can assure you, I get paid the same five-figure salary regardless of how many medications I prescribe or problems I diagnose). When pressed on their apprehension, most often I hear something along the lines of "ignorance is bliss." People would rather not know they have breast or colon or lung cancer if it's not causing them problems, or so they think.

"Someone must have been telling lies about Joseph K., for without having done anything wrong he was arrested one fine morning."[12] In Franz Kafka's novel *The Trial*, K. finds himself arrested and ultimately facing a death sentence without the faintest clue why. After all, "It's in the nature of this judicial system that one is condemned not only in innocence but also in ignorance."[13] Such was the practice of medicine as recently as 50 years ago; patients would awake one morning to a new symptom that would promptly take their life, without the faintest idea of what was going on or why. Today, instead, we can catch these conditions years before they cause problems. Knowledge, rather than ignorance, can empower patients to act while cancers are operable and before cancer symptoms begin to cause them distress. "Ignorance is bliss" seems to fly out the window as soon as there's pain, or jaundice (yellowing of the skin), or blood in the urine.

BREAST CANCER SCREENING

Perhaps the most well-known cancer screening is the mammogram. Digital breast tomosynthesis (DBT), also known as 3D mammography, is considered the "gold standard." Breast MRI is utilized for people with higher-risk or denser breast tissue, which decreases the sensitivity of mammography.[14] All the women in my life dread their annual or biannual mammogram, not only due to the pain, but also the subsequent anxiety. I have been on both sides of the process. For moral support, I've accompanied my mother to her mammogram appointment and seen her pace the room waiting to get the preliminary result. I've also sat in the darkroom in the back with the radiologists and witnessed how they systematically go through dozens of scans, taking no more than a few minutes on each, but dissecting figments and pixels that would drive me mad. They taught me the "rule of tens" in mammography: about 10% of women get called back for additional scanning (further mammography, which is just a specialized x-ray, ultrasound, or MRI), and fewer than 10% of those actually have breast cancer. Fewer than 1% of women scanned actually get diagnosed with cancer. When looking at mortality, nearly 3,000 women need to get screened to save just 1 life.[15] Of course, every life counts. As rabbinical scholars (apocryphally) put it, "To save a life is to save the world." But the lives also add up when considered across millions of people, and the results are staggering. Between 384,000 and 614,500 lives have been saved by mammography since 1989.[16]

However, the survival benefit of the screening clearly increases with age, as cancer risk grows. When cost and psychological distress is weighed against the marginal benefit of screening younger women, the recommendations become controversial. The USPSTF, which tends to be more "conservative," recommends screening *every other* year, but as of 2024, has decreased its recommended starting age to 40, while the ACS recommends screening every year starting at age 45. Women aged 40 to 55 are stuck deciding with their provider whether they prefer a more aggressive (that is, screening every year) or conservative approach.[17]

Access to, and knowledge of, mammography remains a significant contributor to disparities in breast cancer survival. Patients in rural and low socioeconomic status zip codes have lower rates of breast cancer screening. African American and Hispanic women are significantly less likely to receive DBT, the latest x-ray technology, which is associated with superior breast cancer detection. African American and non-English-speaking patients are also less likely to receive timely notification and follow-up of abnormal mammography results, which poses a higher risk for disease and mortality. COVID-19 has only exacerbated this problem. During the peak of the pandemic in 2020, breast cancer screenings across the US decreased by as much as 90%, and new diagnoses decreased by between 24%–50% in countries across the developed world. There were not fewer cases of breast cancer arising. Instead, thousands of women with low-stage tumors lost their opportunity to catch the disease earlier. In particular, Asian American and Hispanic women in the US seemed to have the greatest decline in cancer screening in 2020 during COVID-19. The picture has improved, but has not completely recovered, in the years since.[18]

CERVICAL CANCER SCREENING

Mammograms are not alone in causing women discomfort. Another cancer screening test recommended for women is the

Pap smear for cervical cancer. The Pap smear is named after Greek American gynecologist Georgios Papanicolaou, who first reported the procedure in 1928, although a Romanian physician named Aurel Babes was already doing a similar screening using a platinum loop in 1927.[19] Papanicolaou immigrated to the US as a doctor during the first Balkan war but spent years working in menial jobs until he finally found his way back into medicine as a lab technician (much like my father). He dedicated decades of his life to examining cells of the guinea pig, then human reproductive systems, characterizing the subtle changes that occurred with menstruation. Once he got a sense of what looked normal, he was able to identify cells that appeared abnormal, and found that women who had these abnormal cells would be diagnosed with cervical cancer years later.

Today, the Pap smear is based on the same principle. A Pap test samples cells from the cervix to look at under the microscope for dysplastic changes, that is, changes in the cell structure that suggest it has started on a path to become cancerous. This screening is recommended by the USPSTF for anyone with a cervix, every 3 years, beginning at age 21, until age 65. The old-fashioned microscopy can also be combined with molecular testing for HPV, the virus that causes cervical cancer. This combined approach can be started at age 30, and only needs to be done every 5 years instead of every 3. The ACS recommends HPV testing every 5 years beginning at age 25, without the need for cervical sampling. Before ages 25–30, HPV testing is not recommended, although many women may have the infection. When young, the immune system is robust enough to clear the infection, and thus the risk of cancer being caused by HPV is much lower.

Screenings have reduced cervical cancer death rates by over 70% since the 1960s. In addition, high-risk HPV cases have been declining significantly in the developed world because of vaccination, and cervical cancer risk is expected to plummet in the coming decades as well. Unfortunately, studies around the US found a huge reduction, up to 80%, in cervical cancer screening rates during COVID-19 as well, affecting Asian Americans and Pacific Islanders most severely.[20]

However, opportunities are bred in a storm. The pandemic spurred the US to fast-track the development of self-sampling HPV tests that can be performed by women in the privacy of their own homes. Swiss pharmaceutical company Roche launched a self-sampling product in June of 2022, and it is now being used in countries around the world. In particular, low- to middle-income countries account for 90% of cervical cancer deaths due to limited access to screenings and vaccination; if the home HPV test is made available, this technology could greatly improve their health outcomes.[21]

COLORECTAL CANCER SCREENING

Colorectal cancer screening is another dreaded procedure for men and women alike. The USPSTF recently lowered its recommendation for starting screening to age 45 for the people at average risk, in response to an "epidemic" of cases in younger adults, like actor Chadwick Boseman (and there's now discussion about lowering the age to 40).[22] The screenings should continue until at least 75 years, at which age the data on survival benefit is less clear, and patients can decide with their physicians whether to continue. People with risk factors like family history, inflammatory bowel disease, or being exposed to pelvic/abdominal radiation may need to start earlier. The most common screening for colorectal cancer is colonoscopy, when a camera and instrument are threaded through the colon to identify and cut out polyps that may turn cancerous. This procedure is done under sedation, but the preparation leading up to it can be downright awful. Patients must drink a very salty, diarrhea-inducing concoction, or 24 laxative pills, to clear out their colon so that any polyps can be more easily visualized. Thankfully, if nothing significant is found from the colonoscopy, it only needs to be repeated every 10 years.

Other screening modalities for colorectal cancer that do not involve prep or discomfort have grown in popularity in recent years. High-sensitivity guaiac fecal occult blood test (HSgFOBT) or fecal immunochemical test (FIT) are tests of the stool for blood and tumor markers that can be conducted every year in place of colonoscopy. Unfortunately, they are not quite as good at detecting cancer, and when they do come up positive (with cancer or benign polyps), a colonoscopy is still required to get a tissue sample and confirm that diagnosis. A newer version of this technology is Cologuard, which combines the old-fashioned chemical stool test with a DNA analysis of the stool, looking for markers of cancer. This technology is much more sensitive for detecting cancer, consistently detecting between 92%–100% of cancers, far more than the FIT test alone, but slightly less than the colonoscopy. Unlike colonoscopy, Cologuard only detects around 42% of small polyps, but the cancer risk of those polyps is low. Thanks to its improved sensitivity and specificity, Cologuard is now approved to be safely used every three years, instead of every year. However, as it is proprietary, it is more expensive (over $500 per test), and not all insurers cover the cost. Similarly, any positive result must be followed up with colonoscopy, though the rate of false positives is only 2%–4%.[23]

With screenings as with some family members, they are most appreciated in their absence. Black Americans have a 35% greater chance of dying of colorectal cancer, in part due to difference in screening rates. At its peak in 2020, the COVID-19 lockdowns caused a nearly 80% reduction in colorectal screenings, with harrowing results. One modeling study from England estimated that due to the missed colonoscopies, the five-year survival rate from colorectal cancer would decrease by 6.4%, resulting in nearly 1,500 more deaths, the most of any tumor.[24] While these numbers may pale in comparison to the lives saved by quarantine, they cannot be simply brushed aside, especially considering that colorectal screening had multiple viable alternatives that we failed to maximally utilize in place of colonoscopy. One study suggested that making the stool-based tests readily available could increase screening rates among Black Americans by up to 13 times. Perhaps with the next pandemic, we will be better prepared. In the meanwhile, both colonoscopy and stool testing are proven and safe options, as long as they are done at the recommended time intervals.[25]

LUNG AND PROSTATE CANCER SCREENING

Unlike the other screenings, lung cancer screening with low-dose CT scan is *not* recommended for all adults, but rather those aged 50–80 with a 20 pack-year smoking history, who currently smoke or quit within the last 15 years. (A pack-year is equivalent to smoking one pack a day for a year, or two packs a day for half a year, etc.) The last piece of the guideline, on how recently the person quit smoking, is up for debate. The ACS, which tends to be more aggressive about cancer screening than the government-sponsored USPSTF, recommends that *all* former 20 pack-year smokers, regardless of how long ago they quit, should be screened. Yet many government and commercial insurers still refuse to cover the screening CT, given the discrepancy even though it is the only cancer screening proven to improve overall survival.[26]

Low-dose CT delivers less than a fifth of the radiation of a regular CT scan, mitigating the dangers discussed earlier. Due to the recency and complexity of this guideline, lung cancer screening is the most underutilized of the screening tests, although lung cancer remains the leading cause of death from cancer. The low-dose CT was found to reduce cancer death by 20% in appropriate patients. While Black Americans have the highest lung cancer risk, over 4%, they are the least likely to receive the screening CT. Merely 5% of white patients in the US who are indicated for lung cancer screening actually get the scan, but the figure drops to a paltry 1.7% for Black patients.[27] The disparity is due to multiple factors, likely a combination of systemic racism in health care, and the sheer complexity of the screening recommendations. Despite the low uptake by those who meet screening criteria, doctors are debating whether the guidelines for screening ought to be made less rigid, which could help reduce some of the complexity and increase utilization among Black Americans. Nonetheless, as with the other screening tests, COVID-19 significantly reduced lung cancer screening; this is expected to result in approximately a 3.5% decrease in lung cancer survival over the next decade, due to late detection.[28]

Finally, prostate cancer screening with the blood test for PSA is now controversial, and carries rather ambivalent recommendations. The USPSTF gives it a grade C recommendation (that is, discuss pros and cons with your doctor) for men aged 55–69, and recommends against it for anyone older. The ACS recommends having this discussion at age 50 for average-risk men, and at age 45 for those with high risk, such as Black Americans or men with significant family history of this cancer.

The danger with PSA testing is that levels naturally go up with age. Back when testing was universally recommended, many men would undergo invasive biopsies due to false positive screens, or have their prostate gland removed or receive radiation for low-risk prostate cancer, which in all likelihood would not have led to their deaths. These procedures carry a high risk of problems with urinating, having a bowel movement, or maintaining an erection. Although prostate cancer is the most common cancer in men, and around 1 in every 41 men will die of it, the adage still rings true: "You are much more likely to die *with* prostate cancer than because of it."

In fact, among autopsies of men who died of all causes, around 30% of men 70 or older had cancer in their prostate, which increases to over 50% of men 90 and older.[29] The vast majority of these tumors were early-stage, low-grade cancers, which would never have hurt anyone but could have been caught with PSA testing. The challenges of PSA testing is a prime example of medicine recognizing its own overconfidence. In our aim to treat, we have medicalized many benign aspects of growing older. This has led older adults to get unnecessary and often dangerous procedures in pursuit of lab values and test results deemed "normal," based on younger adults. Perhaps it is "normal" for older men to have a slightly elevated PSA level or a low-grade prostate cancer. It is possible to recognize prostate cancer as deadly and preventable, but also common and often benign, like we do with high blood pressure or blood sugar level. I believe the gravity of the word "cancer" has done many prostate cancer patients an injustice. Nonetheless, the decision about whether to test PSA level ought to be made with your doctor, based on your individual risk factors and "risk tolerance." To screen or not to screen will be the question of the coming decades.

THE FUTURE IS NOW: VACCINES
AND CELL-FREE DNA

While the four screenings explored above are today's standard of care, the future of cancer screening is taking on a very different look. The advent of blood tests for cell-free DNA, released by tumor cells anywhere in the body, is revolutionizing how we detect cancer, and what it means to have it. While this technology is already being used for mutation analysis or monitoring for those with cancer, the question now is whether it could be employed as a screening modality for everyone.

Cell-free DNA is currently in use for screening fetuses for genetic mutations like Down syndrome earlier than by conventional methods. A number of companies are now exploring the technology for its relevance to cancer. One study found that among thousands of blood samples, of both normal persons and people who had cancer, the test could identify the presence of cancer, and the type of cancer, in about 82% of patients.[30] Many of these cancers were at "stage 0," meaning they haven't even grown large enough to be detected on a CT scan. These results are phenomenal, and if replicated in larger studies, could revolutionize cancer screening. But they also beg the question: What then? Will we prescribe toxic chemotherapy for patients without a tissue sample, or even without any recognizable disease on a scan? Or will we tell patients, now anxious that they probably have cancer somewhere, to just "wait and see" whether it grows? Knowledge is power, but only if you can act upon it. Perhaps with the development of better-tolerated immunotherapies and targeted therapies, it may one day be reasonable to treat even people with stage 0 cancer. But today's anticancer arsenal simply isn't sufficient. Even our most successful new therapies carry an immense burden of side effects, which makes most doctors bristle at the idea of using them before it's necessary. Cell-free DNA for screening is a Pandora's box that must be thoroughly studied before it is opened for the general public. But on Wall Street, the flood gates are open, and investors are projected to pour in over $20 billion.[31]

Another tantalizing innovation in the oncology space are vaccines specific for cancer. We previously discussed vaccination against viruses like HPV or hepatitis, which by helping our immune system stave off the virus, reduce one's risk of cancer. But what if we could use the same technology to help our immune system recognize and kill cancer cells *before* they cause problems?

An innovative researcher at the University of Pennsylvania has been studying a vaccine against breast cancer among women with the BRCA1/2 mutations, which as we've discussed, significantly increase their risk of disease. While incredibly dangerous, these mutations also provide scientists with an easy DNA target for a vaccine. So far, they've launched one trial with 16 BRCA+ patients who have previously had breast cancer, to see if it can reduce the risk of recurrence; they began an additional trial of 28 BRCA+ women who haven't had breast cancer, to see if the vaccine can prevent breast cancer entirely. The data will take a few years to come to fruition,[32] but when it does, it could dramatically change the landscape for people with heightened cancer risk.[33]

Similar techniques of harvesting the power of the immune system across cancer types have proven fruitful, but dangerous and expensive. The solid tumor world was revolutionized about 10 years ago with the approval of immunotherapies, like pembrolizumab (Keytruda) and nivolumab (Opdivo), which work across tumor types by taking the brakes off our immune cells (T cells) to help them recognize and kill cancer cells.[34] New combinations of immunotherapies, like programmed cell death protein 1 (PD-1) and cytotoxic T-lymphocyte–associated antigen 4 (CTLA-4) or lymphocyte-activation gene 3 (LAG-3) inhibitors (pardon the alphabet soup), are showing additional promise, though with more side effects. These drugs can cause dysfunction of any organ, most commonly the thyroid, adrenal glands, and colon, but when they affect vital organs like the heart or lungs, they can prove deadly.[35] The latest research suggests that the current doses and schedules we use for these drugs may be far greater than necessary to keep cancers under control.[36] But pharmaceutical companies have little incentive to study less frequent dosing, which could mean lower profits and marginally worse survival, relative to their competitors.

In the liquid cancer world, chimeric antigen receptor T cell (CAR-T) therapy, which involves harvesting and genetically modifying a patient's T cells to fight cancer, has proved curative at times.[37] More recently, we've seen the rise of "bispecific" antibodies across tumor types, which bind both T cells and cancer cells to kick the immune system into gear. Even a virus has been developed to specifically infect melanoma cells and bring about an immune response.[38] All of these therapies are improving survival, but at a cost. Many are associated with various immune-related side effects, and even life-threatening "cytokine release syndrome"; this is when the immune response against the cancer is so powerful it overwhelms the body, resulting in fever, low blood pressure, neurotoxicity, and even death. Furthermore, the cost of developing and manufacturing these products has proven astronomical. CAR-T therapy costs an average of around half a million dollars per person, and even then, drug companies are losing money on it. The immune system is a powerful tool, but it may contain more potential for prevention rather than treatment.

Many cancers, and their recurrence, can be prevented and now even predicted. What may be less predictable is whether early detection technologies and novel approaches like cancer vaccines will actually save money, or just exacerbate our ballooning, unsustainable health care costs.

In summary:

- Anyone who has had cancer has a heightened risk of their cancer returning, and the radiation and chemotherapy used to treat one cancer increase the risk of further cancers years later.

- By detecting cancer when it can be cut out, four cancer screenings—colorectal (colonoscopy or stool test), breast (mammograms), cervical (Pap smears), and lung (CT scans for current or former smokers)—prevent millions of cancer deaths.

- PSA testing for prostate cancer increases early detection, but leads to many false positive results, and may not actually improve survival for everyone.

- Cancer vaccines and testing for cell-free cancer DNA are on the cutting edge of prevention.

CHAPTER 12

Some Are More Equal

Cancer Disparities and Health Care Reform

All are created equal, but some are more equal than others.
—George Orwell, *Animal Farm*

Injustice anywhere is a threat to justice everywhere.
—Reverend Martin Luther King, Jr.

Black and American Indian and Alaska Native (AIAN) people live on average seven years less than white people in the US. Their babies are twice as likely to die in infancy. Their children are twice as likely to face food insecurity. The average wealth of a white household is *10* times greater than that of a Black household.[1] Black people in the US are also *less* likely to be diagnosed early with and *more* likely to die of cancer.[2] These differences represent millions of *real* life-years lost to racism.

I was born a white male into a well-off, educated family. I cannot speak to the experience of being a racial minority, or being poor, in the US, and I would not try. But I can share the experiences of the many underprivileged patients I have had the privilege of taking care of. In fact, I believe it's my duty.

America has given me far more than most. My parents were granted citizenship as religious refugees from the Soviet Union. They came over with nothing—less than $200 to their name—but discovered unparalleled opportunity, which they've passed on to me. Had it not been for the US, I would be a young man in Ukraine today, facing about a 20% chance of death, injury, or displacement due to war. America has literally saved my life. But for many people of color, and people with lesser means, the US has been far less welcoming. Many people who belong to marginalized groups live in a war zone in the US every day, battling historic prejudices, economic inequality, and the inertia of racism. We live in a country that claims all are created equal, but treats some as more equal than others. We cannot grow and innovate without acknowledging and rectifying the mistakes baked into the very fabric of our nation and our health care system.

HISTORIC INJUSTICES IN CANCER

This history of racial injustice in medicine is as old as medicine itself. Phrenology, a nineteenth-century pseudoscience, posited that an individual's character and intelligence could be determined by the shape and contours of their skull. Doctors claimed that certain races had "superior" or "inferior" skull shapes, which they associated with intelligence, morality, and social capability. This led to the categorization of non-European races as "less evolved," reinforcing existing prejudices and legitimizing colonialism, slavery, and social inequalities.

Many of our greatest innovations in medicine have come from experiments on the poor and defenseless. The Tuskegee Study, conducted from 1932 to 1972, was a notorious public health study in which the US Public Health Service enrolled 600 Black men, mostly impoverished and uneducated, under the guise of providing free health care. They were told they were being treated for "bad blood," but in reality, they were being observed for the natural progression of untreated syphilis.[3]

Despite the availability of effective treatment (penicillin) by the 1940s, the participants were deliberately denied care and misled about their health status. Almost 400 men who were promised free health care were actually *never* told they had syphilis, leaving their brains and bones to rot from an entirely treatable disease.[4] This study was so egregious that it served as the inspiration for federal laws and institutional review boards governing clinical trials. But even with safeguards in place, questionable experiments and deep-seated racism in medicine continued for decades.

In the early 1950s, Henrietta Lacks, an African American woman, sought treatment for a lump on her cervix at Johns Hopkins Hospital. Without her knowledge or consent (which was, however, normal procedure at the time), doctors took samples of her tumor cells. Although most cancer cells did not survive when grown in culture during this time period, Lacks's cells, dubbed "HeLa" cells after the first two letters of her names, long outlived her. She died several months after diagnosis. In fact, her cells became the first "immortalized" cell line, and they were cultured into millions of copies, becoming the cornerstone for biomedical research around the country, to this day. Lacks's cells have contributed immensely to medical research, leading to advancements in vaccines, cancer treatments, and more.[5] I remember running experiments with her cells as a laboratory assistant in high school, with no knowledge of where they came from or how. I wasn't the only one in the dark. Lacks and her family were not informed about the use of her cells, nor did they receive any compensation or recognition for all of the innovations they enabled. Stories such as these are why so many of my patients, especially those of color, often voice frustration about being treated like "Guinea pigs" and "experimented upon." These seeds of distrust have been sown over decades and may take equally long, or longer, to heal.

While previously the subjects of questionable experiments, today Black, Hispanic, and AIAN patients are frequently *under*-represented in lifesaving clinical cancer trials. For instance, while 25% of all bladder cancer cases in the US occur in Black patients, less than 2% of all bladder cancer clinical trial participants are Black.[6] And clinical trials are just the tip of the iceberg when it comes to health care disparities.

CURRENT DISPARITIES

The present is a product of the past. Although we've made progress, we're still plagued by the long shadows of our historic failures. With less access to medicine, and less "buy-in" from providers, racial and ethnic minoritized groups and women are less likely to have their cancer found early. With breast cancer, Black and Hispanic women are about 20% more likely to be diagnosed at later stages, and almost 30% less likely to receive surgery.[7] Black women are also twice as likely to suffer delays in treatment or surgery, compared to white women. Lower rates of early diagnosis and delay in treatment have also been observed for Black patients who have liver,[8] gastrointestinal,[9] and lung cancers[10] as well. These disparities in diagnosis and treatment may account for some, but not all, of the disparity in survival. Across all cancers, Black patients have poorer outcomes. For instance, the risk of death is 50% higher among hormone-positive (meaning that it responds to hormones) breast cancer in Black women compared to white women.[11] Other studies found that five-year survival was 10% lower for colon cancer[12] and 20% lower for lung cancer in Black patients compared to white patients.[13]

With prostate cancer, Black men are **twice** as likely to die than white men, and this disparity is exacerbated by genetic as well as social factors.[14]

Women are much less likely to be diagnosed with cancer early than men are, and often more likely to die than men. A study of all cancer patients in the United Kingdom, where the single-payer health care system allows for broader data analysis, found that for all 15 cancer types analyzed, it took doctors longer to diagnose women.[15]

This isn't surprising. For decades, doctors labeled women "hysterical" and discounted their symptoms. Today, thousands of women still die every year because their heart attacks or strokes are ignored by doctors.[16] This dismissal of women goes back centuries. Instead of addressing the inherent injustices in our sexist society, "hysteria" was used as a catch-all diagnosis for women who showed any symptoms such as anxiety, mood swings, or sexual desire. These diagnoses were used to control or institutionalize women who defied societal norms, such as John F. Kennedy's younger sister, who was lobotomized for being a free spirit and defying the family's expectations.

To add insult to injury, historically, women were excluded from medical schools, professional societies, and medical research, so they had no means to contribute their perspectives to the discipline. When they did enter the field, women were often confined to nursing or midwifery roles, with limited opportunities for advancement. Thankfully today, more female than male students are studying medicine across the country. However, after centuries of exclusion and dismissal, women still suffer disparate outcomes in medicine and cancer care.

These disparities are awful and inexcusable. But to us working in medicine, they are sometimes partly explainable. For instance, women are more likely to have nonspecific abdominal or pelvic pain due to their anatomy and menstrual cycles, which can cause doctors to overlook abdominal pain caused by colon or endometrial cancer. Women are also more likely to have blood in their urine due to urinary tract infections, which may explain why they are less likely to have their bladder cancer diagnosed early. Consequently, we've found women are more likely to die of bladder cancer, even in the era of new-fangled therapies (and even though they are more likely to receive surgery).[17] Women of color are in a situation of "double jeopardy" because of their race and sex, having their cancer not diagnosed or their statements not taken seriously, leading to worse survival in breast, ovarian, endometrial, and cervical cancer.[18]

The best thing we can do, as doctors, is set aside our pride and listen to women when they say something feels different. After all, patients know their body best. As patients, all of us, but particularly women and people of color, must advocate for ourselves and call our doctors immediately if we have a persistent fever or weight loss, post-menopausal bleeding, or any new lumps or bumps. Unfortunately, cultural differences and inadequate health care access pose additional barriers to timely diagnosis and treatment.

CULTURAL COMPETENCY

Racial disparities are fueled by a disconnect between patients and their doctors. Practicing in Philadelphia, over half the patients I treat are Black. But in my residency program, less than 10% of the doctors are Black. This is far from an anomaly. Around the country, medical practitioners are predominantly white and Asian and used to be predominantly male, although this is rapidly changing. If we want to truly understand and address the issues our patients face, we need more voices from their communities represented in medicine. We also need to learn to listen.

I once cared for a lady who had seen numerous doctors and heart specialists, but nobody could figure out why she kept accumulating fluid and ending up in the hospital. After taking the time to go through her daily routine, I uncovered that she never realized that "water restriction" applies to other fluids too, like juice or milk. Had anyone taken the time to listen to her, we could have saved needless time and money. I will admit that, as a doctor, I find fully listening to patients incredibly hard. People will often start sharing their whole life story, instead of answering the specific questions asked. In fact, the average doctor interrupts their patient after just 18 seconds![19] With patients scheduled every 15 minutes in the clinic, and the growing burden of documentation in electronic medical records, there simply isn't the time to let people prattle on uninterrupted. But at the same time, I've found that *feeling* heard is paramount to a successful doctor–patient relationship. Whenever I must interrupt my patients, I do so while examining them, and repeat the last thing they said to me, so that they *feel* heard. I also try to explain why I am pressed for time, so people don't take interruptions personally. I suggest that patients write down their questions and concerns, so everything gets discussed during a visit efficiently but comprehensively. Little things, like eye contact or a reassuring touch, can make all the difference.

But if bridging the patient–doctor divide is hard, bridging the divides between ethnic groups, generations, and gender identities is so much harder. For instance, we should definitely be working toward getting more Black doctors (the US decision on affirmative action likely won't help). But while we do, we could all benefit from more education in cultural competency. I've treated elderly Asian patients whose families asked me *not* to tell them they have cancer. Our medical training would call that unethical, but cultural sensitivity would argue otherwise. As a polyglot, I've learned that older, immigrant patients appreciate it when you speak even a few words in their language, while younger, first-generation Americans often find it offensive. When it comes to culturally informed communication, the list of "dos" and "do nots" is limitless.

While keeping up with cultural competency often feels burdensome, it pays dividends. Studies show that when patients feel like their doctors understand them, they are more likely to follow their advice. Unsurprisingly, patients prefer doctors who look and sound like them.[20] This effect transcends the clinic. Black men are the population least likely to receive preventative health care, and they have some of the highest mortality. One study found that engaging barbershops, a cornerstone of the Black community, to help spread the word about treating high blood pressure helped reduce blood pressure *more* than if doctors or pharmacists tried.[21] We all feel more comfortable among our peers, and it can be jarring if a doctor tells you to change your lifestyle or take a new medicine, especially in the context of centuries of racial persecution. Similar initiatives in Black barbershops and churches have been successful in encouraging colonoscopies[22] and prostate cancer screening,[23] which among Black men in particular is a disproportionate cause of early death. Engaging communities in public health initiatives is paramount to their success.

HEALTH SYSTEM REFORM

US World War II General Omar Bradley once said, "Amateurs talk strategy and professionals talk logistics." So far, we've discussed medicine, one of the strategies of health care. But at the root of all these disparities and missed opportunities for prevention lie the failing logistics of health care: our broken health system. I've seen patients ration life-sustaining pills because they couldn't afford them, tough it out with a heart attack to avoid the ambulance charge, or even be denied life-saving surgeries because our hospital was "out of network." The amount that finances influence health outcomes is unquantifiable, and yet most doctors are woefully ignorant of them. This ignorance is, in part, deliberate. We are taught to provide the same, top-tier medical care regardless of a patient's finances, so that rich and poor are treated equally. But when a patient leaves the hospital and can't afford any of the medicines we've recommended, that commitment to equal treatment rings hollow.

In recent years, US health care spending has ballooned, with little to show for it. The US spends $4.5 trillion, nearly $13,500 per person per year, on health care (double that of other developed countries),[24] and yet our citizens live about 10 years less than our compatriots in other developed countries.[25] Seventy-nine million Americans, or over 40% of all working-age adults, struggle with paying medical bills,[26] and 20 million Americans (about 6%) owe a combined total of over $220 billion of medical debt (over $10,000 per person).[27] Because of our fragmented, nonintuitive system, we often spend billions on hospitalizations and procedures that could have been prevented with a fraction of the spending on affordable medicines or preventative care. The ballooning costs of health care have fueled a wave of populism, empowering politicians like Donald Trump and Bernie Sanders, who promise to upend the entire system (the former with nebulous "concepts of a plan"). Everyone, on both sides of the political aisle, recognizes that our health care system is broken and unsustainable, but people have vastly different opinions on how to fix it.

The root of our failures is that nobody can fix something they don't understand, and few care to understand the whole picture. Cancer care can be broken down into four major players (or stakeholders), each of whom depend on the others. First are patients. Whether they're hoping to live longer with cancer or seeking to prevent it, laypeople spend billions on medicines, over-the-counter products, and even books (like this one), while raising millions in donations for cancer research, and also "hiring" the payers (the government or insurance companies) to cover the cost of most of their care. These payers are the second player. Their goal is to turn a profit (or, in the case of the government, minimize a loss) by only paying for treatments deemed "worthwhile." That's where the third players—the doctors and research institutions—come in. All oncologists recommend cancer treatments, and some, at academic centers, run basic research to identify new treatments and clinical trials to prove these treatments actually work. They are the gatekeepers that payers rely upon to only recommend worthwhile treatment. Doctors can be motivated by money, but with salaries that have dramatically fallen behind inflation, I believe more and more people are going into medicine either to truly help patients, or for the "prestige" that comes with academia. Finally, the fourth player is the pharmaceutical industry, which takes the research from academic doctors and invests millions to develop drugs, prove that they work so that payers pay for them (by running large, multimillion-dollar clinical trials), market these drugs to consumers and doctors, and then reap a profit.

While everyone aspires to improve survival for cancer patients, many of these players have conflicting goals. Every dollar of pharmaceutical profit is a loss for patients or for an insurer or the government (that is, Medicare and Medicaid). Doctors, seeking the prestige of pioneering medicines, and patients, seeking to maximize their survival, usually find their interests aligned with the pharmaceutical companies developing new drugs—or so patients think, until they're forced to pay thousands of dollars out of pocket, and taxpayers find themselves footing most of the bill (since most people who have cancer are old enough to be covered by Medicare). Among each of the four major players, different subgroups also often find themselves at odds, like doctors prescribing expensive medicines to the chagrin of cost-cutting hospital administrators. The system relies on a delicate balance between the power of all the players involved, but recent shifts in this power have resulted in neglecting prevention, in higher costs, and in poorer outcomes for patients. Nowhere is this imbalance more evident than when we look at the payers.

SINGLE-PAYER HEALTH CARE

The US is the only developed nation with a fully private health care system (barring the VA), and mostly private health insurance sector. This means for-profit companies make up the bulk of payers for health care. Other nations have "single-payer" health care, where the government pays for, and provides, all health care (imagine VA hospitals, but for everyone). Proponents of single-payer point to cost savings from eliminating the middleman (for-profit health insurance companies) and streamlining health care for everyone, improving affordability and reducing disparities. Critics point to the inefficiencies and poor performance of government-provided services, as seen with the scandals that have rocked the VA.

The United Kingdom, Spain, and New Zealand deliver health care through the Beveridge model, named after the creator of the National Health Service in Britain. These countries have a fully socialized health care system, where taxpayer dollars allow the government to run hospitals and hire doctors, cutting out all private insurance and private hospitals. However, as countries like the United Kingdom have experienced austerity and cost-cutting in their health care systems, they've developed a two-tiered system, where the wealthy pay out of pocket for better care and the standard for everyone else drifts downward.[28] Other countries, like Canada and Australia, have chosen to split the difference with a National Health Insurance model, where the government provides health insurance for everyone, but hospitals and doctors remain private rather than owned or paid by the government.[29] This model is closest to the Medicare-for-all proposal in the US. However, this middle ground also means that Canadians and Australians are two to three times less likely to be able to afford their medicine compared to the British (Americans are eight times less likely!).[30] Also, Canadians often have to wait longer for certain procedures, although as American wait times have worsened, the two have become comparable.[31] Moreover, while a single payer has helped raise health care standards for the poor and underserved in Europe and Canada, it may also stoke the flames of racism and xenophobia, with many healthy, majority-group voters perceiving their resources as being siphoned toward caring for refugees and immigrants.[32] Lord knows, the US already has enough racism and xenophobia as things stand now.

The truth is, at least from my cynical perspective, private insurance isn't going anywhere, whether we like it or not. The insurance industry has grown into a trillion-dollar industry, with some of the largest expenditures among industries on lobbying our government. To eliminate private insurance, we'd have to "pry it from their cold, dead hands." Nonetheless, we can still learn many lessons from single-payer systems, even while maintaining the status quo.

Working in the VA, I am perpetually astonished by the ease with which I can provide my patients with medicines, tests, or services at home. I don't face the countless hurdles of insurance prior authorization, copays, or network restrictions. Medicines are either available for everyone, or not at all; everyone in the VA gets the same care. The facilities may not be the gleaming, glass towers that I'm used to practicing in, but the VA gets the same job done at a fraction of the price.

Unlike the VA, other hospitals aren't particularly invested in prevention. When you are admitted to a non-VA hospital, it receives a lump sum based on your condition. Hospitals do get financially penalized if you come back within 30 days, but beyond that, hospital administrators don't particularly care what happens to you after you leave. Private insurers may be *more* invested in keeping their customers healthy, but only up to a point. Unlike the VA system, they don't have the same incentive to reduce "lifetime" health expenditures by investing in preventive care early. As long as you don't get sick during the year you buy their insurance, they make a profit. Customers often switch insurers from one year to the next, and nearly everyone switches to Medicare at age 65, so insurers have no incentive to try to keep you healthy for the decades ahead. In fact, private insurers rely on the fact most Americans will get diagnosed with their expensive, chronic issues after age 65, leaving Medicare (i.e., taxpayers) to foot the bill. In recent years, many private insurers have made it their mission to maximize profits by creating barriers and denying as much care as they legally can. Doctors are left unable to prescribe the medicines their patients need, and patients unable to afford what their doctors prescribe. Patients in poor communities are hit hardest, with an increasing number of health systems around the country refusing Medicaid patients because of low reimbursements and bureaucratic obstacles to billing.[33] In fact, while the COVID-19 pandemic left most hospital systems in the red, health insurance companies have posted record profits,[34] stemming from decreased consumer utilization of preventive care and more barriers to treatments for patients and doctors.

Here is where legislation must come in. If we can't eliminate private insurance, we must at least ensure that it provides affordable, accessible, and prevention-oriented care for everyone. First, private insurers must be held accountable for denying life-saving care. The murder of United Healthcare CEO Brian Thomas brought to light the anger boiling over around the nation, with about one in five medicines recommended by doctors being denied by a private insurer.[35] Just as doctors can get sued for failing to provide life-saving care, tort (civil wrongdoing) reform should be introduced to hold private insurers accountable for their denials. Then there's the matter of skyrocketing costs. The Affordable Care Act (ACA, also known as Obamacare) has made strides toward increasing spending on prevention. The balancing act of eliminating surcharges for pre-existing conditions, while adding a penalty for not buying insurance, should have driven additional sick as well as healthy people into the insurance market. Unfortunately, the penalty clause was struck down by a Republican-controlled Congress, and the ACA ended up bringing in a lot of sick people without a balance of healthy people to counterweight the costs. With the rising costs of drugs, the COVID-19 and opioid epidemics, and many majority-Republican states refusing Medicaid expansion, the past years have spelled disaster for health care costs.

Today, even with the subsidies provided by the ACA marketplace, over half of Americans struggle to pay their health care bills.[36] Any additional regulations to cover more preventive care would probably only increase insurance costs in the short term (unless insurers grew willing to accept less than record-breaking profits), and thus have little buy-in from shortsighted politicians. Moreover, the ACA currently finds itself in jeopardy of being eliminated entirely by the Republican-controlled legislature and executive branch. Millions of patients with low-income or pre-existing conditions could find themselves losing access to insurance and preventative care, resulting in a costly spiral of preventable hospitalizations and expanding health care costs. Without insurance, these patients are usually unable to pay for their hospital stays, accruing debt that ruins their lives. Meanwhile, hospitals (most of which run at a loss) turn to the government to bail them out, so taxpayers actually end up paying more in the long run.

Long story short, innovative solutions are needed, and fast. Mandating spending on prevention has only gotten us so far. Perhaps private insurers could be required to take on a per-capita government contract to cover all the people in a given geographic area for a certain period, thus incentivizing preventative spending. In economics, as in personal relations, carrots are always more effective at getting things done than sticks. And while divvying up regions would stifle free-market competition, one could argue that no affordable, high-quality health insurance currently exists for most Americans, and thus the free market has already failed.

MONOPOLIZATION OF HEALTH CARE DELIVERY

Across the country, as in my hometown of Pittsburgh, insurers and health care systems are already merging to create "single-payer" entities. These "integrated delivery networks" (IDNs) have both an insurance and a health care delivery arm, which means the same company that sells your health insurance operates the hospital where you get seen. These IDNs function sort of like a government single-payer system, and are incentivized to keep costs down by investing in prevention.

While this structure has the potential to reduce costs, it also represents the increasing monopolization and corporatization of health care (and the American economy in general). These supercharged health care systems often register as nonprofit entities to avoid paying taxes, but pay their top executives salaries that rival Wall Street's, in the tens of millions.[37] They've also been the subjects of ongoing lawsuits surrounding limiting access to health care for patients with rival insurances that are not part of their system, thus making life-saving care inaccessible. And if that sounds dystopian, in addition, a flood of private equity money from Wall Street has bought private practices, ERs, and hospitals. Some 25% of all ERs in the country are now owned by investors (as opposed to doctors or hospitals). Owning large shares of the market allows these investors to drive salaries for health care workers down, drive prices for health care procedures up, and sacrifice high-quality care for efficiency, all in the name of record-setting profits.[38] While vertical integration (the merging of companies that produce different products within a sector) can promote efficiency, it also allows for monopolistic practices, which are being increasingly abused across health care, to the detriment of patients and doctors alike.

MEDICAL TRAINING AND PRACTICE

Technology and reform provide opportunities and challenges. We are just entering the era where artificial intelligence can help radiologists read scans faster, or help doctors type their notes and make medical decisions with ease. But technology has also separated patients from their doctors, with screen time replacing patient interaction. Another cost-cutting practice that's increased over the past several years is the replacement of doctors with advanced practice providers (APPs). This catchall term refers mostly to nurse practitioners and physician assistants who have been granted more autonomy, such as prescribing medicines, without requiring a doctor's direct supervision. From clinics to emergency rooms to hospital wards, APPs are being hired to ostensibly do the same jobs as doctors at a fraction of the cost to the system. Many APPs now even carry the title of doctor (such as a doctor of nursing), and often wear white coats, making them indistinguishable from medical doctors to lay people. In a funny twist, most inpatient doctors I've seen have since taken to wearing scrubs and Patagonia fleece jackets to distinguish themselves from the APPs, who are clad in full professional attire with the once-revered white coat.

Certain aspects of physicians' practice these days are very amenable to APPs, who typically do not have as many years of training, particularly in the foundations of biology underlying medicine (some egregious examples exist of online APP training with next to no real-world experience). For instance, one does not need many years of training to do primary care wellness checkups and counsel on prevention and lifestyle changes. APPs can also serve to alleviate much of the busy work behind the ever-bloating requirements of electronic medical records imposed on doctors by insurance companies (part of a maddening cat-and-mouse game in which insurers try to avoid paying for services due to insufficient documentation, and health systems respond by requiring a laundry list of inputs from doctors, after which the patient's medical record requires a Rosetta stone to decipher). For such purposes, APPs are a blessing.

The problem arises in scenarios where providers must identify unwell from well, and manage acutely and appropriately. For every 10 seemingly mind-numbing wellness checks in the clinic, I'm likely to encounter one serious medical problem that a patient may not have even suspected. An APP with fewer years of training, and a lack of understanding of underlying principles, may not pick up on those subtle signs of impending doom. Certain fields that are critically dependent on timely diagnosis, such as the ER, are particularly dangerous for independent practice by nondoctors. While APPs have been shown to have similar outcomes and even better patient satisfaction in the primary care clinic,[39] many studies have shown they are *more* likely to make life-threatening mistakes[40] and waste resources in the ER.[41]

The future of cost-conscious health care delivery will undoubtedly incorporate APPs in roles where they can encourage preventative care, conduct wellness exams, contribute to chart-bloat for billing's sake, and facilitate chronic disease management,[42] but consumers must be wary not to let a hospital's bottom line affect their health and safety. Patients should have no shame in demanding to see a medical doctor if unsatisfied or concerned about their care, particularly in acute settings like the ER or with complicated decisions, like in oncology. Only consumer pushback, and litigation for poor outcomes, will convince health systems to use APPs appropriately and judiciously. Despite what administrators may claim, there's no way to replace decades of medical training without jeopardizing patient safety.

These discussions of how to supplant doctors miss the root of the issue with medical training—the national shortage of doctors, which limits patient access and drives the cost of health care up. The American Association of Medical Colleges estimates that by 2036, the US will face a shortage of 86,000 physicians, particularly affecting primary care in rural areas.[43] A multitude of reasons explain why physicians are in short supply, from the nearly $300,000 average price tag of medical school, to years of grueling training in residency (a form of apprenticeship), during which hours may exceed 80 per week and "real" hourly pay approaches minimum wage in some localities.

The lifestyle of medical training is equally unforgiving. My mother had to attend her interview for residency the day after giving birth to me. She sat in a conference room in excruciating pain, profusely sweating and lactating, for a once-a-year opportunity to work as an underpaid apprentice in a field she had already studied for years. In fact, all doctors, in order to practice independently, must go through a taxing and nerve-racking match system where they rank their preferred institutions, and then get matched accordingly. Once matched to a hospital, they have no choice to train anywhere else. I've known colleagues who were sent far and wide by the "match," sometimes to their last choice. I've seen relationships torn up by the distance imposed by the match (I was thankful to match in Philadelphia, the same city where my then-girlfriend lived). Medical education and training are arduous and pose significant barriers to entry into medicine, particularly to people of poorer backgrounds who cannot afford the schooling (thus limiting diversity) and to family-oriented individuals. Students and residents are often forced to choose between their careers and their loved ones (not to mention delay having children by years, so much so that many residency programs now cover fertility preservation).

Yet hope for reform exists. Top medical schools, such as New York University and Johns Hopkins, have adopted programs that eliminate tuition for all, or nearly all, students. Residents (apprentice doctors) around the country, including at my program at Penn Medicine, have unionized to advocate for a living wage and acceptable work conditions. This trend promises the biggest improvement in residency conditions since the 80-hour workweek limit (!) was introduced in 2003, which some doctors still argue is too *few* hours to properly train a doctor.[44] To me, the rigor required by medical training further highlights the disparities in knowledge and experience between medical doctors and APPs, and serves as the chief argument for why physicians must be compensated sufficiently to attract the best minds to such an austere career. Without a doubt, medical education is by necessity taxing, but it must be reformed to ensure an adequate number and a diverse group of competent future doctors.

PHARMACEUTICAL PRICING

The final piece of the puzzle, the largest contributor to growing costs in health care, particularly in oncology, is the pharmaceutical industry. The global drug industry rakes in over $1.5 trillion dollars in profit annually. Pharma company profits are greater, and have grown faster, than those of companies in other sectors of the economy.[45] Over the past decades, the US government has dropped the ball and paid pharmaceutical companies however much they asked, leaving patients in the US with far greater medical expenditure (and debt) than people in any other developed country. At long last, the Biden administration's 2024 policy will allow Medicare to negotiate drug prices with pharmaceutical companies, saving taxpayers billions of dollars (but for now, the policy is limited to a handful of medicines, to assuage pharmaceutical lobbyists).[46] A similar program, called 340B, has allowed many safety-net hospitals around the country to buy medications at a discounted price.[47] If these initiatives could be expanded, patients would benefit, to the chagrin of pharma companies.

Further cost savings could come from cutting out the middlemen of the middlemen—pharmacy benefit managers (PBM), who negotiate between insurance companies and drug companies. Four of these PBM companies have consolidated 80% of the entire industry,[48] and have been raking in unheard-of profits while driving up costs. Thankfully, the Federal Trade Commission is actively engaged in lawsuits against PBMs for their monopolistic business practices, although dismantling the industry will be difficult. The disorganized, noncentralized combination of middlemen and pharmaceuticals is part of the reason why the US ends up spending far more on drugs than all other countries, where the single-payer government insurance entity negotiates with drug companies directly. We in the US pay the bulk of the pharmaceutical industry's profits, funding the medical research (along with a lot of advertisements) that the rest of the world benefits from but pays less for. Reducing spending may mean slower drug development, but bankrupting our health care system would mean no development at all.

The US is straining under the weight of its $36 trillion debt (the figure is likely to be much greater by the time you read this). Americans are sick and tired of spending more on health care than any other nation, with nothing to show for it. The path forward is controversial. But setting aside political and economic disagreements, we can start to make health care reforms around a few common-sense principles:

- Health care systems, pharma companies, and health policies should be spearheaded by doctors and public health professionals, not bureaucrats and Wall Street businesspeople.

- "Nonprofit" health care systems should not be allowed to pay their executives exorbitant salaries[49] and should be mandated to reinvest their revenue into serving their communities and lowering costs for consumers, rather than hoarding assets.

- Insatiable greed for profits among private insurers, pharmaceutical companies, and for-profit hospitals and health systems are monopolistic and unsustainable, and must be curtailed either by stronger regulation or by increasing free-market competition.

- More resources should be invested in prevention and patient education, especially for rural and urban underserved populations, as each dollar *more than* pays for itself in improved health outcomes.

There's an old Soviet joke about a plumber who ends up in the gulag. When the fellow inmates ask him how he got there, he explains, "They called me to take a look at a leak in the Kremlin. I told them, 'Comrades, you're gonna have to change the whole system here.'" Our health care system stinks. To prevent disease and suffering and provide high-quality health care while avoiding financial catastrophe, we must fundamentally rethink our entire health care system, if not our society and culture as a whole. I don't have the perfect answer, and anyone who claims they do is lying. We live in a patchwork system that has been crafted over centuries and built on the backs of poor minorities and immigrants, but has yielded most of the world's cutting-edge innovations. It will require many strings and countless tailors to find new weaves and hold those patches together against the increasing weight of our health care costs. Change is slow and painful, and even if we commit to reforming US health care, it will take us decades to unlearn our addiction to profit, sex discrimination, and racial/ethnic prejudices. Unfortunately, in prevention as in treatment, time is a precious commodity.

In summary:

- Cancer survival is highly disparate: Black women are 50% more likely to die of breast cancer than white women are, and Black men are twice as likely to die of prostate cancer than white men are.

- Limited access to health care and distrust of physicians are leading causes of survival disparities; public outreach programs, and a more diverse population of doctors, are essential.

- US health care is broken; we have the highest costs and yet the worst life expectancy of all developed nations.

- Single-payer health care to replace private insurances could save millions of dollars, but also runs the risk of government inefficiency.

- Private equity is forcing hospitals and doctors to maximize profits at the expense of patients; even nonprofit hospitals pay their executives millions, while paying nothing in taxes.

- Americans pay more for the same drugs than other countries; allowing Medicare to negotiate prices with pharmaceutical companies for a limited number of medications is a small step in the right direction.

CHAPTER 13

The Art of Living and Dying Well

Palliative and End-of-Life Care

Grief is just love with no place to go.
—JAMIE ANDERSON

What tormented Ivan Ilyich most was the deception,
the lie, which for some reason they all accepted,
that he was not dying but was simply ill, and that he
only need keep quiet and undergo a treatment and then
something very good would result.
—LEO TOLSTOY, *THE DEATH OF IVAN ILYICH*

Loss is as old as life itself. As long as there has been joy, there has been loss. We've spent hundreds of pages discussing the optimal lifestyle to reduce the risk of cancer and live longer. But we must also recognize that death is inevitable. The secret to happy living is not to live in fear of death, but to live with a healthy acceptance of it. Most importantly, we should each think about what we would want our final months or days to look like and communicate these preferences to our families. Making those decisions in advance, for yourself, empowers you to take control of your own passing and also relieves the burden of doubt or guilt that family members may feel if left to make such decisions on their own.

PALLIATIVE AND END-OF-LIFE CARE

I hear the damned question constantly: "Are they going to die?" I never know how to answer. Everyone's going to die, it's just a matter of how soon. Likewise, sure, "Everything happens for a reason," but the outcome may well have been predictable and preventable. The terminology we use around death deliberately obscures its proximity and causality. Doctors usually approach death with a stigma, a sheepishness borne of our own discomfort, doing our patients and their families a serious disservice. Instead, death ought to be discussed as plainly and concretely as any other medical topic. We should provide patients with specific statistics, even when they're demoralizing, if requested.

Patients should know the ways in which they're likely to die. Most often, people dying from cancer suffocate from fluid in their lungs or undergo a heart attack. Receiving chest compressions for a heart attack usually results in broken ribs and punctured lungs, with a slim chance of recovery. An unexpected death is rarely a peaceful once. Only with this knowledge can people make informed decisions. Even with patients and families who refuse to accept the direness of their situation, sometimes lashing out at the messenger, we must hold fast and suppress the urge to acquiesce with false reassurances. Death is unavoidable, and close for many. Patients have the right to believe they're invincible until the very end; doctors do not have this luxury. We must reconsider how we speak, and think, of death, in ways large and small.

I hear hesitancy, shock, and even odious resentment from cancer patients when I recommend that they speak to a palliative care specialist. I believe many patients, misled by antiquated misconceptions, confuse palliative care with hospice. This is simply not true. Not all palliative care is hospice.

Palliative care is specialized medical care designed to provide relief from the symptoms, pain, and emotional stress of a serious illness. Simple tweaks, like medicines for appetite loss or nausea, have been proven to improve the quality of life for both the patient and their family. Palliative care practitioners work alongside other members of a care team, so patients can receive active cancer treatment from their oncologist while having a separate doctor dedicated to making sure their other needs are met.

End-of-life care, or hospice, is a form of palliative care that focuses specifically on the care of patients for whom death is expected within six months. It aims to ensure that patients live their remaining days with dignity, as comfortably as possible, and according to their wishes. End-of-life care includes managing symptoms, providing emotional and spiritual support, and making decisions about life-sustaining treatments. This final decision about life-sustaining care can be particularly important but also traumatic for families if done poorly. When families are left to make decisions on their own, without any advance directives (without the patient having expressed their wishes in advance), they are more likely to feel guilt afterward about their decisions. One can achieve acceptance without resignation, and one can still appreciate life while bracing for death.

I remember that when my grandfather was diagnosed, my father took it upon himself to manage all aspects of his treatment plan. I imagine the control helped him feel that he was doing his very best to save his dad. But when my grandfather's condition suddenly deteriorated and he died shortly thereafter, my dad was left with years of guilt about the decisions he had made. The kindest thing any of us can do for our next of kin is provide them with a concrete plan on what we would and would not want done to us in the final days—most importantly: Would we want chest compressions if we died; would we want to be kept alive on a breathing tube (intubated), and for how long; and would we want to be treated in an intensive care unit? Saying yes to question 1 requires saying yes to questions 2 and 3. You cannot get chest compressions and be "brought back" from death if you are not then willing to be kept alive artificially on a breathing tube. Other questions involve placement of a permanent feeding tube, if your loved one is unable to swallow, or placement in a nursing facility if they're unable to care for themselves.

Ideally, these conversations should take place, and be regularly reevaluated, years before these events come to pass. In oncology, we often neglect these conversations because we fear our patients will interpret the focus on dying as "giving up" on keeping them alive. But nothing could be further from the truth. Our goal should be to maintain a patient's quality of life for as long as possible. This goal is particularly jeopardized in the final months, when patients sometimes undergo numerous painful and traumatizing interventions to be brought back from the brink of death, only to find themselves spiraling closer and closer with every hospitalization and having next to no quality life outside the hospital. Everyone wants to think they'll be among the very small percentage that will recover from each acute episode, and some of the life-sustaining marvels we've developed in recent years perpetuate this thinking. In American society, many people think fighting till the last breath and "raging against the dying of the light" signifies valor. In the intensive care unit, I hear platitudes like "She's a fighter" repeated until families convince themselves they can defy the odds. But too often, the numbers play out exactly as expected, and families are left in disbelief at an entirely predictable outcome. Even in the *best-case* scenarios, the quality of life that people have in the extra few months they eke out is far from how they wanted to live. I personally would not want to live unable to eat, get out of bed, or wipe my own behind. But that's me, and everyone's different.

Sometimes it's patients who refuse to accept their coming demise, but more often, it's family members. Doctors often make macabre jokes that the further removed a family member is from their dying loved one (for example, the niece who last saw her uncle five years ago), the more likely they are to insist on full restorative care. There's probably a kernel of truth in that. When you haven't actively been taking care of or been seeing a dying person every day, you remember them in their healthy state, and you think, "I'm not ready to let them go." But when faced with the reality of the state of their loved one, families often reconsider. When they see a lifeless body hooked up to countless tubes and IVs, with bloodshot eyes and pale, gangrenous fingers (which often happens, due to the medicines used to artificially maintain blood pressure), family members often realize the selfishness of keeping a loved one in this state. It's unfair to the health care system to waste millions of dollars, but moreover, it's unfair to your loved one to keep them in a half-alive state against their wishes.

Equally as important as having end-of-life conversations is designating a decision-maker, or legal power of attorney (POA). Per US law, when a patient is incapacitated, the hierarchy for making decisions is POA (if you designated one), spouse (if not divorced), adult child (or children), parent, sibling, known relatives, or finally, court-appointed decision-maker. I've seen patients languish on artificial life support for weeks as we attempt to track down relatives or muddle through legal red tape. Having no POA can be miserable, as can having too many. I once cared for a terminally ill man who had designated both his wife and mom as his POAs. Of course, we always hope for consensus among family, but in the rare cases one can't be struck, we defer to the POA. In this instance there were two equal POAs, with opposite opinions. As the man lay dying from his cancer, his wife and mother squabbled; the wife wanted to make him comfortable and bring him home to pass with his family around him; the mother, still in denial, wanted everything done. The arguments grew heated, accusations of cheating and abuse were flung, and finally the tension devolved into a fist fight at the foot of a dying man's bed. Ultimately, the patient passed in the hospital, uncomfortable and without family (as they'd been banned). He was far from the first, or the last, victim of familial disagreements I've seen, particularly when it comes to the end of life. "All happy families are alike; each unhappy family is unhappy in its own way," wrote Tolstoy. The same could be said about dying. All meaningful deaths I've seen have been alike in the support and sanity of family and decision-makers; each traumatic death is obscene in its own way.

"THE DECEPTION . . . THAT HE WAS NOT DYING BUT WAS SIMPLY ILL"[1]

Preventing suffering from cancer also means accepting death when it's time. I've seen far too many frail, lifeless bodies brutalized by futile resuscitations—ribs broken, blood spewing, families traumatized because nobody knew when to stop. There is an art to living, and an art to dying.

I once took care of an elderly Russian man whose brain and body had been ravaged by late-stage aggressive lymphoma. He'd progressed on everything from chemo to CAR-T therapy. I had seen him many times on and off over his month-long hospital stay. With his immune system destroyed by chemo, he suffered numerous infections and complications, finding himself in and out of the intensive care unit and on every broad-spectrum (meaning acting on a range of bacterial types) antibiotic available. His leg was as red and thick as a watermelon, with a ravaging infection, and he had numerous drains and tubes sticking out. At first, he was lucid, and I would have conversations with him and his wife in the late hours of the night while all my other patients slept. They reminded me of my grandparents, and they even hailed from a town near my hometown of Dnipro in Ukraine. But as the weeks went by, the cancer slowly consumed his mind. In the end, the gentleman could no longer eat, because everything swallowed would go down the wrong pipe and cause recurrent bouts of pneumonia. The nation's experts had no treatments left to offer. I was invited to translate during another goals-of-care discussion with the family.

As I entered the room, I saw a shadow of the man I once recognized. He was frail, and could barely sit up. But he was vocally upset that he was no longer allowed to drink. "Give me water," he shouted in Russian, as I tried to explain it was dangerous for him and we were trying to do what's best. Up to this point, his family had wanted to do *everything*, including restricting his drinking to avoid another life-threatening pneumonia. This was a story I'd seen play out time and again in inpatient cancer treatment. The care team had had many conversations with them about the futility of further treatment, and we didn't expect to change their minds this time around. But quite frankly, there was nothing else left to do. As the conversation dragged on, the patient got more and more confused and furious. At the mention of hospice, he shouted, "How much is it, you swindlers?" As I tried to calm him, he faced me and yelled, "Give me water, fucking Zhid!" He had called me an antisemitic name. How did he know I was Jewish? I didn't recall ever mentioning my religion. I knew that in Russian, "fucking Jew" was synonymous with "cheapskate," but that didn't make the slur feel any less jarring. Had he hated me for my religion all these months, or were these just the delusional outbursts of a dying man?

Of course, no one else in the room, save his wife and son, understood what he had said. One of them said, "Dad, that's not nice," a rather tepid rebuke. I kept my composure and continued to translate for the team (omitting that part, of course), but deep down I wasn't sure if I wanted to laugh or cry. It was comically absurd, to hear an old-world antisemitic slur in a new-fangled hospital in Philadelphia. Like the legacy of racism in medicine, history could not be outrun. But it was also tragic. These would be some of the last memories his family would have of their father and grandfather, as a delirious bigot in a dark hospital room.

Afterward, outside the room, the family came to apologize, saying, "He just wanted some water." I'm not sure what I would've said had it been my dad. It was this shared awkwardness that I believe finally convinced the family to let us make him comfortable, or as the patient had put it, "Let a dying man have his champagne." He was allowed to drink, the antibiotics were stopped, and he died the next day. I never saw the family again. But these were my final memories of this man, whom I once viewed as another of my grandfathers, calling me a "fucking Jew." Perhaps, had we read the writing on the wall weeks or days earlier, we could've spared this man and his family some indignity. In a twisted way, maybe he had been "swindled" after all.

On the flip side, I've seen many cases of successful hospice care. Of course, the patients died. That outcome was inescapable. But they died peacefully at home, or comfortable in the hospital, with their entire family by their side. I remember one family that hosted a grandchild's birthday party in the hospital room, stuffing it to the brim with loved ones. Others have even hosted weddings in the hospital (we once had two in a week!).

Doctors are notoriously bad at predicting the timing of death. We spend so much time learning how to prolong life that we learn little about how it is ultimately extinguished. Oftentimes, dying patients live for weeks after we withdraw all life-supporting care. But at least they're not being poked, prodded, wheeled for scans, or woken up early with a barrage of questions. Perhaps it's macabre or cynical, but people dying in hospice often appear a lot more comfortable than people dying while we are still trying to save them.

RELIGION AND DEATH

I've seen many patients and families at the end of life turn to religion, for comfort or for reassurance of an afterlife. Perhaps we seek a sense of cosmic justice—a reason for tragedy, or a sense that we'll be rewarded for our good deeds. I view this as a further example that at death, many people regret not having fulfilled their own needs in life. To prevent this, we must each live our lives to the fullest, so that if a fatal diagnosis strikes, we don't find ourselves mired in regrets.

I've caught myself holding hands with families and participating in Catholic last rites, and silently swaying along with a Muslim Salat. Of all these practices, ironically, I feel most out of place during Jewish rituals. They remind me of past beliefs I no longer hold. It's hard to believe in a God that allows so much death. Today, I'm far from religious, but I can appreciate the value religion brings to people. The origin of the name "Israel" in the Bible is "one who wrestles with God." Everyone, regardless of faith (or lack thereof), should seek ways to wrestle with God or circumstance, to question the way they have lived and evaluate what needs of theirs may be unfulfilled. Religion is one of many ways we care for our mental health, while a healthy lifestyle is how we care for our physical health. Both aspects of health are essential for preventing cancer, living with cancer, and ultimately, dying well of cancer.

The art of living well is the art of dying well. Optimizing our lives to live more healthfully and reduce our risk of cancer or early death should not mean repressing the fact that we *will* die. Instead, we ought to focus on and appreciate the parts of living that matter to us, while healthy and while sick. "Live each day as your last," is a trite platitude, and obviously there are countless things we do on a daily basis that we wouldn't do if we were imminently dying. As much as I love oncology, I wouldn't spend my last days treating patients, and yet I still go to work every morning. Nonetheless, trying to minimize any unnecessary burdens we carry can help us feel more fulfilled in life, and, I hope, more prepared for death. There are no good deaths, but there are peaceful ones.

> Life is real! Life is earnest!
> And the grave is not its goal;
> Dust thou art, to dust returnest,
> Was not spoken of the soul.
> . . .
> Let us, then, be up and doing,
> With a heart for any fate;
> Still achieving, still pursuing,
> Learn to labor and to wait.
>
> (Longfellow, "A Psalm of Life")

In summary:

- Palliative care and hospice are *not* the same: Palliative care focuses on relieving pain and increasing the quality of life, while hospice deals with end-of-life care.

- People who have cancer, and their families, should be aware of the likely outcome; talking to a palliative care practitioner early can help improve quality of life and help you better plan for the end of life.

- Patients and families who refuse to acknowledge their imminent demise prolong pain and suffering for the patient and lead to additional trauma and grief for the family.

Conclusion

'Tis a fearful thing to love what death can touch.
—Yehuda HaLevi, Sephardic physician and poet, 1075–1141

Decoding, and possibly curing, cancer is medicine's moon landing. Former president Joe Biden called his initiative to fund more cancer research a moonshot, because quite honestly, that's what it is. Cancer is thousands of complicated processes, far too numerous to understand, working in tandem on a scale far too small to see. We have learned to read our own instructions in DNA and engineer cells to identify and destroy cancers, but we've only begun to scratch the surface of the complexity at play. It will take many more years, and billions more dollars, to "cure" cancer, if that's even possible. But preventing it for thousands of people is very much in reach.

Many of my patients struggle with *why* they got cancer, and often, we'll never know for certain. Sometimes, "there is no why," and we truly are just "bugs trapped in amber." But sometimes there is a reason. And too often, in our health care system, we get so caught up thinking "What now?" that we don't stop to wonder or address the reason why. Doctors sometimes neglect to counsel our patients on healthy lifestyle choices, or advocate for public health initiatives, to address the many known preventable causes of cancer. "How?" is a flashy question; *How* do we engineer immune cells to attack cancer cells, *how* do we match precision medicines with driver mutations?

But in the long run, "Why?" will be the question that matters most. In the 1960s, everyone was obsessed with the *how* of landing a man on the moon, and few stopped to question *why*. But once we had solved the how, the lack of a reason came into sharper focus. We haven't attempted a manned moon landing again, because we recognize that it served little purpose beyond symbolism, and the cost was, quite literally, astronomical. I'm afraid we're repeating the same mistakes in the fight against cancer today, at the expense of affordable and accessible health care for future generations. Only *prevention* can rescue our unsustainable health care system and avert tremendous suffering and death.

Regarding prevention, we've reviewed dozens of modifiable (things people can change about their lives) risk factors, which together may account for nearly 50% of all cancer cases worldwide. The relative importance of these risk factors differs drastically across the world, with developing countries struggling more with infections and pollution, and less with obesity. For the US, below are ranked the cancer risk factors, reported with the estimated relative percentage of each risk factor, out of all approximately 700,000 preventable cancer cases diagnosed each year. Bear in mind, many risk factors overlap, so the total adds up to more than 100%.

Risk factor[1] (Percentage of all preventable cancer diagnoses): Common cancer types

- Smoking/chewing tobacco (48%): Lung, bladder, throat
- Obesity (19%): Breast, colorectal, stomach, esophageal
- Alcohol (14%): Liver, esophagus, breast, colorectal

- UV radiation (12%, counting only melanoma): Melanoma, other skin cancers
- Diet (low fiber and red, smoked, and processed meats) (11%): Colorectal, stomach
- Occupational exposures (10%): Lung, bladder
- Infections: HPV, HIV, hepatitis B, hepatitis C, Epstein-Barr virus, *H. pylori* (9%): Stomach, liver, blood (lymphoma), cervical, anal, throat
- Pollution (8%, but likely higher due to microplastics): Lung, bladder, kidney
- Physical inactivity (8%): Esophageal, stomach, colorectal, breast
- Radon (3%): Lung
- Secondhand smoke (1%): Lung, bladder

Extrapolating from this ranking, below I list proven lifestyle recommendations to minimize cancer risk (and decrease overall risk of death), in order of importance:

1. Stop smoking.
2. Maintain a healthy weight.
3. Minimize alcohol intake.
4. Apply sunscreen.
5. Eat a diet high in fiber, fruits, and vegetables and low in red, processed, and smoked meats and ultra-processed foods.
6. Wear protective equipment on the job, and advocate for yourself if you feel unsafe.
7. Get vaccinated against HPV.

8. Use protection when having sex, and get tested regularly.

9. Exercise 5 times a week (at least 150 minutes total per week).

10. Try to live in greener areas with less traffic (and if you can't, utilize home air filters).

11. Test your basement for high levels of radon.

Recommendations, for which we don't yet have strong data showing they prevent cancer, but which I believe are likely to appear in the next several years, include:

- Don't vape (edible marijuana does not carry cancer risk but may lead to long-term cognitive dysfunction).

- Don't microwave food in plastic containers, and avoid Teflon cookware and plastic utensils, cutting boards, and single-use water bottles.

- Minimize antibiotic use, and embrace a little dirt, especially for kids.

- Minimize life stress, and focus on mental health and wellness.

Of course, all these recommendations are intertwined with societal changes that must also take place to promote public health, including: improved public transportation; easier access to health care screenings and vaccines; the elimination of food deserts; the provision of free, healthy foods to schoolchildren and marginalized groups; combatting misinformation; regulating pollution more strongly; decreasing the availability of tobacco, vapes, and processed foods; improving access to substance rehabilitation centers and harm reduction measures; and overall, reducing life stressors.

These laundry lists of personal and societal changes are daunting. Our lives are the products of decades of bad habits as well as good ones, and society carries the inertia of centuries of exploitation and persecution. Things won't change in a day. But we can each aspire to make one small change, every day that we feel up for it. Before you know it, you'll be checking boxes off left and right. I've seen countless patients succeed in improving their lives, and it's never through shame, but through determination, optimism, and strong social support networks. I've also seen countless patients miss the mark, and it's almost never due to weakness or lack of willpower, but because of the social and psychological barriers stacked against them. There's no magic bullet. There's no herb to prevent cancer, and no one drug to cure it. It takes work, and grit, and love, and self-respect, and a healthy fear of death. Death is guaranteed, but the length and quality of life that precedes it is in our control as individuals and as a society.

A FEARFUL THING TO LOVE
WHAT DEATH CAN TOUCH

When my grandfather rapidly succumbed to his cancer, my parents scrambled to make funeral arrangements. I was only 13 years old at the time, and I had never before seen my father so unnerved. He was the kind of person to plan everything months ahead, accounting for every contingency. Losing his dad so suddenly was the one thing he hadn't planned for.

My grandfather, born in a Jewish village and raised speaking Yiddish, was the last religious member of our family. My dad wanted him to have a Jewish funeral, but we didn't know any rabbis, let alone one who spoke Russian (more than 90% of the people at the funeral were my grandfather's elderly Ukrainian diaspora friends, none of whom spoke English). Having just studied for my bar mitzvah, I was "voluntold" to deliver some prayers in Hebrew and Russian.

To the best of my ability, I recited the Mourner's Kaddish, a millennia-old prayer praising God for peace in this world and the next. During the prayer, the speaker recites the blessings, and the congregation responds with "Amen" (Hebrew for "We agree"). Unfortunately, none of the attendants knew what to say, or when, but I somehow stifled tears and fumbled through the prayer. I followed the prayer with a Jewish poem I had found that read, "It's a fearful thing to love what death can touch." Since then, I've had too many occasions to recite the Kaddish and this poem, both with other loved ones I've lost and with Jewish patients of mine who passed in the hospital. Every time, I'm taken back to the time of my grandfather's funeral.

Looking back, this was the moment in which I had come full circle. When I was born, my grandfather had accompanied me to my mikvah, a ritual bath to "convert" to Judaism (since Judaism is matrilineal and my mother was Ukrainian orthodox). Now here I was 13 years later, on the heels of my bar mitzvah, burying my grandfather with a Jewish prayer.

My grandfather had grown up on the run from the Nazis, his parents murdered, and his village razed to the ground. Even after the war, he was a victim of the antisemitic Soviet state, where he was persecuted for his name and his looks (I've always been told I inherited his big, Jewish nose). He never learned Hebrew and never connected with Judaism, until decades later, when he immigrated and found himself with ample time and religious freedom. When I was born, he insisted that his grandson get to be a part of his faith in a way that he never could. I imagine he would have been proud to hear me recite a prayer for him. Like the rest of our friends and family, he would not have known a word of it, but he would have poignantly understood its meaning.

Judaism describes its teachings as "a tree of life to those who hold fast to it" and its prognosis as "those who study it are fulfilled and happy." On the one hand, studying Judaism and following its rituals has helped me connect to generations of ancestors, many of whom I never got to meet, or even know about, because of the bloody culmination of millennia of persecution. But in a broader interpretation, I've learned to draw fulfillment from the study of one of the other trees of life: medicine.

The Jewish scholars of the past sought answers to the questions of our existence and our suffering. They did not have the tools and knowledge we do now, but they found other paths, like prayer and ritual, to imbue the lives of their communities with meaning. Today, we are faced with different existential questions, and are armed with far more complex tools, but the pursuit of knowledge remains the same. One of the monumental questions of our time, and the one I've dedicated much of my life to, is "What causes cancer, and how do we prevent it?"

I wonder what my grandparents would have said, some 40 years ago, if I could go back in time to tell them the air they were breathing, the water they were drinking, was irradiating them, laying the seeds of cancer deep within their cells. Would they have moved? Did they have the ability to do so? Would they have believed me? Then I think about all the people today, many with the means to change their toxic way of life, many more without the means, and countless people entirely ignorant of the looming fallout. Processed diets. Seas of plastic. Vaccine denial. Will future generations think of us with disbelief and astonishment? Will my grandchildren bury me not as a close family member but as a distant memory, a victim of a backward time?

* * *

The story of cancer encompasses history, religion, science, and humanity. It is the story of disturbed, nefarious cells, who can feed off their neighbors and spread like wildfire, much like the hateful ideologies that exploited and murdered my great-grandparents. Cancer is also the story of ongoing social inequities, of the exploitation of workers and consumers by large corporations, and the failure of governments to protect their constituents. It can arise from greed, lust, wrath, pride, gluttony, and sloth. It can also arise randomly, or as a curse hidden deep within a family's genes. At its core, cancer is the tree of life gone awry. On this tree hang billions of lives, begging to be saved.

Today, we are just beginning to unravel the molecular and social underpinnings of humanity's most complex, and often most deadly, killer. Just as I fumbled through the Mourner's Kaddish, we must fumble and learn everything we can about cancer, and be brave enough to translate our learning into personal and societal action. Only then can we prevent innumerable needless deaths, and learn to find fulfillment in life. Only then can we honor the memories of the countless loved ones we've lost.

Those many years ago, as funeral attendants lowered my grandfather's casket into the earth, I said my final goodbyes and sprinkled a fistful of soil from Israel onto the coffin. The body in that coffin was scarred on a cellular level by decades of radiation, hardship, and persecution. But externally, it just looked like my grandfather. My larger-than-life, but now lifeless, grandfather.

For a year until that date came around again, the headstone remained covered, in keeping with Jewish tradition. When it was finally unveiled, my grandmother and all their friends would come to leave pebbles on the gravestone, as the ancient Israelites had done in the desert. Soon, many pebbles were stacked there, each a reminder of the many lives my grandfather had touched. The pebbles awaited my grandmother when she joined him in the earth some five years later. Her life was beautiful, cultured, yet mired in grief, denied a lifetime of opportunity and a peaceful retirement with her husband.

Flowers wilt, people wither, and memories fade, but the pebbles remain. They stand firm against time and live on in the meaning they harbor. They both ask and answer "Why?"

> "He who creates peace in the heavens,
> may he create peace for us and all people;
> and we shall say, Amen."
>
> (Mourner's Kaddish)

Acknowledgments

The essence of all beautiful art is gratitude.
—Friedrich Nietzsche

I express my deepest gratitude to my inspiring parents, encouraging sister, and amazing wife for their unwavering love and support. I hope to dedicate books to them in the years to come.

Special thanks to my agent Nick Mullendore for taking a chance on my first book and to my editor Suzanne Silva and her team, Jennifer D'Urso and Debby Bors, for their patience and diligence.

Lastly, I'd like to acknowledge all my stellar mentors, colleagues, and teachers at the University of Pennsylvania Hospital, in particular Lin Mei, Charu Aggarwal, Melina Marmarelis, and Corey Langer. I feel honored to have worked with such brilliant minds and kind hearts.

Notes

Introduction

1. "Percivall Pott (1714–1788)." Embryo Project Encyclopedia. May 31, 2017. https://embryo.asu.edu/pages/percivall-pott-1714-1788.

2. Islami, F., E. C. Marlow, B. Thomson, M. L. McCullough, H. Rumgay, S. M. Gapstur, et al. "Proportion and number of cancer cases and deaths attributable to potentially modifiable risk factors in the United States, 2019." *CA: A Cancer Journal for Clinicians* 74, no. 5 (July 11, 2024): 405–32. https://doi.org/10.3322/caac.21858.

3. Ades, F., K. Tryfonidis, and D. Zardavas. "The past and future of breast cancer treatment—from the papyrus to individualised treatment approaches." *Ecancermedicalscience* 11 (June 8, 2017). https://doi.org/10.3332/ecancer.2017.746.

Chapter 1. Why Us? Cancer Risk and Prevention

1. Ades, F., K. Tryfonidis, and D. Zardavas. "The past and future of breast cancer treatment—from the papyrus to individualised treatment approaches." *Ecancermedicalscience* 11 (June 8, 2017). https://doi.org/10.3332/ecancer.2017.746.

2. Dagenais, G. R., D. P. Leong, S. Rangarajan, F. Lanas, P. Lopiz-Jaramillo, R. Gupta, et al. "Variations in common diseases, hospital admissions, and deaths in middle-aged adults in 21 countries from five continents (PURE): a prospective cohort study." *Lancet* 395, no. 10226 (2020): 785–94. https://doi.org/10.1016/S0140-6736(19)32007-0.

3. Vonnegut, K. *Slaughterhouse-Five.* Delacorte. 1969. 77.

4. American Cancer Society. "Lifetime risk of developing or dying from cancer." n.d. https://www.cancer.org/cancer/risk-prevention/understanding-cancer-risk/lifetime-probability-of-developing-or-dying-from-cancer.html.

5. UC Health. "Never-smokers: why are they being diagnosed more frequently with lung cancer?" n.d. https://www.uchealth.com/en/media-room/articles/never-smokers-why-are-they-being-diagnosed-more-frequently-with-lung-cancer.

6. Ma, Y., Y. Yang, F. Wang, P. Zhang, C. Shi, Y. Zou, et al. "Obesity and risk of colorectal cancer: a systematic review of prospective studies." *PLoS ONE* 8, no. 1 (January 17, 2013): e53916. https://doi.org/10.1371/journal.pone.0053916.

7. Ma, Y., Y. Yang, F. Wang, P. Zhang, C. Shi, Y. Zou, et al. "Obesity and risk of colorectal cancer: a systematic review of prospective studies." *PLoS ONE* 8, no. 1 (January 17, 2013): e53916. https://doi.org/10.1371/journal.pone.0053916.

8. Dubin, S., and D. Griffin. "Lung cancer in non-smokers." *Missouri Medicine* 117, no. 4 (July–August, 2020): 375–79. https://www.ncbi.nlm.nih.gov/pmc/articles/PMC7431055/.

9. World Health Organization. "Vaccines and immunization." October 29, 2019. https://www.who.int/topics/immunization/en/.

10. Worldometer. "Life expectancy by country and in the world (2024)." n.d. https://www.worldometers.info/demographics/life-expectancy/.

11. Hollowell, A. "Just 4 in 10 Americans trust physicians, hospitals, study says." n.d. https://www.beckershospitalreview.com/public-health/just-4-in-10-americans-trust-physicians-hospitals-study-says.html.

12. Centers for Medicare and Medicaid Services. December 18, 2024. "Historical." https://www.cms.gov/data-research/statistics-trends-and-reports/national-health-expenditure-data/historical.

Chapter 2. What Goes Around: Viruses, Bacteria, and Other Microbes

1. Watts, G. "Nobel prize is awarded to doctors who discovered *H pylori*." *BMJ* 331, no. 7520 (October 6, 2005): 795. https://doi.org/10.1136/bmj.331.7520.795.

2. Weintraub, P. "The doctor who drank infectious broth, gave himself an ulcer, and solved a medical mystery." *Discover Magazine*. April 17, 2023. https://www.discovermagazine.com/health/the-doctor-who-drank-infectious-broth-gave-himself-an-ulcer-and-solved-a-medical-mystery.

3. Watts, G. "Nobel prize is awarded to doctors who discovered *H pylori*." *BMJ* 331, no. 7520 (October 6, 2005): 795. https://doi.org/10.1136/bmj.331.7520.795.

4. Salih, B. A. "*Helicobacter pylori* infection in developing countries: the burden for how long?" *Saudi Journal of Gastroenterology* 15, no. 3 (January 1, 2009): 201. https://doi.org/10.4103/1319-3767.54743.

5. Arnold, C. "The viruses that made us human." *NOVA*. September 28, 2016. https://www.pbs.org/wgbh/nova/article/endogenous-retroviruses/.

6. Briggs, H. "Neanderthals 'self-medicated' for pain." BBC News. March 8, 2017. https://www.bbc.com/news/science-environment-39205530.

7. Cara, E. "These germs are a major cancer risk, new report highlights." Gizmodo. September 20, 2024. https://gizmodo.com/these-germs-are-a-major-cancer-risk-new-report-highlights-2000501401.

8. Zdilla, M. J., A. M. Aldawood, A. Plata, J. A. Vos, and H. W. Lambert. "Troisier sign and Virchow node: the anatomy and pathology of pulmonary adenocarcinoma metastasis to a supraclavicular lymph node." *Autopsy and Case Reports* 9, no. 1 (January 1, 2019). https://doi.org/10.4322/acr.2018.053.

9. Rawla, P., and A. Barsouk. "Epidemiology of gastric cancer: global trends, risk factors and prevention." *Gastroenterology Review* 14, no. 1 (January 1, 2019): 26–38. https://doi.org/10.5114/pg.2018.80001.

10. Balakrishnan, M., R. George, A. Sharma, and D. Y. Graham. "Changing trends in stomach cancer throughout the world." *Current Gastroenterology Reports* 19, no. 8 (July 20, 2017). https://doi.org/10.1007/s11894-017-0575-8.

11. Mukaisho, K.-I., T. Nakayama, T. Hagiwara, T. Hattori, and H. Sugihara. "Two distinct etiologies of gastric cardia adenocarcinoma: interactions among pH, *Helicobacter pylori*, and bile acids." *Frontiers in Microbiology* 6 (May 11, 2015). https://doi.org/10.3389/fmicb.2015.00412.

12. Arnold, M., S. P. Moore, S. Hassler, L. Ellison-Loschmann, D. Forman, and F. Bray. "The burden of stomach cancer in indigenous populations: a systematic review and global assessment." *Gut* 63, no. 1 (October 23, 2013): 64–71. https://doi.org/10.1136/gutjnl-2013-305033.

13. Boysen, T., M. Mohammadi, M. Melbye, S. Hamilton-Dutoit, B. Vainer, A. V. Hansen, et al. "EBV-associated gastric carcinoma in high- and low-incidence areas for nasopharyngeal carcinoma." *British Journal of Cancer* 101, no. 3 (July 14, 2009): 530–33. https://doi.org/10.1038/sj.bjc.6605168.

14. Rawla, P., and A. Barsouk. "Epidemiology of gastric cancer: global trends, risk factors and prevention." *Gastroenterology Review* 14, no. 1 (January 1, 2019): 26–38. https://doi.org/10.5114/pg.2018.80001.

15. Ahmed, N. "23 years of the discovery of *Helicobacter pylori*: is the debate over?" *Annals of Clinical Microbiology and Antimicrobials* 4, no. 1 (October 31, 2005). https://doi.org/10.1186/1476-0711-4-17.

16. Seeras, K., R. N. Qasawa, and S. Prakash. "Truncal Vagotomy." StatPearls. December 11, 2022. https://www.ncbi.nlm.nih.gov/books/NBK526104/.

17. World Health Organization. "Schistosomiasis." February 1, 2023. https://www.who.int/news-room/fact-sheets/detail/schistosomiasis.

18. Inobaya, M., R. Olveda, T. Chau, D. Olveda, and A. Ross. "Prevention and control of schistosomiasis: a current perspective." *Research and Reports in Tropical Medicine* 5 (October 1, 2014): 65–75. https://doi.org/10.2147/rrtm.s44274.

19. Inobaya, M., R. Olveda, T. Chau, D. Olveda, and A. Ross. "Prevention and control of schistosomiasis: a current perspective." *Research and*

Reports in Tropical Medicine 5 (October 1, 2014): 65–75. https://doi.org/10
.2147/rrtm.s44274.

20. World Health Organization. "Schistosomiasis." February 1, 2023.
https://www.who.int/news-room/fact-sheets/detail/schistosomiasis.

21. Saginala, K., A. Barsouk, J. S. Aluru, P. Rawla, S. A. Padala, and
A. Barsouk. "Epidemiology of bladder cancer." *Medical Sciences* 8, no. 1
(March 13, 2020): 15. https://doi.org/10.3390/medsci8010015.

22. Inobaya, M., R. Olveda, T. Chau, D. Olveda, and A. Ross. "Prevention and control of schistosomiasis: a current perspective." *Research and
Reports in Tropical Medicine* 5 (October 1, 2014): 65–75. https://doi.org/10
.2147/rrtm.s44274.

23. Elgharably, A., A. I. Gomaa, M. M. E. Crossey, P. J. Norsworthy, I.
Waked, and S. D. Taylor-Robinson. "Hepatitis C in Egypt—past, present,
and future." *International Journal of General Medicine* 10 (December 1,
2016): 1–6. https://doi.org/10.2147/ijgm.s119301.

24. Elgharably, A., A. I. Gomaa, M. M. E. Crossey, P. J. Norsworthy, I.
Waked, and S. D. Taylor-Robinson. "Hepatitis C in Egypt—past, present,
and future." *International Journal of General Medicine* 10 (December 1,
2016): 1–6. https://doi.org/10.2147/ijgm.s119301.

25. Elgharably, A., A. I. Gomaa, M. M. E. Crossey, P. J. Norsworthy, I.
Waked, and S. D. Taylor-Robinson. "Hepatitis C in Egypt—past, present,
and future." *International Journal of General Medicine* 10 (December 1,
2016): 1–6. https://doi.org/10.2147/ijgm.s119301.

26. Elgharably, A., A. I. Gomaa, M. M. E. Crossey, P. J. Norsworthy, I.
Waked, and S. D. Taylor-Robinson. "Hepatitis C in Egypt—past, present,
and future." *International Journal of General Medicine* 10 (December 1,
2016): 1–6. https://doi.org/10.2147/ijgm.s119301.

27. Elgharably, A., A. I. Gomaa, M. M. E. Crossey, P. J. Norsworthy, I.
Waked, and S. D. Taylor-Robinson. "Hepatitis C in Egypt—past, present,
and future." *International Journal of General Medicine* 10 (December 1,
2016): 1–6. https://doi.org/10.2147/ijgm.s119301.

28. Fattovich, G., T. Stroffolini, I. Zagni, and F. Donato. Hepatocellular
carcinoma in cirrhosis: incidence and risk factors. *Gastroenterology* 127 (5),
S35–S50. https://doi.org/10.1053/j.gastro.2004.09.014.

29. Fattovich, G., T. Stroffolini, I. Zagni, and F. Donato. Hepatocellular
carcinoma in cirrhosis: incidence and risk factors. *Gastroenterology* 127 (5),
S35–S50. https://doi.org/10.1053/j.gastro.2004.09.014.

30. Smith, B. D., R. L. Morgan, G. A. Beckett, Y. Falck-Ytter, D. Holtzman,
C.-G. Teo, et al. "Recommendations for the identification of chronic

Hepatitis C Virus infection among persons born during 1945–1965." *Morbidity and Mortality Weekly Report* 61 (August 17, 2012): 1–18. https://www.cdc.gov/mmwr/preview/mmwrhtml/rr6104a1.htm.

31. CDC. September 21, 2022. "Too few people treated for hepatitis C." https://www.cdc.gov/vitalsigns/hepc-treatment/index.html.

32. CDC. "Clinical screening and diagnosis for Hepatitis C." December 19, 2023. https://www.cdc.gov/hepatitis-c/hcp/diagnosis-testing/index.html#:~:text=CDC%20recommends%20universal%20hepatitis%20C,C%20complications%20and%20interrupt%20transmission.

33. U.S. Department of Health and Human Services. "Viral hepatitis in the United States: data and trends." June 7, 2016. https://www.hhs.gov/hepatitis/learn-about-viral-hepatitis/data-and-trends/index.html.

34. Florko, N. "Prisons say they can't afford to cure everyone with hepatitis C. But some are figuring out a way." *STAT.* July 25, 2023. https://www.statnews.com/2022/12/15/prisons-cant-afford-hep-c-drugs-but-some-figured-out-a-way/.

35. CDC. "Fast facts: global Hepatitis B vaccination." July 30, 2024. https://www.cdc.gov/global-hepatitis-b-vaccination/data-research/?CDC_AAref_Val=https://www.cdc.gov/globalhealth/immunization/diseases/hepatitis-b/data/fast-facts.html.

36. National Cancer Institute. April 30, 2025. Liver (hepatocellular) cancer screening (PDQ®)–health professional version. NIH. https://www.cancer.gov/types/liver/hp/liver-screening-pdq.

37. Weng, M. K., M. Doshani, M. A. Khan, S. Frey, K. Ault, K. L. Moore, et al. "Universal Hepatitis B vaccination in adults aged 19–59 years: updated recommendations of the Advisory Committee on Immunization Practices—United States, 2022." *Morbidity and Mortality Weekly Report* 71, no. 13 (March 31, 2022): 477–83. https://doi.org/10.15585/mmwr.mm7113a1.

38. Larson, H. J., E. Gakidou, and C. J. L. Murray. "The vaccine-hesitant moment." *New England Journal of Medicine* 387, no. 1 (June 29, 2022): 58–65. https://doi.org/10.1056/nejmra2106441.

39. Cleveland Clinic. "Blood transfusion." Accessed May 1, 2024. https://my.clevelandclinic.org/health/treatments/14755-blood-transfusion.

40. Kimanya, M. E., M. N. Routledge, E. Mpolya, C. N. Ezekiel, C. P. Shirima, and Y. Y. Gong. "Estimating the risk of aflatoxin-induced liver cancer in Tanzania based on biomarker data." *PLoS ONE* 16, no. 3 (March 11, 2021): e0247281. https://doi.org/10.1371/journal.pone.0247281.

41. Warnatzsch, E. A., D. S. Reay, M. Camardo Leggieri, and P. Battilani. "Climate change impact on aflatoxin contamination risk in Malawi's maize

crops." *Frontiers in Sustainable Food Systems* 4 (November 25, 2020). https://doi.org/10.3389/fsufs.2020.591792.

42. Food Insight. "Aflatoxins in the U.S. food supply." n.d. https://foodinsight.org/all-about-aflatoxins/.

43. LaMotte, S. "Dirty Dozen 2022: produce with the most and least pesticides." CNN. April 7, 2022. https://www.cnn.com/2022/04/07/health/dirty-dozen-produce-2022-wellness/index.html.

44. Tsao, S. W., C. M. Tsang, and K. W. Lo. "Epstein–Barr virus infection and nasopharyngeal carcinoma." *Philosophical Transactions of the Royal Society B Biological Sciences* 372, no. 1732 (September 11, 2017): 20160270. https://doi.org/10.1098/rstb.2016.0270/.

45. Cao, S. M., M. J. Simons, and C. N. Qian. "The prevalence and prevention of nasopharyngeal carcinoma in China." *Chinese Journal of Cancer* 30, no. 2 (February 5, 2011): 114–19. https://doi.org/10.5732/cjc.010.10377.

46. Healthdirect Australia. "HTLV-1 infection." n.d. https://www.healthdirect.gov.au/htlv-1-infection.

47. Penn Wharton University of Pennsylvania. "Mortality in the United States: past, present, and future." December 13, 2023. https://budgetmodel.wharton.upenn.edu/issues/2016/1/25/mortality-in-the-united-states-past-present-and-future.

48. Tulchinsky, T. H. "John Snow, cholera, the Broad Street pump; waterborne diseases then and now." *Case Studies in Public Health* (March 30, 2018): 77–99. https://doi.org/10.1016/b978-0-12-804571-8.00017-2.

49. CDC. "History of Smallpox". October 23, 2024. https://www.cdc.gov/smallpox/history/history.html.

50. CDC. "History of Smallpox". October 23, 2024. https://www.cdc.gov/smallpox/history/history.html.

51. Bleakley, H. "Disease and development: evidence from hookworm eradication in the American South." *Quarterly Journal of Economics* 122, no. 1 (February 1, 2007): 73–117. https://doi.org/10.1162/qjec.121.1.73.

Chapter 3. You Are What You Eat: Foods and Toxins

1. Kelly, D. B. "The untold truth of ketchup." Mashed. March 15, 2017. https://www.mashed.com/49274/untold-truth-ketchup/.

2. Balakrishnan, M., R. George, A. Sharma, and D. Y. Graham. "Changing trends in stomach cancer throughout the world." *Current Gastroenterology Reports* 19, no. 8 (July 20, 2017). https://doi.org/10.1007/s11894-017-0575-8.

3. Zhang, Y., Y. Zhang, J. Jia, H. Peng, Q. Qian, Z. Pan, et al. "Nitrite and nitrate in meat processing: functions and alternatives." *Current Research in*

Food Science 6 (January 1, 2023): 100470. https://doi.org/10.1016/j.crfs.2023 .100470.

4. Barsouk, A., K. C. Thandra, K. Saginala, P. Rawla, and A. Barsouk. "Chemical risk factors of primary liver cancer: an update." *Hepatic Medicine Evidence and Research* 12 (January 1, 2021): 179–88. https://doi.org/10 .2147/hmer.s278070.

5. *Guardian* staff. "Charcuterie's link to colon cancer confirmed by French authorities." *Guardian*. July 13, 2022. https://www.theguardian.com/world /2022/jul/12/charcuterie-link-colon-cancer-confirmed-french-authorities.

6. Balakrishnan, M., R. George, A. Sharma, and D. Y. Graham. "Changing trends in stomach cancer throughout the world." *Current Gastroenterology Reports* 19, no. 8 (July 20, 2017). https://doi.org/10.1007/s11894-017-0575-8.

7. Patil, P. S., A. Saklani, P. Gambhire, S. Mehta, R. Engineer, A. De'Souza, et al. "Colorectal cancer in India: an audit from a tertiary center in a low prevalence area." *Indian Journal of Surgical Oncology* 8, no. 4 (April 22, 2017): 484–90. https://doi.org/10.1007/s13193-017-0655-0.

8. Orlich, M. J., P. N. Singh, J. Sabaté, K. Jaceldo-Siegl, J. Fan, S. Knutsen, et al. Vegetarian dietary patterns and mortality in Adventist Health Study 2. *JAMA Internal Medicine* 173, no. 13 (2013): 1230–38. https://doi.org/10 .1001/jamainternmed.2013.6473.

9. Howarth, T. "This diet can reverse your biological age in 8 weeks, claims bold new study." *BBC Science Focus Magazine*. July 28, 2024. https://www.sciencefocus.com/news/going-vegan-for-eight-weeks -reduces-your-biological-age.

10. Landry, M. J., C. P. Ward, K. M. Cunanan, L. R. Durand, D. Perelman, J. J. Robinson, et al. Cardiometabolic effects of omnivorous vs vegan diets in identical twins: a randomized clinical trial. *JAMA Network Open* 6, no. 11 (2023): e2344457. https://doi.org/10.1001/jamanetworkopen.2023.44457.

11. Bir, C., and F. B. Norwood. "1 in 10 Americans say they don't eat meat—a growing share of the population." The Conversation. March 1, 2022. https://theconversation.com/1-in-10-americans-say-they-dont-eat -meat-a-growing-share-of-the-population-176948.

12. Sekiguchi, M., I. Oda, T. Matsuda, and Y. Saito. "Epidemiological trends and future perspectives of gastric cancer in Eastern Asia." *Digestion* 103, no. 1 (September 7, 2021): 22–28. https://doi.org/10.1159/000518483.

13. Ren, J.-S., F. Kamangar, D. Forman, and F. Islami. "Pickled food and risk of gastric cancer—a systematic review and meta-analysis of English and Chinese literature." *Cancer Epidemiology Biomarkers & Prevention* 21, no. 6 (June 1, 2012): 905–15. https://doi.org/10.1158/1055-9965.epi-12-0202.

14. Tsugane, S., S. Sasazuki, M. Kobayashi, and S. Sasaki. "Salt and salted food intake and subsequent risk of gastric cancer among middle-aged Japanese men and women." *British Journal of Cancer* 90, no. 1 (January 1, 2004): 128–34. https://doi.org/10.1038/sj.bjc.6601511.

15. Ertuglu, L. A., F. Elijovich, C. L. Laffer, and A. Kirabo. Salt-sensitivity of blood pressure and insulin resistance. *Frontiers in Physiology* 12 (December 13, 2021): 793924. https://doi.org/10.3389/fphys.2021.793924.

16. Tovosia, S., P.-H. Chen, A. M.-J. Ko, H.-P. Tu, P.-C. Tsai, and Y.-C. Ko. "Prevalence and associated factors of betel quid use in the Solomon Islands: a hyperendemic area for oral and pharyngeal cancer." *American Journal of Tropical Medicine and Hygiene* 77, no. 3 (September 1, 2007): 586–90. https://pubmed.ncbi.nlm.nih.gov/17827384/.

17. Barsouk, A., J. S. Aluru, P. Rawla, K. Saginala, and A. Barsouk. "Epidemiology, risk factors, and prevention of head and neck squamous cell carcinoma." *Medical Sciences* 11, no. 2 (June 13, 2023): 42. https://doi.org/10.3390/medsci11020042.

18. Reichart, P. A., T. Dietrich, P. Khongkhunthian, and S. Srisuwan. "Decline of oropharyngeal cancer in Chiangmai province, Thailand, between 1988 and 1999." *Oral Oncology* 39, no. 6 (June 2, 2003): 569–73. https://doi.org/10.1016/s1368-8375(03)00039-3.

19. Little, M. A., P. Pokhrel, K. L. Murphy, C. T. Kawamoto, G. S. Suguitan, and T. A. Herzog. "Intention to quit betel quid: a comparison of betel quid chewers and cigarette smokers." *Oral Health and Dental Management* 13, no. 2 (June 1, 2014): 512–18. https://pubmed.ncbi.nlm.nih.gov/24984674/.

20. Tseng, M.-F., S. C.-S. Tsai, C.-Y. Wu, C.-C. Lin, and R.-H. Wong. "The effectiveness of betel quid cessation among workers through the adoption of the five action areas of the Ottawa Charter." *Substance Use & Misuse* 56, no. 5 (March 15, 2021): 718–27. https://doi.org/10.1080/10826084.2021.1892141.

21. UK Tea & Infusions Association. "The History of Tea." n.d. https://www.tea.co.uk/history-of-tea#:~:text=The%20story%20of%20tea%20begins,his%20servant%20had%20accidentally%20created.

22. Fernandez, R. "Discover the surprising origins of coffee: a history of coffee." Good Cuppa Coffee. June 26, 2023. https://goodcuppacoffee.com/blogs/best-coffee-blog-for-coffee-lovers/a-history-of-coffee.

23. Luo, H., and H. Ge. "Hot tea consumption and esophageal cancer risk: a meta-analysis of observational studies." *Frontiers in Nutrition* 9 (April 10, 2022): 831567. https://doi.org/10.3389/fnut.2022.831567.

24. UN News. "UN health agency group finds coffee poses no cancer risk; issues warning on 'very hot' drinks." June 15, 2016. https://news.un.org/en/story/2016/06/532202-un-health-agency-group-finds-coffee-poses-no-cancer-risk-issues-warning-very#:~:text=Studies%20in%20places%20such%20as,which%20the%20beverage%20was%20drunk.

25. Mayne, S. T., H. A. Risch, R. Dubrow, W.-H. Chow, M. D. Gammon, T. L. Vaughan, et al. "Carbonated soft drink consumption and risk of esophageal adenocarcinoma." *Journal of the National Cancer Institute* 98, no. 1 (January 4, 2006): 72–75. https://doi.org/10.1093/jnci/djj007.

26. Chokshi, N. "That wasn't Mark Twain: how a misquotation is born." April 26, 2017. https://www.nytimes.com/2017/04/26/books/famous-misquotations.html.

27. Osto, M., M. Farshchian, A. Alnabolsi, S. A. Smidi, M. Baiyasi, and G. A. Potts. "Aluminum-containing antiperspirants are not associated with breast cancer." *Journal of Cosmetic Dermatology* 21, no. 10 (2022): 5244–45. https://doi.org/10.1111/jocd.14796.

28. Wang, C., K. Ding, X. Xie, J. Zhou, P. Liu, S. Wang, et al. "Soy product consumption and the risk of cancer: a systematic review and meta-analysis of observational studies." *Nutrients* 16, no. 7 (March 28, 2024): 986. https://doi.org/10.3390/nu16070986.

29. Xie, J., K. L. Terry, E. M. Poole, K. M. Wilson, B. A. Rosner, W. C. Willett, et al. "Acrylamide hemoglobin adduct levels and ovarian cancer risk: a nested case-control study." *Cancer Epidemiology Biomarkers & Prevention* 22, no. 4 (February 16, 2013): 653–60. https://doi.org/10.1158/1055-9965.epi-12-1387.

30. Wang, L., M. Du, K. Wang, N. Khandpur, S. L. Rossato, J. Drouin-Chartier, et al. "Association of ultra-processed food consumption with colorectal cancer risk among men and women: results from three prospective US cohort studies." *BMJ* 378 (2022): e068921. https://doi.org/10.1136/bmj-2021-068921.

31. Griel, A. E., E. H. Ruder, and P. M. Kris-Etherton. "The changing roles of dietary carbohydrates: from simple to complex." *Arteriosclerosis, Thrombosis, and Vascular Biology* 26, no. 9 (2006): 1958–65. https://doi.org/10.1161/01.ATV.0000233384.97125.bd.

32. Hofmann, S. M., and M. H. Tschöp. "Dietary sugars: a fat difference." *Journal of Clinical Investigation* 119, no. 5 (2009): 1089–92. https://doi.org/10.1172/jci39332.

Chapter 4. The Gift of Living Well: Diet, Exercise, and Obesity

1. Wideman, C. H., G. R. Nadzam, and H. M. Murphy. "Implications of an animal model of sugar addiction, withdrawal and relapse for human health." *Nutritional Neuroscience* 8, no. 5–6 (October 1, 2005): 269–76. https://doi.org/10.1080/10284150500485221.

2. World Health Organization. "Obesity and overweight." March 1, 2024. https://www.who.int/news-room/fact-sheets/detail/obesity-and -overweight.

3. Anto, L., and C. N. Blesso. "Interplay between diet, the gut microbiome, and atherosclerosis: role of dysbiosis and microbial metabolites on inflammation and disordered lipid metabolism." *Journal of Nutritional Biochemistry* 105 (2022): 108991. https://doi.org/10.1016/j.jnutbio.2022.108991.

4. Mauri, G., A. Sartore-Bianchi, A.-G. Russo, S. Marsoni, A. Bardelli, and S. Siena. "Early-onset colorectal cancer in young individuals." *Molecular Oncology* 13, no. 2 (December 6, 2018): 109–31. https://doi.org/10.1002/1878 -0261.12417.

5. Zhao, J., L. Xu, J. Sun, M. Song, L. Wang, S. Yuan, et al. "Global trends in incidence, death, burden and risk factors of early-onset cancer from 1990 to 2019." *BMJ Oncology* 2, no. 1 (July 1, 2023): e000049. https://doi .org/10.1136/bmjonc-2023-000049.

6. Cavallo, J. "Generation X and millennials have higher risk for many cancers compared to older generations." *The ASCO Post*. August 1, 2024. https://ascopost.com/news/august-2024/generation-x-and-millennials -have-higher-risk-for-many-cancers-compared-to-older-generations/?utm _source=TAP%2DEN%2D081324&utm_medium=email&utm_term =ccb13fc4c345d78cbc9f07b968c66a3f.

7. ScienceDaily. "What made humans 'the fat primate'?" June 19, 2019. https://www.sciencedaily.com/releases/2019/06/190626160337.htm #:~:text=While%20other%20primates%20have%20less,related%20 monkey%20species%2C%20rhesus%20macaques.

8. Iyengar, N. M., A. Gucalp, A. J. Dannenberg, and C. A. Hudis. Obesity and cancer mechanisms: tumor microenvironment and inflammation. *Journal of Clinical Oncology* 34, no. 35 (December 2016): 4270–76. https:// doi.org/10.1200/jco.2016.67.4283.

9. National Institutes of Health. "How brown fat improves metabolism." September 17, 2019. https://www.nih.gov/news-events/nih-research -matters/how-brown-fat-improves-metabolism.

10. Zhang, X., N. Ma, Q. Lin, K. Chen, F. Zheng, J. Wu, et al. "Body Roundness Index and all-cause mortality among US adults." *JAMA Net-*

work Open 7, no. 6 (June 5, 2024): e2415051. https://doi.org/10.1001/jamanetworkopen.2024.15051.

11. Bendix, A. "People who got colon cancer in their 20s or 30s describe what it was like and the signs that were ignored." December 18, 2023. NBC News. https://www.nbcnews.com/health/cancer/colon-cancer-young-people-describe-signs-ignored-rcna129838#.

12. Abraham Lincoln Online. "The Gettysburg address." n.d. https://www.abrahamlincolnonline.org/lincoln/speeches/gettysburg.htm.

13. Lynn, A. "Why 97% of oncology clinical trials fail to receive FDA approval." Technology Networks. November 27, 2019. https://www.technologynetworks.com/drug-discovery/articles/why-97-of-oncology-clinical-trials-fail-to-receive-fda-approval-327724#:~:text=However%2C%20FDA%20approval%20currently%20has,Siah%20and%20Lo%2C%202019.

14. Clark, J. E. "Diet, exercise or diet with exercise: comparing the effectiveness of treatment options for weight-loss and changes in fitness for adults (18–65 years old) who are overfat, or obese; systematic review and meta-analysis." *Journal of Diabetes & Metabolic Disorders* 14, no. 1 (April 16, 2015). https://doi.org/10.1186/s40200-015-0154-1.

15. Belluz, J., and C. Haubursin. "The science is in: exercise won't help you lose much weight." *Vox.* January 2, 2019. https://www.vox.com/2018/1/3/16845438/exercise-weight-loss-myth-burn-calories.

16. National Institutes of Health. "Calorie restriction in humans builds strong muscle and stimulates healthy aging genes." October 13, 2023. https://www.nih.gov/news-events/news-releases/calorie-restriction-humans-builds-strong-muscle-stimulates-healthy-aging-genes.

17. Centers for Disease Control and Prevention. "Adult activity: an overview." December 20, 2023. https://www.cdc.gov/physical-activity-basics/guidelines/adults.html.

18. Institute of Medicine. "Lessons from the Blue Zones®: workshop summary." National Academies Press. 2015. https://www.ncbi.nlm.nih.gov/books/NBK298903/.

19. Shmerling, R. H. "When dieting doesn't work." Harvard Health. May 26, 2020. https://www.health.harvard.edu/blog/when-dieting-doesnt-work-2020052519889.

20. World Health Organization. "Shortages impacting access to glucagon-like peptide 1 receptor agonist products; increasing the potential for falsified versions." January 29, 2024. https://www.who.int/news/item/29-01-2024-shortages-impacting-access-to-glucagon-like-peptide-1-receptor-agonist-products--increasing-the-potential-for-falsified-versions.

21. Mayo Clinic. "GLP-1 agonists: diabetes drugs and weight loss." June 29, 2022. https://www.mayoclinic.org/diseases-conditions/type-2-dia betes/expert-answers/byetta/faq-20057955#:~:text=Weight%20loss%20 can%20vary%20depending,or%20kg)%20when%20using%20liraglutide.

22. Wang, L., R. Xu, D. C. Kaelber, and N. A. Berger. "Glucagon-like peptide 1 receptor agonists and 13 obesity-associated cancers in patients with type 2 diabetes." *JAMA Network Open* 7, no. 7 (2024): e2421305. https:// doiorg/10.1001/jamanetworkopen.2024.21305.

23. Bezin, J., A. Gouverneur, M. Pénichon, C. Mathieu, R. Garrel, D. Hillaire-Buys, et al. "GLP-1 receptor agonists and the risk of thyroid cancer." *Diabetes Care* 46, no. 2 (2023): 384–90. https://doi.org/10.2337/dc22 -1148.

24. Newman, J. "Forget cutting sugar—new tech makes it healthier instead." *Wall Street Journal.* July 31, 2024. https://www.wsj.com/science /biology/healthier-sugar-fiber-enzyme-harvard-scientists-a8bb2dce?mod =e2fb&fbclid=IwZXh0bgNhZW0BMAABHdlHI _tEdgJPnI0fysXoigkKfXlWjiWFPVDri_m0Ft5v886lA3WxlCGCUQ_aem _cfa1QGXDo1AhtnbYyZVM-Q&utm_campaign=23862284081830105&utm _content=120211699040190106&utm_id=23862284081830105&utm _medium=paid&utm_source=fb&utm_term=120211663749960106.

25. Lamotte, S. "Common low calorie sweetener linked to heart attack and stroke." CNN. https://www.cnn.com/2024/06/06/health/xylitol-heart -attack-stroke-wellness/index.html#:~:text=A%20low%2Dcalorie%20 sweetener%20called,sweetener%2C%20a%20new%20study%20found.

26. Cohut, M. "How exercise tells the brain to curb appetite." *Medical News Today*. April 29, 2018. https://www.medicalnewstoday.com/articles /321660#:~:text=Studies%20have%20now%20shown%20that,drive%20 our%20state%20of%20hunger.

27. Goodreads. "Lewis Carroll." n.d. https://www.goodreads.com /quotes/57223-now-here-you-see-it-takes-all-the-running-you.

28. Barsouk, A. "Animals reveal their secrets to cheating death." *Forbes.* November 25, 2018. https://www.forbes.com/sites/adambarsouk/2018/11 /25/animals-reveal-their-secrets-to-cheating-death/.

29. Szczepanski, K. "The invention of gunpowder: a history." ThoughtCo. July 3, 2019. https://www.thoughtco.com/invention-of-gunpowder-195160.

30. Kenyon, C. "Aging in *C. elegans*." In C. elegans *II*, 2nd ed., ed. D. L. Riddle, T. Blumenthal, B. J. Meyer, and J. R. Priess (Cold Spring Harbor Press, 1997). https://www.ncbi.nlm.nih.gov/books/NBK20213/.

31. Lord, S. R., and A. L. Harris. "Is it still worth pursuing the repurposing of metformin as a cancer therapeutic?" *British Journal of Cancer* 128, no. 6 (February 23, 2023): 958–66. https://doi.org/10.1038/s41416-023 -02204-2.

32. The Nutrition Source. "Antioxidants." Accessed May 9, 2024. Harvard T. H. Chan School of Public Health. https://nutritionsource.hsph .harvard.edu/antioxidants/.

33. Szabo, E., J. T. Mao, S. Lam, M. E. Reid, and R. L. Keith. "Chemoprevention of lung cancer: Diagnosis and management of lung cancer, 3rd ed: American College of Chest Physicians evidence-based clinical practice guidelines." *Chest* 143, no. 5 (Suppl): e40S–e60S. https://doi.org/10.1378 /chest.12-2348.

34. BBC Science Focus Magazine. "Will you die if you eat a polar bear's liver?" n.d. https://www.sciencefocus.com/the-human-body/will-you-die -if-you-eat-a-polar-bears-liver.

35. Szabo, E., J. T. Mao, S. Lam, M. E. Reid, and R. L. Keith. "Chemoprevention of lung cancer: Diagnosis and management of lung cancer, 3rd ed: American College of Chest Physicians evidence-based clinical practice guidelines." *Chest* 143, no. 5 (Suppl): e40S–e60S. https://doi.org/10.1378 /chest.12-2348.

36. Sui, J., J. Guo, D. Pan, Y. Wang, G. Sun, and H. Xia. "The efficacy of dietary intake, supplementation, and blood concentrations of carotenoids in cancer prevention: insights from an umbrella meta-analysis." *Foods* 13, no. 9 (2024): 1321. https://doi.org/10.3390/foods13091321.

37. Cui, A., P. Xiao, Y. Ma, Z. Fan, F. Zhou, J. Zheng, et al. "Prevalence, trend, and predictor analyses of vitamin D deficiency in the US population, 2001–2018." *Frontiers in Nutrition* 9 (October 3, 2022). https://doi.org /10.3389/fnut.2022.965376.

38. National Institutes of Health. "Vitamin D: fact sheet for health professionals." Office of Dietary Supplements. July 26, 2024. https://ods.od .nih.gov/factsheets/VitaminD-HealthProfessional/.

39. National Institutes of Health. "Vitamin D: fact sheet for health professionals." Office of Dietary Supplements. July 26, 2024. https://ods.od .nih.gov/factsheets/VitaminB12-HealthProfessional/.

40. Starr, P. "Oral nicotinamide prevents common skin cancers in high-risk patients, reduces costs." Special issue. *American Health & Drug Benefits* 8, (2015): 13–14. https://pmc.ncbi.nlm.nih.gov/articles /PMC4570055/.

41. Mayo Clinic. "St. John's wort." August 10, 2023. https://www.mayoclinic.org/drugs-supplements-st-johns-wort/art-20362212.

42. Hopkins Tanne, J. "US consumer group names 'dirty dozen' dietary supplements." *BMJ* 328, no. 7446 (April 22, 2004): 975. https://doi.org/10.1136/bmj.328.7446.975-c.

43. Knoops, K. T. B., L. C. P. G. M. De Groot, D. Kromhout, A.-E. Perrin, O. Moreiras-Varela, A. Menotti, et al. "Mediterranean diet, lifestyle factors, and 10-year mortality in elderly European men and women." *JAMA* 292, no. 12 (September 21, 2004): 1433. https://doi.org/10.1001/jama.292.12.1433.

44. Griswold, M. G., N. Fullman, C. Hawley, N. Arian, S. R. M. Zimsen, H. D. Tymeson, et al. "Alcohol use and burden for 195 countries and territories, 1990–2016: a systematic analysis for the Global Burden of Disease Study 2016." *Lancet* 392, no. 10152 (2018): 1015–35. https://doi.org/10.1016/S0140-6736(18)31310-2.

45. Lowe, D. "The Sirtris compounds: worthless? Really?" January 12, 2010. *Science*. https://www.science.org/content/blog-post/sirtris-compounds-worthless-really.

46. Damgaard, M. V., and J. T. Treebak. "What is really known about the effects of nicotinamide riboside supplementation in humans." *Science Advances* 9, no. 29 (July 21, 2023). https://doi.org/10.1126/sciadv.adi4862.

Chapter 5. On and Off the Clock: Occupational Exposures, Pollution, and Plastic

1. Brain, J. "Chimney sweeps and climbing boys." April 7, 2021. https://www.historic-uk.com/CultureUK/History-Boy-Chimney-Sweep/.

2. Brain, J. "Chimney sweeps and climbing boys." April 7, 2021. https://www.historic-uk.com/CultureUK/History-Boy-Chimney-Sweep/.

3. Brain, J. "Chimney sweeps and climbing boys." April 7, 2021. https://www.historic-uk.com/CultureUK/History-Boy-Chimney-Sweep/.

4. GBD 2016 Occupational Carcinogens Collaborators. "Global and regional burden of cancer in 2016 arising from occupational exposure to selected carcinogens: a systematic analysis for the Global Burden of Disease Study 2016." *Occupational and Environmental Medicine* 77, no. 3 (February 13, 2020): 151–59. https://doi.org/10.1136/oemed-2019-106012.

5. Alberg, A. J., M. V. Brock, J. G. Ford, J. M. Samet, and S. D. Spivack. "Epidemiology of Lung Cancer." *CHEST* 143, no. 5 (May 1, 2013): e1S–e29S. https://doi.org/10.1378/chest.12-2345.

6. U.S. Consumer Product Safety Commission. "Asbestos in the home." https://www.cpsc.gov/safety-education/safety-guides/home/asbestos-home.

7. Attanoos, R. L., A. Churg, F. Galateau-Salle, A. R. Gibbs, and V. L. Roggli. "Malignant mesothelioma and its non-asbestos causes." *Archives of Pathology & Laboratory Medicine* 142, no. 6 (February 26, 2018): 753–60. https://doi.org/10.5858/arpa.2017-0365-ra.

8. US Environmental Protection Agency. "Ambler asbestos piles." https://cumulis.epa.gov/supercpad/cursites/csitinfo.cfm?id=0300445.

9. American Cancer Society. "Talcum powder and cancer." n.d. https://www.cancer.org/cancer/risk-prevention/chemicals/talcum-powder-and-cancer.html.

10. Poinen-Rughooputh, S., M. S. Rughooputh, Y. Guo, Y. Rong, and W. Chen. "Occupational exposure to silica dust and risk of lung cancer: an updated meta-analysis of epidemiological studies." *BMC Public Health* 16, no. 1 (November 4, 2016). https://doi.org/10.1186/s12889-016-3791-5.

11. Steenland, K., and L. Stayner. "Silica, asbestos, man-made mineral fibers, and cancer." *Cancer Causes & Control* 8, no. 3 (January 1, 1997): 491–503. https://doi.org/10.1023/a:1018469607938.

12. Consonni, D., S. De Matteis, A. C. Pesatori, P. A. Bertazzi, A. C. Olsson, H. Kromhout, et al. "Lung cancer risk among bricklayers in a pooled analysis of case–control studies." *International Journal of Cancer* 136, no. 2 (May 27, 2014): 360–71. https://doi.org/10.1002/ijc.28986.

13. Steenland, K., and W. Sanderson. "Lung cancer among industrial sand workers exposed to crystalline silica." *American Journal of Epidemiology* 153, no. 7 (2001): 695–703. https://doi.org/10.1093/aje/153.7.695.

14. Li, N., Z. Zhai, Y. Zheng, S. Lin, Y. Deng, G. Xiang, J. Yao, et al. "Association of 13 occupational carcinogens in patients with cancer, individually and collectively, 1990–2017." *JAMA Network Open* 4, no. 2 (February 18, 2021): e2037530. https://doi.org/10.1001/jamanetworkopen.2020.37530.

15. 't Mannetje, A., V. Bencko, P. Brennan, D. Zaridze, N. Szeszenia-Dabrowska, P. Rudnai, et al. "Occupational exposure to metal compounds and lung cancer. Results from a multi-center case–control study in Central/Eastern Europe and UK." *Cancer Causes & Control* 22, no. 12 (September 29, 2011): 1669–80. https://doi.org/10.1007/s10552-011-9843-3.

16. Behrens, T., C. Ge, R. Vermeulen, B. Kendzia, A. Olsson, J. Schüz, et al. "Occupational exposure to nickel and hexavalent chromium and the risk of lung cancer in a pooled analysis of case-control studies (SYNERGY)." *International Journal of Cancer* 152, no. 4 (September 2, 2022): 645–60. https://doi.org/10.1002/ijc.34272.

17. Dryson, E., A. 't Mannetje, C. Walls, D. McLean, F. McKenzie, M. Maule, et al. "Case-control study of high risk occupations for bladder

cancer in New Zealand." *International Journal of Cancer* 122, no. 6 (November 20, 2007): 1340–46. https://doi.org/10.1002/ijc.23194.

18. Takkouche, B., C. Regueira-Mendez, and A. Montes-Martinez. "Risk of cancer among hairdressers and related workers: a meta-analysis." *International Journal of Epidemiology* 38, no. 6 (September 14, 2009): 1512–31. https://doi.org/10.1093/ije/dyp283.

19. Veterans of Foreign Wars. "Nearly 40 percent of vets report toxic exposure." April 25, 2023. https://www.vfw.org/media-and-events/latest -releases/archives/2023/4/nearly-40-percent-of-vets-report-toxic -exposure.

20. US Department of Veterans Affairs. *The PACT Act and your VA benefits*. n.d. https://www.va.gov/resources/the-pact-act-and-your-va -benefits/.

21. Chang, G.-C., C.-H. Chiu, C.-J. Yu, Y.-C. Chang, Y.-H. Chang, K.-H. Hsu, et al. "Low-dose CT screening among never-smokers with or without a family history of lung cancer in Taiwan: a prospective cohort study." *Lancet Respiratory Medicine* 12, no. 2, 141–52. https://doi.org/10.1016/S2213 -2600(23)00338-7.

22. International Atomic Energy Agency. "Radiological conditions in the Dnieper River basin." 2006. https://www-pub.iaea.org/MTCD /Publications/PDF/Pub1230_web.pdf.

23. Clarence Borel, plaintiff-appellee, v. Fibreboard Paper Products Corporation et al., defendants-appellants, National Surety Corporation, intervenor-appellee, 493 F.2d 1076 (5th Cir. 1973). https://law.justia.com /cases/federal/appellate-courts/F2/493/1076/4552/.

24. Clarence Borel, plaintiff-appellee, v. Fibreboard Paper Products Corporation et al., defendants-appellants, National Surety Corporation, intervenor-appellee, 493 F.2d 1076 (5th Cir. 1973). https://law.justia.com /cases/federal/appellate-courts/F2/493/1076/4552/.

25. Mesothelioma Hope. "Mesothelioma and asbestos trust funds." June 3, 2025. https://www.mesotheliomahope.com/legal/asbestos-trust -funds/#:~:text=Bankrupt%20asbestos%20companies%20established%20 asbestos,court%20or%20filing%20a%20lawsuit.

26. Zhang, L., I. Rana, R. M. Shaffer, E. Taioli, and L. Sheppard. "Exposure to glyphosate-based herbicides and risk for non-Hodgkin lymphoma: a meta-analysis and supporting evidence." *Mutation Research/Reviews in Mutation Research* 781 (February 11, 2019): 186–206. https://doi.org/10.1016 /j.mrrev.2019.02.001.

27. Johnson v. Monsanto Co. 16-cv-01244-MMC. (California Ct App. July 20, 2020). https://law.justia.com/cases/california/court-of-appeal/2020/a155940.html.

28. Raymond, N., and J. Stempel. "Judge slashes Bayer $1.56 billion Roundup verdict to $611 million." April 5, 2024. https://www.reuters.com/legal/judge-slashes-bayer-156-billion-roundup-verdict-611-million-2024-04-05/

29. Rich, N. "The lawyer who became DuPont's worst nightmare." January 6, 2016. https://www.nytimes.com/2016/01/10/magazine/the-lawyer-who-became-duponts-worst-nightmare.html.

30. Wee, S. Y., and A. Z. Aris. Revisiting the "forever chemicals", PFOA and PFOS exposure in drinking water. *npj Clean Water 6*, 57 (2023). https://doi.org/10.1038/s41545-023-00274-6.

31. Rich, N. "The lawyer who became DuPont's worst nightmare." January 6, 2016. https://www.nytimes.com/2016/01/10/magazine/the-lawyer-who-became-duponts-worst-nightmare.html.

32. Rich, N. "The lawyer who became DuPont's worst nightmare." January 6, 2016. https://www.nytimes.com/2016/01/10/magazine/the-lawyer-who-became-duponts-worst-nightmare.html.

33. Rich, N. "The lawyer who became DuPont's worst nightmare." January 6, 2016. https://www.nytimes.com/2016/01/10/magazine/the-lawyer-who-became-duponts-worst-nightmare.html.

34. Steenland, K., J. N. Hofmann, D. T. Silverman, and S. M. Bartell. "Risk assessment for PFOA and kidney cancer based on a pooled analysis of two studies." *Environment International* 167 (July 22, 2022): 107425. https://doi.org/10.1016/j.envint.2022.107425.

35. Steenland, K., T. Fletcher, C. R. Stein, S. M. Bartell, L. Darrow, M.-J. Lopez-Espinosa, et al. "Review: evolution of evidence on PFOA and health following the assessments of the C8 Science Panel." *Environment International* 145 (September 18, 2020): 106125. https://doi.org/10.1016/j.envint.2020.106125.

36. Rich, N. "The lawyer who became DuPont's worst nightmare." January 6, 2016. https://www.nytimes.com/2016/01/10/magazine/the-lawyer-who-became-duponts-worst-nightmare.html

37. Agency for Toxic Substances and Disease Registry. "Fast facts: PFAS in the U.S. population." November 12, 2024. CDC. https://www.atsdr.cdc.gov/pfas/data-research/facts-stats/index.html#:~:text=Nearly%20all%20people%20in%20the,with%20reduced%20production%20and%20use.

38. Lerner, S. "PFAS chemical associated with severe COVID-19." December 7, 2020. https://theintercept.com/2020/12/07/pfas-pfba-severe-covid-study/.

39. Tarapore, P., and B. Ouyang. "Perfluoroalkyl chemicals and male reproductive health: Do PFOA and PFOS increase risk for male infertility?" *International Journal of Environmental Research and Public Health 18*, no. 7 (April 5, 2021): 3794. https://doi.org/10.3390/ijerph18073794.

40. Rich, N. "The lawyer who became DuPont's worst nightmare." January 6, 2016. https://www.nytimes.com/2016/01/10/magazine/the-lawyer-who-became-duponts-worst-nightmare.html.

41. Hawke, E. "New Hollywood film 'Dark Waters' highlights the shocking reality of PFAS pollution." February 4, 2020. https://chemtrust.org/dark-waters-film-pfas/.

42. Beck, E. C. "The Love Canal tragedy." *EPA Journal* (January 1979). https://www.epa.gov/archive/epa/aboutepa/love-canal-tragedy.html.

43. Beck, E. C. "The Love Canal tragedy." *EPA Journal* (January 1979). https://www.epa.gov/archive/epa/aboutepa/love-canal-tragedy.html.

44. Beck, E. C. "The Love Canal tragedy." *EPA Journal* (January 1979). https://www.epa.gov/archive/epa/aboutepa/love-canal-tragedy.html.

45. Beck, E. C. "The Love Canal tragedy." *EPA Journal* (January 1979). https://www.epa.gov/archive/epa/aboutepa/love-canal-tragedy.html.

46. Beck, E. C. "The Love Canal tragedy." *EPA Journal* (January 1979). https://www.epa.gov/archive/epa/aboutepa/love-canal-tragedy.html.

47. Beck, E. C. "The Love Canal tragedy." *EPA Journal* (January 1979). https://www.epa.gov/archive/epa/aboutepa/love-canal-tragedy.html.

48. Environmental Protection Agency. "Superfund Site: Love Canal." n.d. https://cumulis.epa.gov/supercpad/SiteProfiles/index.cfm?fuseaction=second.cleanup&id=0201290.

49. Beck, E. C. "The Love Canal tragedy." *EPA Journal* (January 1979). https://www.epa.gov/archive/epa/aboutepa/love-canal-tragedy.html.

50. Environmental Protection Agency. "Superfund history." November 25, 2024. https://www.epa.gov/superfund/superfund-history.

51. Environmental Protection Agency. "East Palestine, Ohio Train Derailment." October 17, 2024. https://www.epa.gov/east-palestine-oh-train-derailment.

52. Isidore, C. "Deliberate toxic burn following Norfolk Southern derailment was not necessary, safety regulator testifies." March 6, 2024. CNN. https://www.cnn.com/2024/03/06/business/norfolk-southern-derailment-controlled-burn-unecessary-ntsb.

53. Kielhorn, J., C. Melber, U. Wahnschaffe, A. Aitio, and I. Mangelsdorf. "Vinyl chloride: still a cause for concern." *Environmental Health Perspectives* 108, no. 7 (July 1, 2000): 579–88. https://doi.org/10.1289/ehp.00108579.

54. Isidore, C. "Deliberate toxic burn following Norfolk Southern derailment was not necessary, safety regulator testifies." March 6, 2024. CNN. https://www.cnn.com/2024/03/06/business/norfolk-southern -derailment-controlled-burn-unecessary-ntsb.

55. Isidore, C. "Deliberate toxic burn following Norfolk Southern derailment was not necessary, safety regulator testifies." March 6, 2024. CNN. https://www.cnn.com/2024/03/06/business/norfolk-southern -derailment-controlled-burn-unecessary-ntsb.

56. Kroll Settlement Administration. "East Palestine." June 13, 2025. https://eastpalestinetrainsettlement.com.

57. Weisbrod, K. "Their lives were ruined by oil pollution, and a court awarded them $9.5 billion. But Ecuadorians have yet to see a penny from Chevron." *Inside Climate News*. December 18, 2022. https://insideclimate news.org/news/18122022/steven-donziger-chevron-ecuador-oil-pollution/.

58. Arif, I., M. D. Adams, and M. T. J. Johnson. "A meta-analysis of the carcinogenic effects of particulate matter and polycyclic aromatic hydro- carbons." *Environmental Pollution* 351, no. 15 (April 1, 2024): 123941. https://doi.org/10.1016/j.envpol.2024.123941.

59. Li, W., and W. Wang. "Causal effects of exposure to ambient air pollution on cancer risk: insights from genetic evidence." *Science of the Total Environment* 912 (February 1, 2024): 168843. https://doi.org/10.1016/j .scitotenv.2023.168843.

60. Brown, J. A., J. L. Ish, C.-J. Chang, D. B. Bookwalter, K. M. O'Brien, R. R. Jones, et al. "Outdoor air pollution exposure and uterine cancer incidence in the sister study." *Journal of the National Cancer Institute* 116, no.6 (February 12, 2024): 948–56. https://doi.org/10.1093/jnci/djae031.

61. Kioumourtzoglou, M.-A. "Do air fresheners impact our health?" February 5, 2024. https://www.columbiadoctors.org/news/do-air-fresheners -impact-our-health#:~:text=And%20there%20is%20growing%20evidence, to%20numerous%20adverse%20health%20outcomes.

62. Natural Resources Defense Council. "Flint Water Crisis: Everything You Need to Know." October 8, 2024. https://www.nrdc.org/stories/flint -water-crisis-everything-you-need-know.

63. Weisman, R. J., A. Heinrich, F. Letkiewicz, M. Messner, K. Studer, L. Wang, et al. "Estimating national exposures and potential bladder cancer cases associated with chlorination DBPs in U.S. drinking water."

Environmental Health Perspectives 130, no. 8 (August 1, 2022). https://doi
.org/10.1289/ehp9985.

64. Shi, J., K. Zhang, T. Xiao, J. Yang, Y. Sun, C. Yang, et al. "Exposure to
disinfection by-products and risk of cancer: a systematic review and
dose-response meta-analysis." *Ecotoxicology and Environmental Safety* 270
(January 1, 2024): 115925. https://doi.org/10.1016/j.ecoenv.2023.115925.

65. Shi, J., K. Zhang, T. Xiao, J. Yang, Y. Sun, C. Yang, et al. "Exposure to
disinfection by-products and risk of cancer: a systematic review and
dose-response meta-analysis." *Ecotoxicology and Environmental Safety* 270
(January 1, 2024): 115925. https://doi.org/10.1016/j.ecoenv.2023.115925.

66. Leonard, S. V. L., C. R. Liddle, C. A. Atherall, E. Chapman,
M. Watkins, S. D. J. Calaminus, et al. "Microplastics in human blood:
polymer types, concentrations and characterisation using μFTIR." *Environment International* 188 (May 14, 2024): 108751. https://doi.org/10.1016/j
.envint.2024.108751.

67. Zhang, N., Y. B. Li, H. R. He, J. F. Zhang, and G. S. Ma. "You are what
you eat: microplastics in the feces of young men living in Beijing." *Science
of the Total Environment* 767 (December 31, 2020): 144345. https://doi.org
/10.1016/j.scitotenv.2020.144345.

68. Goswami, S., S. Adhikary, S. Bhattacharya, R. Agarwal, A. Ganguly,
S. Nanda, et al. "The alarming link between environmental microplastics
and health hazards with special emphasis on cancer." *Life Sciences* 355
(August 3, 2024): 122937. https://doi.org/10.1016/j.lfs.2024.122937.

69. Ju, G., X. Zhan, X. Chen, T. Zhang, X. Zhai, C. Chu, et al. "Bisphenol
S enhances the cell proliferation ability of prostate cancer cells by regulating the expression of SDS." *Toxicology in Vitro* 98 (June 2024): 105827.
https://doi.org/10.1016/j.tiv.2024.105827.

70. Hu, Y., M. Shen, C. Wang, Q. Huang, R. Li, G. Dorj, et al. "A meta-
analysis-based adverse outcome pathway for the male reproductive
toxicity induced by microplastics and nanoplastics in mammals." *Journal of
Hazardous Materials* 465 (March 1, 2024): 133375. https://doi.org/10.1016/j
.jhazmat.2023.133375.

71. Cohen, N. J., M. Yao, V. Midya, S. India-Aldana, T. Mouzica, S. S.
Andra, et al. "Exposure to perfluoroalkyl substances and women's fertility
outcomes in a Singaporean population-based preconception cohort."
Science of The Total Environment, 873 (2023): 162267. https://doi.org/10
.1016/j.scitotenv.2023.162267.

72. Tarapore, P., and B. Ouyang. "Perfluoroalkyl chemicals and male
reproductive health: Do PFOA and PFOS increase risk for male infertility?"

International Journal of Environmental Research and Public Health 18, no. 7 (April 5, 2021): 3794. https://doi.org/10.3390/ijerph18073794.

73. Li, J., Y. Zhang, and X. Wang. (2023). "Effects of Microplastic Exposure on Human Digestive, Reproductive, and Respiratory Health: A Rapid Systemic Review." *Environmental Science & Technology, 57*(12), 4796–4805. https://doi.org/10.1021/acs.est.3c09524

74. Okamoto, Katie. "Your laundry sheds harmful microfibers. Here's what you can do about it." *Wirecutter.* August 5, 2021. https://www.nytimes.com/wirecutter/blog/reduce-laundry-microfiber-pollution/.

75. Okamoto, Katie. "Black plastic kitchen tools might expose you to toxic chemicals. Here's what to use instead." *Wirecutter.* November 23, 2024. https://www.nytimes.com/wirecutter/reviews/toxic-black-plastic-kitchen-alternatives/.

76. Romanello, M., M. Walawender, S. C. Hsu, et al. "The 2024 report of the *Lancet* Countdown on health and climate change: facing record-breaking threats from delayed action." *Lancet* 404 (2024): 10465: 1847–96. https://doi.org/10.1016/S0140-6736(24)01822-1.

77. Burke, M., A. Driscoll, S. Heft-Neal, J. Xue, J. Burney, and M. Wara. "The changing risk and burden of wildfire in the United States." *Proceedings of the National Academy of Science U S A* 118, no. 2 (2021): e2011048118. https://doi.org/10.1073/pnas.2011048118.

78. Chen, K., Y. Ma, M. L. Bell, and W. Yang. "Canadian wildfire smoke and asthma syndrome emergency department visits in New York City." *JAMA* 330, no. 14 (2023): 1385–87. https://doi.org/10.1001/jama.2023.18768.

79. Neumann, J. E., M. Amend, S. Anenberg, et al. "Estimating PM2.5-related premature mortality and morbidity associated with future wildfire emissions in the western US." *Environmental Research Letters* 16, no. 3 (2021): 035019. https://doi.org/10.1088/1748-9326/abe82b.

80. Merriam-Webster.com Dictionary. "eppur si muove." n.d. https://www.merriam-webster.com/dictionary/eppur%20si%20muove.

81. Vonnegut, Kurt. *Slaughterhouse-Five.* Delacorte. 1969. 18.

Chapter 6. Infinite Reproduction: Sex and Cancer

1. Rider, J. R., K. M. Wilson, J. A. Sinnott, R. S. Kelly, L. A. Mucci, and E. L. Giovannucci. "Ejaculation frequency and risk of prostate cancer: updated results with an additional decade of follow-up." *European Urology* 70, no. 6 (March 28, 2016): 974–82. https://doi.org/10.1016/j.eururo.2016.03.027.

2. Giles, G. G., G. Severi, D. R. English, M. R. E. McCredie, R. Borland, P. Boyle, et al. "Sexual factors and prostate cancer." *BJU International* 92,

no. 3 (July 23, 2003): 211–16. https://doi.org/10.1046/j.1464-410x.2003 .04319.x.

3. Wu, A. H., C. L. Pearce, A. W. Lee, C. Tseng, A. Jotwani, P. Patel, et al. "Timing of births and oral contraceptive use influences ovarian cancer risk." *International Journal of Cancer* 141, no. 12 (July 27, 2017): 2392–99. https://doi.org/10.1002/ijc.30910.

4. Jordan, S. J., R. Na, E. Weiderpass, H.-O. Adami, K. E. Anderson, P. A. Van Den Brandt, et al. "Pregnancy outcomes and risk of endometrial cancer: a pooled analysis of individual participant data in the Epidemiology of Endometrial Cancer Consortium." *International Journal of Cancer* 148, no. 9 (October 26, 2020): 2068–78. https://doi.org/10.1002 /ijc.33360.

5. La Vecchia, C., A. Decarli, S. Franceschi, M. Regallo, and G. Tognoni. "Age at first birth and the risk of epithelial ovarian cancer." *Journal of the National Cancer Institute* 73, no. 3 (1984): 663–66. https://pubmed.ncbi.nlm .nih.gov/6590912/.

6. Blake, E. A., M. Y. De Zoysa, E. B. Morocco, S. B. Kaiser, M. Kodama, B. H. Grubbs, et al. "Teenage pregnancy complicated by primary invasive ovarian cancer: association for oncologic outcome." *Journal of Gynecologic Oncology* 29, no. 5 (2018): e79. https://doi.org/10.3802/jgo.2018.29.e79.

7. Fu, S., H. Ke, H. Yuan, H. Xu, W. Chen, and L. Zhao. "Dual role of pregnancy in breast cancer risk." *General and Comparative Endocrinology* 352 (March 26, 2024): 114501. https://doi.org/10.1016/j.ygcen.2024.114501.

8. Karlsson, T., T. Johansson, J. Höglund, W. E. Ek, and Å. Johansson. "Time-dependent effects of oral contraceptive use on breast, ovarian, and endometrial cancers." *Cancer Research* 81, no. 4 (February 15, 2021): 1153–62. https://doi.org/10.1158/0008-5472.can-20-2476.

9. Karlsson, T., T. Johansson, J. Höglund, W. E. Ek, and Å. Johansson. "Time-dependent effects of oral contraceptive use on breast, ovarian, and endometrial cancers." *Cancer Research* 81, no. 4 (February 15, 2021): 1153–62. https://doi.org/10.1158/0008-5472.can-20-2476.

10. Guo, C., B. Zhan, M.-Y. Li, L. Yue, and C. Zhang. "Association between oral contraceptives and cervical cancer: a retrospective case–control study based on the National Health and Nutrition Examination Survey." *Frontiers in Pharmacology* 15 (July 17, 2024): 1 400667. https://doi .org/10.3389/fphar.2024.1400667.

11. Iversen, L., S. Sivasubramaniam, A. J. Lee, S. Fielding, and P. C. Hannaford. "Lifetime cancer risk and combined oral contraceptives: the Royal College of General Practitioners' Oral Contraception Study."

American Journal of Obstetrics and Gynecology 216, no. 6 (February 8, 2017): 580.e1–580.e9. https://doi.org/10.1016/j.ajog.2017.02.002.

12. Mørch, L. S., A. Meaidi, G. Corn, M. Hargreave, and C. W. Skovlund. "Breast cancer in users of levonorgestrel-releasing intrauterine systems." *JAMA*, October 16, 2024. https://doi.org/10.1001/jama.2024.18575.

13. Cochran, S. D., and V. M. Mays. "Risk of breast cancer mortality among women cohabiting with same sex partners: findings from the National Health Interview Survey, 1997–2003." *Journal of Women's Health* 21, no. 5 (February 23, 2012): 528–33. https://doi.org/10.1089/jwh.2011.3134.

14. Center for American Progress. "LGBT Women Are Among Most at Risk of Poverty in America." 13 Mar. 2015, https://www.americanprogress .org/press/release-lgbt-women-are-among-most-at-risk-of-poverty-in -america/.

15. Tundealao, S., A. Sajja, T. Titiloye, I. Egab, and I. Odole. "Prevalence of self-reported cancer based on sexual orientation in the United States: a comparative analysis between lesbian, bisexual, gay, and heterosexual individuals." *Cancer Causes & Control* 34, no. 11 (July 12, 2023): 1027–35. https://doi.org/10.1007/s10552-023-01749-0.

16. Marks, D. H., S. T. Arron, and M. Mansh. "Skin cancer and skin cancer risk factors in sexual and gender minorities." *Dermatologic Clinics* 38, no. 2 (November 23, 2019): 209–18. https://doi.org/10.1016/j.det.2019.10.005.

17. De Blok, C. J. M., C. M. Wiepjes, N. M. Nota, K. Van Engelen, M. A. Adank, K. M. A. Dreijerink, et al. "Breast cancer risk in transgender people receiving hormone treatment: nationwide cohort study in the Nether-lands." *BMJ*, May 14, 2019, l1652. https://doi.org/10.1136/bmj.l1652.

18. de Nie, I., C. J. M. de Blok, T. M. van der Sluis, E. Barbé, G. L. S. Pigot, C. M. Wiepjes, et al. "Prostate cancer incidence under androgen deprivation: nationwide cohort study in trans women receiving hormone treatment." *Journal of Clinical Endocrinology and Metabolism* 105, no. 9 (2020): e3293–e3299.

19. Crowley, F., M. Mihalopoulos, S. Gaglani, A. K. Tewari, C.-K. Tsao, M. Djordjevic, et al. "Prostate cancer in transgender women: consider-ations for screening, diagnosis and management." *British Journal of Cancer* 128, no. 2 (2023): 177–89. https://doi.org/10.1038/s41416-022-01989-y.

20. Grimstad, F. W., K. G. Fowler, E. P. New, C. A. Ferrando, R. R. Pollard, G. Chapman, et al. "Uterine pathology in transmasculine persons on testosterone: a retrospective multicenter case series." *American Journal of Obstetrics and Gynecology* 220, no. 3 (December 21, 2018): 257.e1–257.e7. https://doi.org/10.1016/j.ajog.2018.12.021.

21. Centers for Disease Control and Prevention. "Sexually Transmitted Infections Surveillance, 2023." Accessed September 20, 2024. https://www.cdc.gov/sti-statistics/?CDC_AAref_Val=https://www.cdc.gov/std/statistics/2022/default.htm.

22. Centers for Disease Control and Prevention. "Sexually Transmitted Infections Surveillance, 2022." n.d. https://www.cdc.gov/sti-statistics/?CDC_AAref_Val=https://www.cdc.gov/std/statistics/2022/default.htm.

23. IARC Working Group on the Evaluation of Carcinogenic Risks to Humans. "Molecular mechanisms of HPV-induced carcinogenesis." National Institutes of Health. In *Human papillomaviruses* (International Agency for Research on Cancer, 2007). https://www.ncbi.nlm.nih.gov/books/NBK321762/.

24. Beral, V. "Reprint of 'Cancer of the cervix: A sexually transmitted infection?'" *Cancer Epidemiology* 39, no. 6 (November 5, 2015): 1148–51. https://doi.org/10.1016/j.canep.2015.08.005.

25. Lorincz, A. T., R. Reid, B. A. Jenson, M. D. Greenberg, W. Lancaster, and R. J. Kurman. "Human papillomavirus infection of the cervix." *Obstetrics and Gynecology* 79, no. 3 (March 1, 1992): 328–37. https://doi.org/10.1097/00006250-199203000-00002.

26. Frisch, M., B. Glimelius, A. J. C. Van Den Brule, J. Wohlfahrt, C. J. L. M. Meijer, J. M. M. Walboomers, et al. "Sexually transmitted infection as a cause of anal cancer." *New England Journal of Medicine* 337, no. 19 (November 6, 1997): 1350–58. https://doi.org/10.1056/nejm199711063371904.

27. Laprise, C., S. A. Madathil, N. F. Schlecht, G. Castonguay, D. Soulières, P. F. Nguyen-Tan, et al. "Human papillomavirus genotypes and risk of head and neck cancers: results from the HeNCe Life case-control study." *Oral Oncology* 69 (April 10, 2017): 56–61. https://doi.org/10.1016/j.oraloncology.2017.03.013.

28. LeWine, H. E. "HPV transmission during oral sex a growing cause of mouth and throat cancer." June 4, 2013. Harvard Health Publishing. https://www.health.harvard.edu/blog/hpv-transmission-during-oral-sex-a-growing-cause-of-mouth-and-throat-cancer-201306046346.

29. Mutch, D. "Why annual pap smears are history—but routine ob-gyn visits are not." American College of Obstetricians and Gynecologists. August 2024. https://www.acog.org/womens-health/experts-and-stories/the-latest/why-annual-pap-smears-are-history-but-routine-ob-gyn-visits-are-not.

30. ACOG Committee. "Human papillomavirus vaccination." *Obstetrics and Gynecology* 136, no. 2 (July 23, 2020): e15–21. https://doi.org/10.1097/aog.0000000000004000.

31. Kamolratanakul, S., and P. Pitisuttithum. "Human." *Vaccines* 9, no. 12 (November 30, 2021): 1413. https://doi.org/10.3390/vaccines9121413.

32. Benson, A. B., A. P. Venook, M. M. Al-Hawary, N. Azad, Y.-J. Chen, K. K. Ciombor, et al. "Anal carcinoma, Version 2.2023, NCCN Clinical Practice Guidelines in Oncology." *Journal of the National Comprehensive Cancer Network* 21, no. 6 (June 1, 2023): 653–77. https://doi.org/10.6004/jnccn.2023.0030.

33. Nielsen, K. J., K. K. Jakobsen, J. S. Jensen, C. Grønhøj, and C. Von Buchwald. "The effect of prophylactic HPV vaccines on oral and oropharyngeal HPV infection—a systematic review." *Viruses* 13, no. 7 (July 11, 2021): 1339. https://doi.org/10.3390/v13071339.

34. Benson, A. B., A. P. Venook, M. M. Al-Hawary, N. Azad, Y.-J. Chen, K. K. Ciombor, et al. "Anal carcinoma, Version 2.2023, NCCN Clinical Practice Guidelines in Oncology." *Journal of the National Comprehensive Cancer Network* 21, no. 6 (June 1, 2023): 653–77. https://doi.org/10.6004/jnccn.2023.0030.

35. Nielsen, K. J., K. K. Jakobsen, J. S. Jensen, C. Grønhøj, and C. Von Buchwald. "The effect of prophylactic HPV vaccines on oral and oropharyngeal HPV infection—a systematic review." *Viruses* 13, no. 7 (July 11, 2021): 1339. https://doi.org/10.3390/v13071339.

36. Meites, E., P. G. Szilagyi, H. W. Chesson, E. R. Unger, J. R. Romero, and L. E. Markowitz. "Human papillomavirus vaccination for adults: updated recommendations of the Advisory Committee on Immunization Practices." *Morbidity and Mortality Weekly Report* 68, no. 32 (August 15, 2019): 698–702. https://doi.org/10.15585/mmwr.mm6832a3.

37. Goodman, E., M. Felsher, D. Wang, L. Yao, and Y.-T. Chen. "Early initiation of HPV vaccination and series completion in early and mid-adolescence." *Pediatrics* 151, no. 3 (February 27, 2023). https://doi.org/10.1542/peds.2022-058794.

38. Nielsen, K. J., K. K. Jakobsen, J. S. Jensen, C. Grønhøj, and C. Von Buchwald. "Human papillomavirus vaccination for adults: updated recommendations of the Advisory Committee on Immunization Practices." *Morbidity and Mortality Weekly Report* 68, no. 32 (August 15, 2019): 698–702. https://doi.org/10.15585/mmwr.mm6832a3.

39. Fortner, R. T., K. L. Terry, N. Bender, N. Brenner, K. Hufnagel, J. Butt, et al. "Sexually transmitted infections and risk of epithelial ovarian cancer: results from the Nurses' Health Studies." *British Journal of Cancer* 120, no. 8 (March 21, 2019): 855–60. https://doi.org/10.1038/s41416-019-0422-9.

40. Hamar, B., B. Teutsch, E. Hoffmann, P. Hegyi, A. Váradi, P. Nyirády, et al. "*Trichomonas vaginalis* infection is associated with increased risk of

cervical carcinogenesis: a systematic review and meta-analysis of 470 000 patients." *International Journal of Gynecology & Obstetrics* 163, no. 1 (April 3, 2023): 31–43. https://doi.org/10.1002/ijgo.14763.

41. Taylor, M. L., A. G. Mainous, and B. J. Wells. "Prostate cancer and sexually transmitted diseases: a meta-analysis." *Family Medicine* 37, no. 7 (August 1, 2005): 506–12. https://pubmed.ncbi.nlm.nih.gov/15988645.

42. Workowski, K. A., L. H. Bachmann, P. A. Chan, C. M. Johnston, C. A. Muzny, I. Park, et al. "Sexually Transmitted Infections Treatment Guidelines, 2021." *MMWR Recommendations and Reports* 70, no. 4 (July 22, 2021): 1–187. https://doi.org/10.15585/mmwr.rr7004a1.

43. Altman, L. K. "New homosexual disorder worries health officials." *New York Times*. May 11, 1982. https://www.nytimes.com/1982/05/11 /science/new-homosexual-disorder-worries-health-officials.html.

44. Lopez, G. "The Reagan administration's unbelievable response to the HIV/AIDS epidemic." *Vox*. December 1, 2016. https://www.vox.com /2015/12/1/9828348/ronald-reagan-hiv-aids.

45. Nolan, E. "Fact check: did Rush Limbaugh read a list of gay men who died as an 'AIDS Update'?" *Newsweek*. February 18, 2021. https://www .newsweek.com/fact-check-did-rush-limbaugh-mock-aids-death-radio -show-1570282.

46. GMHC. "History." June 11, 2024. https://www.gmhc.org/history/.

47. Gilbey, R. "The double life of Rock Hudson: 'Let's be frank, he was a horndog!'" *Guardian*. October 6, 2023. https://www.theguardian.com/film /2023/oct/06/rock-hudson-secret-sex-life-all-that-heaven-allowed.

48. Ryan White HIV/AIDS Program. "Who was Ryan White?" February 2022. https://ryanwhite.hrsa.gov/about/ryan-white#:~:text=How%20 could%20he%20have%20AIDS%3F,-Play%20audio&text=Transcription%20 of%20Audio%3A,on%20AIDS%20at%20the%20time.

49. Center for Cancer Research. "The first AIDS drugs." n.d. https://ccr .cancer.gov/news/landmarks/article/first-aids-drugs#:~:text=In%201987%2C %20it%20became%20the,the%20perinatal%20transmission%20of%20HIV.

50. National Institute of Allergy and Infectious Diseases. "Antiretroviral drug discovery and development." February 5, 2024. https://www.niaid.nih .gov/diseases-conditions/antiretroviral-drug-development.

Chapter 7. Virtue and Vice: Smoking, Vaping, Alcohol, and Other Drugs

1. Andrews, E. "Who invented beer?" April 21, 2020. History.com. https://www.history.com/articles/who-invented-beer.

2. Sudhinaraset, M., C. Wigglesworth, and D. T. Takeuchi. "Social and cultural contexts of alcohol use: influences in a social-ecological framework." *Alcohol Research 38,* no. 1 (2016): 35–45. https://pmc.ncbi.nlm.nih .gov/articles/PMC4872611/.

3. Martyn, C. N. "Smoking in British popular culture 1800–2000." *BMJ* 321, no. 7257 (2000): 389. https://pmc.ncbi.nlm.nih.gov/articles /PMC1118355/.

4. Leon, M. E., A. Peruga, A. McNeill, E. Kralikova, N. Guha, S. Minozzi, et al. "European Code Against Cancer, 4th Edition: Tobacco and cancer." *Cancer Epidemiology* 39 (August 11, 2015): S20–33. https://doi.org/10.1016/j .canep.2015.06.001.

5. Schaal, C., and S. P. Chellappan. "Nicotine-mediated cell proliferation and tumor progression in smoking-related cancers." *Molecular Cancer Research* 12, no. 1 (January 8, 2014): 14–23. https://doi.org/10.1158/1541 -7786.mcr-13-0541.

6. Alberg, A. J., M. V. Brock, J. G. Ford, J. M. Samet, and S. D. Spivack. "Epidemiology of lung cancer." *CHEST* 143, no. 5 (May 1, 2013): e1S–e29S. https://doi.org/10.1378/chest.12-2345.

7. Thun, M. J., S. J. Henley, and E. E. Calle. "Tobacco use and cancer: an epidemiologic perspective for geneticists." *Oncogene* 21, no. 48 (October 15, 2002): 7307–25. https://doi.org/10.1038/sj.onc.1205807.

8. Centers for Disease Control and Prevention. "Current cigarette smoking among adults in the United States." September 17, 2024. https:// www.cdc.gov/tobacco/php/data-statistics/adult-data-cigarettes/index .html.

9. World Health Organization. "Tobacco." July 31, 2023. https://www .who.int/news-room/fact-sheets/detail/tobacco.

10. Chaiton, M., L. Diemert, J. E. Cohen, S. J. Bondy, P. Selby, A. Philip-neri, et al. "Estimating the number of quit attempts it takes to quit smoking successfully in a longitudinal cohort of smokers." *BMJ Open* 6, no. 6 (2016): e011045. https://pmc.ncbi.nlm.nih.gov/articles/PMC4908897 /#:~:text=The%20Centers%20for%20Disease%20Control,11%20 attempts%20before%20quitting%20permanently.

11. Doll, R., & Hill, A. B. "Smoking and carcinoma of the lung: preliminary report." *British Medical Journal* 2, no. 4682 (September 30, 1950), 739–48. https://doi.org/10.1136/bmj.2.4682.739.

12. Doll, R., & Hill, A. B. "The mortality of doctors in relation to their smoking habits: a preliminary report." *British Medical Journal* 1, no. 4877 (June 26, 1954), 1451–55. https://doi.org/10.1136/bmj.1.4877.1451.

13. Tobacco Tactics. "Tobacco Industry Research Committee." February 7, 2020. https://www.tobaccotactics.org/article/tobacco-industry-research-committee/.

14. US Surgeon General. "Smoking and health: report of the Advisory Committee to the Surgeon General of the Public Health Service." 1964. https://www.profiles.nlm.nih.gov/spotlight/nn/feature/smoking.

15. Collaborative for Health & Environment. "Tobacco: 'Doubt is their product.'" n.d. https://www.healthandenvironment.org/environmental-health/social-context/history/tobacco-doubt-is-their-product.

16. National Association of Attorneys General. "The Master Settlement Agreement." June 12, 2024. https://www.naag.org/our-work/naag-center-for-tobacco-and-public-health/the-master-settlement-agreement/.

17. O'Connor, A. "Many of today's unhealthy foods were brought to you by Big Tobacco." September 19, 2023. https://lsa.umich.edu/psych/news-events/all-news/faculty-news/many-of-today-s-unhealthy-foods-were-brought-to-you-by-big-tobac.html#:~:text=In%20the%201980s%2C%20tobacco%20giants,Kraft%20Macaroni%20%26%20Cheese%20and%20Lunchables.

18. National Academies of Sciences, Engineering, and Medicine. *Public Health Consequences of E-Cigarettes*. 2018. National Academies Press. https://doi.org/10.17226/24952.

19. Tang, M.-S., X.-R. Wu, H.-W. Lee, Y. Xia, F.-M. Deng, A. L. Moreira, et al. "Electronic-cigarette smoke induces lung adenocarcinoma and bladder urothelial hyperplasia in mice." *Proceedings of the National Academy of Sciences* 116, no. 43 (October 7, 2019): 21727–31. https://doi.org/10.1073/pnas.1911321116.

20. Hashibe, M., H. Morgenstern, Y. Cui, D. P. Tashkin, Z.-F. Zhang, W. Cozen, et al. "Marijuana use and the risk of lung and upper aerodigestive tract cancers: results of a population-based case-control study." *Cancer Epidemiology Biomarkers & Prevention* 15, no. 10 (October 1, 2006): 1829–34. https://doi.org/10.1158/1055-9965.epi-06-0330.

21. Lacson, J. C. A., J. D. Carroll, E. Tuazon, E. J. Castelao, L. Bernstein, and V. K. Cortessis. "Population-based case-control study of recreational drug use and testis cancer risk confirms an association between marijuana use and nonseminoma risk." *Cancer* 118, no. 21 (September 10, 2012): 5374–83. https://doi.org/10.1002/cncr.27554.

22. Coutts, A., F. M. Fouad, A. Abbara, A. M. Sibai, Z. Sahloul, and K. Blanchet. "Responding to the Syrian health crisis: the need for data and research." *Lancet Respiratory Medicine* 3, no. 3 (March 1, 2015): e8–9. https://doi.org/10.1016/s2213-2600(15)00041-7.

23. International Agency for Research on Cancer. *Biological agents: a review of human carcinogens.* 2012. https://publications.iarc.fr/119.

24. Torres-Duque, C., D. Maldonado, R. Perez-Padilla, M. Ezzati, and G. Viegi. "Biomass fuels and respiratory diseases: a review of the evidence." *Proceedings of the American Thoracic Society* 5, no. 5 (July 14, 2008): 577–90. https://doi.org/10.1513/pats.200707-100rp.

25. Hoppe, M. M., R. Sundar, D. S. P. Tan, and A. D. Jeyasekharan. "Biomarkers for homologous recombination deficiency in cancer." *Journal of the National Cancer Institute* 110, no. 7 (April 10, 2018): 704–13. https://doi.org/10.1093/jnci/djy085.

26. Floud, S., C. Hermon, R. F. Simpson, and G. K. Reeves. "Alcohol consumption and cancer incidence in women: interaction with smoking, body mass index and menopausal hormone therapy." *BMC Cancer* 23, no. 1 (August 16, 2023). https://doi.org/10.1186/s12885-023-11184-8.

27. Cao, Y., W. C. Willett, E. B. Rimm, M. J. Stampfer, and E. L. Giovannucci. "Light to moderate intake of alcohol, drinking patterns, and risk of cancer: results from two prospective US cohort studies." *BMJ* 351 (August 18, 2015): h4238. https://doi.org/10.1136/bmj.h4238.

28. Provenzale, D., R. M. Ness, X. Llor, J. M. Weiss, B. Abbadessa, G. Cooper, et al. "NCCN Guidelines insights: colorectal cancer screening, version 2.2020." *Journal of the National Comprehensive Cancer Network* 18, no. 10 (October 1, 2020): 1312–20. https://doi.org/10.6004/jnccn.2020.0048.

29. Ganne-Carrié, N., C. Chaffaut, V. Bourcier, I. Archambeaud, J.-M. Perarnau, F. Oberti, et al. "Estimate of hepatocellular carcinoma incidence in patients with alcoholic cirrhosis." *Journal of Hepatology* 69, no. 6 (August 6, 2018): 1274–83. https://doi.org/10.1016/j.jhep.2018.07.022.

30. Jepsen, P., F. Kraglund, J. West, G. E. Villadsen, H. T. Sørensen, and H. Vilstrup. "Risk of hepatocellular carcinoma in Danish outpatients with alcohol-related cirrhosis." *Journal of Hepatology* 73, no. 5 (June 5, 2020): 1030–36. https://doi.org/10.1016/j.jhep.2020.05.043.

31. Bagnardi, V., M. Rota, E. Botteri, I. Tramacere, F. Islami, V. Fedirko, et al. "Alcohol consumption and site-specific cancer risk: a comprehensive dose–response meta-analysis." *British Journal of Cancer* 112, no. 3 (November 25, 2014): 580–93. https://doi.org/10.1038/bjc.2014.579.

32. Centers for Disease Control and Prevention. "Facts about excessive drinking." Drink Less, Be Your Best. October 7, 2024. https://www.cdc.gov/drink-less-be-your-best/facts-about-excessive-drinking/index.html#:~:text=Financial%20costs,health%20care%20services%20for%20injuries.

33. Solzhenitsyn, A. *The gulag archipelago*, vol. 1. Harper and Ferry. 1974. 87.

34. Editorial Staff. "Alcohol and drug abuse statistics (facts about addiction)." American Addiction Centers. September 5, 2024. https://americanaddictioncenters.org/addiction-statistics#:~:text=Quick%20Facts%20on%20Drug%20Addiction,disorder%20in%20the%20past%20year.&text=10.2%25%20of%20Americans%2012%20and,disorder%20in%20the%20past%20year.

35. Hébert, A. H., and A. L. Hill. "Impact of opioid overdoses on US life expectancy and years of life lost, by demographic group and stimulant co-involvement: a mortality data analysis from 2019 to 2022." *Lancet Regional Health—Americas 36*: 100813 (August 1, 2024). https://doi.org/10.1016/j.lana.2024.100813.

Chapter 8. All the Rays We Cannot See: UV Light and Radiation

1. Broad, W. J. "A glow in the dark, and a lesson in scientific peril." *New York Times.* October 6, 1988. https://www.nytimes.com/1998/10/06/science/a-glow-in-the-dark-and-a-lesson-in-scientific-peril.html.

2. Connell, P. P., and S. Hellman. "Advances in radiotherapy and implications for the next century: a historical perspective." *Cancer Research* 69, no. 2 (January 15, 2009): 383–92. https://doi.org/10.1158/0008-5472.can-07-6871.

3. American Academy of Dermatology Association. "Skin cancer." March 25, 2025. https://www.aad.org/media/stats-skin-cancer.

4. International Agency for Research on Cancer. "Non-melanoma skin cancer fact sheet." Global Cancer Observatory. 2024. https://gco.iarc.fr/today/data/factsheets/cancers/17-Non-melanoma-skin-cancer-fact-sheet.pdf.

5. International Agency for Research on Cancer. "Melanoma." 2024. Global Cancer Observatory. https://gco.iarc.fr/today/data/factsheets/cancers/16-Melanoma-of-skin-fact-sheet.pdf.

6. International Agency for Research on Cancer. "Non-melanoma skin cancer fact sheet." 2024. Global Cancer Observatory. https://gco.iarc.fr/today/data/factsheets/cancers/17-Non-melanoma-skin-cancer-fact-sheet.pdf.

7. Hoeijmakers, Jan H. J. "DNA damage, aging, and cancer." *New England Journal of Medicine* 361, no. 15 (October 7, 2009): 1475–85. https://doi.org/10.1056/nejmra0804615.

8. Saginala, K., A. Barsouk, J. S. Aluru, P. Rawla, and A. Barsouk. "Epidemiology of melanoma." *Medical Sciences* 9, no. 4 (October 20, 2021): 63. https://doi.org/10.3390/medsci9040063.

9. Tubbs, A., and A. Nussenzweig. "Endogenous DNA damage as a source of genomic instability in cancer." *Cell* 168, no. 4 (February 1, 2017): 644–56. https://doi.org/10.1016/j.cell.2017.01.002.

10. Tomlinson, I., P. Sasieni, and W. Bodmer. "How many mutations in a cancer?" *American Journal of Pathology* 160, no. 3 (March 1, 2002): 755–58. https://doi.org/10.1016/s0002-9440(10)64896-1.

11. Media Team. "1 to 10 mutations are needed to drive cancer, scientists find." Wellcome Sanger Institute. October 19, 2017. https://www.sanger.ac.uk/news_item/1-10-mutations-are-needed-drive-cancer-scientists-find/.

12. Brenner, M., and V. J. Hearing. "The protective role of melanin against UV damage in human skin." *Photochemistry and Photobiology* 84, no. 3 (November 16, 2007): 539–49. https://doi.org/10.1111/j.1751-1097.2007.00226.x.

13. Brenner, M., and V. J. Hearing. "The protective role of melanin against UV damage in human skin." *Photochemistry and Photobiology* 84, no. 3 (November 16, 2007): 539–49. https://doi.org/10.1111/j.1751-1097.2007.00226.x.

14. Yu, N., F.-C. Chen, S. Ota, L. B. Jorde, P. Pamilo, L. Patthy, et al. "Larger genetic differences within Africans than between Africans and Eurasians." *Genetics* 161, no. 1 (May 1, 2002): 269–74. https://doi.org/10.1093/genetics/161.1.269.

15. Umar, S. A., and S. A. Tasduq. "Ozone layer depletion and emerging public health concerns - an update on epidemiological perspective of the ambivalent effects of ultraviolet radiation exposure." *Frontiers in Oncology* 12 (March 10, 2022). https://doi.org/10.3389/fonc.2022.866733.

16. World Economic Forum. "The ozone layer is on the right path to recovery: here's how the world made it happen." September 10, 2024. https://www.weforum.org/agenda/2022/12/ozone-layer-hole-update-nasa/.

17. Masters, R., E. Anwar, B. Collins, R. Cookson, and S. Capewell. "Return on investment of public health interventions: a systematic review." *Journal of Epidemiology & Community Health* 71 (2022): 827–34. https://jech.bmj.com/content/71/8/827.

18. Giles-Corti, B., D. R. English, C. Costa, E. Milne, D. Cross, and R. Johnston. "Creating SunSmart schools." *Health Education Research* 19, no. 1 (2004): 98–109. https://doi.org/10.1093/her/cyg003.

19. Saginala, K., A. Barsouk, J. S. Aluru, P. Rawla, and A. Barsouk. "Epidemiology of melanoma." *Medical Sciences* 9, no. 4 (October 20, 2021): 63. https://doi.org/10.3390/medsci9040063.

20. Gould, E. "Economic evaluation of the U.S. Environmental Protection Agency's lead hazard control program." *Pediatric* 121, no. 5 (2008): e1074–1080. https://doi.org/10.1542/peds.2007-1195.

21. Jones, S. E., and G. P. Guy. "Sun safety practices among schools in the United States." *JAMA Dermatology* 153, no. 5 (March 3, 2017): 391. https://doi.org/10.1001/jamadermatol.2016.6274.

22. Holman, D. M., K. R. Ragan, A. K. Julian, and F. M. Perna. "The context of sunburn among U.S. adults: common activities and sun protection behaviors." *American Journal of Preventive Medicine* 60, no. 5 (February 15, 2021): e213–20. https://doi.org/10.1016/j.amepre.2020.12.011.

23. NBC News. "How to choose the best sunscreen, according to these dermatologists." November 11, 2019. https://www.nbcnews.com/better/lifestyle/how-choose-best-sunscreen-according-these-dermatologists-ncna1002451.

24. The Skin Cancer Foundation. "Ask the expert: does a high SPF protect my skin better?" May 23, 2023. https://www.skincancer.org/blog/ask-the-expert-does-a-high-spf-protect-my-skin-better/.

25. NBC News. "Three simple hacks for a better day at the beach." November 11, 2019. https://www.nbcnews.com/better/lifestyle/how-choose-best-sunscreen-according-these-dermatologists-ncna1002451.

26. National Ocean Service. "Sunscreen chemicals and coral reefs." June 20, 2024. https://oceanservice.noaa.gov/news/sunscreen-corals.html.

27. Skin Cancer Foundation. "Sun protective clothing - the Skin Cancer Foundation." Updated May 2025. https://www.skincancer.org/skin-cancer-prevention/sun-protection/sun-protective-clothing/.

28. Gordon, L. G., A. J. Rodriguez-Acevedo, B. Køster, G. P. Guy, C. Sinclair, E. Van Deventer, et al. "Association of indoor tanning regulations with health and economic outcomes in North America and Europe." *JAMA Dermatology* 156, 4 (April 1, 2020): 401–10. https://doi.org/10.1001/jamadermatol.2020.0001.

29. Skin Cancer Foundation. "Spray, don't bake: the Skin Cancer Foundation suggests indoor tanning alternatives for young women this spring." July 23, 2024. https://www.skincancer.org/press/spray-dont-bake-the-skin-cancer-foundation-suggests-indoor-tanning-alternatives-for-young-women-this-spring/.

30. Choukas-Bradley, S., S. R. Roberts, A. J. Maheux, and J. Nesi. "The perfect storm: a developmental–sociocultural framework for the role of social media in adolescent girls' body image concerns and mental health."

Clinical Child and Family Psychology Review 25, no. 4 (July 16, 2022): 681–701. https://doi.org/10.1007/s10567-022-00404-5.

31. Moodycliffe, A. M., D. Nghiem, G. Clydesdale, and S. E. Ullrich. "Immune suppression and skin cancer development: regulation by NKT cells." *Nature Immunology* 1, no. 6 (December 2000): 521–25. https://doi .org/10.1038/82782.

32. González Maglio, D. H., M. L. Paz, and J. Leoni. "Sunlight effects on immune system: is there something else in addition to UV-induced immunosuppression?" *BioMed Research International* 2016, (2016): 1934518. https://doi.org/10.1155/2016/1934518.

33. Schwarz, T. "25 Years of UV-induced immunosuppression mediated by T Cells—from disregarded T suppressor cells to highly respected regulatory T cells." *Photochemistry and Photobiology* 84, no. 1 (2008): 10–18. https://doi.org/10.1111/j.1751-1097.2007.00223.x.

34. US Preventive Services Task Force, K. Bibbins-Domingo, D. C. Grossman, S. J. Curry, K. W. Davidson, M. Ebell, et al. "Screening for skin cancer: US Preventive Services Task Force recommendation statement." *JAMA* 316, no. 4 (2016): 429–35. https://doi.org/10.1001/jama.2016.8465.

35. Hoorens, I., K. Vossaert, L. Pil, B. Boone, S. De Schepper, K. Onge-nae, et al. "Total-body examination vs lesion-directed skin cancer screen-ing." *JAMA Dermatology* 152, no. 1 (2016): 27–34. https://doi.org/10.1001 /jamadermatol.2015.2680.

36. Weinstock, M.A., P. M. Risica, R. A. Martin, W. Rakowski, K. J. Smith, M. Berwick, et al. "Reliability of assessment and circumstances of performance of thorough skin self-examination for the early detection of melanoma in the Check-It-Out Project." *Preventive Medicine* 38, no. 6 (June 2004): 761–65. https://doi.org/10.1016/j.ypmed.2004.01.020.

37. Gandini, S., F. Sera, M. S. Cattaruzza, P. Pasquini, D. Abeni, P. Boyle, et al. "Meta-analysis of risk factors for cutaneous melanoma: I. Common and atypical naevi." *European Journal of Cancer* 41, no. 1 (January 2005): 28–44. https://doi.org/10.1016/j.ejca.2004.10.015.

38. Terushkin, V., E. Ng, J. A. Stein, S. Katz, D. E. Cohen, S. Meehan, et al. "A prospective study evaluating the utility of a 2-mm biopsy margin for complete removal of histologically atypical (dysplastic) nevi." *Journal of the American Academy of Dermatology* 77, no. 6 (December 2017): 1096–99. https://doi.org/10.1016/j.jaad.2017.07.016.

39. Muse, M. E., and J. S. Crane. "Actinic cheilitis." StatPearls. July 31, 2023. https://www.ncbi.nlm.nih.gov/books/NBK551553.

40. NHS. "Bowen's disease." Reviewed October 6, 2022. https://www
.nhs.uk/conditions/bowens-disease/.

41. Berwick, M., E. Erdei, and J. Hay. "Melanoma epidemiology and
public health." *Dermatological Clinics* 27, no. 2 (April 2009): 205–14.
https://doi.org/10.1016/j.det.2008.12.002.

42. Lucero, R., and D. Horowitz. "Xeroderma pigmentosum." Stat-
Pearls. July 4, 2023. https://www.ncbi.nlm.nih.gov/books/NBK551563/.

43. Saginala, K., A. Barsouk, J. S. Aluru, P. Rawla, and A. Barsouk.
"Epidemiology of melanoma." *Medical Sciences* 9, no. 4 (October 20, 2021):
63. https://doi.org/10.3390/medsci9040063.

44. Saginala, K., A. Barsouk, J. S. Aluru, P. Rawla, and A. Barsouk.
"Epidemiology of melanoma." *Medical Sciences* 9, no. 4 (October 20, 2021):
63. https://doi.org/10.3390/medsci9040063.

45. Saginala, K., A. Barsouk, J. S. Aluru, P. Rawla, and A. Barsouk.
"Epidemiology of melanoma." *Medical Sciences* 9, no. 4 (October 20, 2021):
63. https://doi.org/10.3390/medsci9040063.

46. Saginala, K., A. Barsouk, J. S. Aluru, P. Rawla, and A. Barsouk.
"Epidemiology of melanoma." *Medical Sciences* 9, no. 4 (October 20, 2021):
63. https://doi.org/10.3390/medsci9040063.

47. Moan, J., E. Cicarma, R. Setlow, A. C. Porojnicu, W. B. Grant, and
A. Juzeniene. "Time trends and latitude dependence of uveal and cutaneous
malignant melanoma induced by solar radiation." *Dermato-Endocrinology* 2,
no. 1 (January 1, 2010): 3–8. https://doi.org/10.4161/derm.2.1.11745.

48. US Bureau of Labor Statistics. "Mining (except oil and gas): NAICS
212. Industries at a glance." Retrieved June 13, 2025, from https://www.bls
.gov/iag/tgs/iag212.htm.

49. Klemic, H. "Uranium occurrences in sedimentary rocks of Pennsylvania." *Geological Survey Bulletin* 1107-D (1962): 243–88. https://pubs.usgs
.gov/bul/1107d/report.pdf.

50. Eidy, M., A. C. Regina, and K. Tishkowski. "Radon toxicity." StatPearls.
January 26, 2024. https://www.ncbi.nlm.nih.gov/books/NBK562321/.

51. Zdrojewicz, Z., and J. Strzelczyk. "Radon treatment controversy."
Dose-Response 4, no. 2 (April 1, 2006). https://doi.org/10.2203/dose
-response.05-025.zdrojewicz.

52. Eidy, M., A. C. Regina, and K. Tishkowski. "Radon toxicity." Stat-
Pearls. January 26, 2024. https://www.ncbi.nlm.nih.gov/books/NBK562321/.

53. EPA. "Overview of EPA's State Indoor Radon Grants program: a focus
on activities conducted during 2021." n.d. https://www.epa.gov/system/files
/documents/2022-02/final-2021-annual-sirg-activities-report-508c.pdf.

54. Eidy, M., A. C. Regina, and K. Tishkowski. "Radon toxicity." Stat-Pearls. January 26, 2024. https://www.ncbi.nlm.nih.gov/books/NBK562321/.

55. EPA. "Overview of EPA's State Indoor Radon Grants program: a focus on activities conducted during 2021." n.d. https://www.epa.gov/system/files /documents/2022-02/final-2021-annual-sirg-activities-report-508c.pdf.

56. Merck. "Cost, insurance & financial help." n.d. https://www .keytruda.com/financial-support/.

57. World Health Organization. "Cost-effectiveness of radon control." WHO Handbook on Indoor Radon. 2009. https://www.ncbi.nlm.nih.gov /books/NBK143215/.

58. Canadian Nuclear Safety Commission. "Types and sources of radiation." Government of Canada. Retrieved June 14, 2025, from http:// nuclearsafety.gc.ca/eng/resources/radiation/introduction-to-radiation /types-and-sources-of-radiation.

59. Di Trolio, R., G. Di Lorenzo, B. Fumo, and P. A. Ascierto. "Cosmic radiation and cancer: is there a link?" *Future Oncology* 11, no. 7 (March 25, 2015): 1123–35. https://doi.org/10.2217/fon.15.29.

60. Liu, T., C. Zhang, and C. Liu. "The incidence of breast cancer among female flight attendants: an updated meta-analysis." *Journal of Travel Medicine* 23, no. 6 (November 2016): taw055. https://doi.org/10.1093 /jtm/taw055.

61. Martin, C. J., and M. Barnard. "How much should we be concerned about cumulative effective doses in medical imaging?" *Journal of Radiological Protection* 42, no. 1 (October 21, 2021): 011514. https://doi.org/10.1088 /1361-6498/ac31c1.

62. Jorgensen, T. J. "Air travel exposes you to radiation—how much health risk comes with it?" *Scientific American*. February 20, 2024. https:// www.scientificamerican.com/article/air-travel-exposes-you-to-radiation -how-much-health-risk-comes-with-it/.

63. Canadian Nuclear Safety Commission. "Types and sources of radiation." Government of Canada. Retrieved June 14, 2025, from http:// nuclearsafety.gc.ca/eng/resources/radiation/introduction-to-radiation /types-and-sources-of-radiation.

64. Harvard Health. "Radiation risk from medical imaging." September 30, 2021. https://www.health.harvard.edu/cancer/radiation-risk-from -medical-imaging.

65. Harvard Health. "Radiation risk from medical imaging." September 30, 2021. https://www.health.harvard.edu/cancer/radiation-risk-from -medical-imaging.

66. Jewish Virtual Library. "The Pale of Settlement." n.d. https://www.jewishvirtuallibrary.org/the-pale-of-settlement.

67. European Parliament. "Forsmark: how Sweden alerted the world about the danger of the Chernobyl disaster." n.d. https://www.europarl.europa.eu/news/en/headlines/society/20140514STO47018/forsmark-how-sweden-alerted-the-world-about-the-danger-of-chernobyl-disaster.

68. Centers for Disease Control and Prevention. "Physician fact sheet: acute radiation syndrome (ARS)." National Center for Environmental Health. Retrieved June 14, 2025, from https://www.cdc.gov/nceh/radiation/emergencies/arsphysicianfactsheet.htm.

69. Centers for Disease Control and Prevention. "Potassium iodide (KI)." National Center for Environmental Health. January 30, 2025. https://www.cdc.gov/nceh/radiation/emergencies/ki.htm.

70. World Health Organization. "World Health Organization report explains the health impacts of the world's worst-ever civil nuclear accident." April 13, 2006. https://web.archive.org/web/20110404181327/http://www.who.int/mediacentre/news/releases/2006/pr20/en/index.html.

71. Bellona. "The Prydniprovsky Chemical Plant—Ukraine's uranium heritage." 2020. https://bellona.org/publication/the-prydniprovksy-chemical-plant-ukraines-uranium-heritage.

72. OECD Nuclear Energy Agency. "The INES Scale: the International Nuclear and Radiological Event Scale." 2008. https://www.iaea.org/sites/default/files/ines.pdf.

73. Horton, A. "'Dodged a bullet': how whistleblowers averted a second US nuclear disaster." *Guardian*. May 6, 2022. https://www.theguardian.com/tv-and-radio/2022/may/05/meltdown-three-mile-island-netflix-us-nuclear-accident.

74. Horton, A. "'Dodged a bullet': how whistleblowers averted a second US nuclear disaster." *Guardian.* May 6, 2022. https://www.theguardian.com/tv-and-radio/2022/may/05/meltdown-three-mile-island-netflix-us-nuclear-accident.

75. K=1 Project. "Hiroshima and Nagasaki: the long term health effects." Columbia University. Retrieved June 14, 2025, from https://k1project.columbia.edu/news/hiroshima-and-nagasaki.

76. Radiation Effects Research Foundation. "Solid cancer risks among atomic-bomb survivors." n.d. https://www.rerf.or.jp/en/programs/roadmap_e/health_effects-en/late-en/cancrisk.

77. Ron, E., D. L. Preston, K. Mabuchi, D. E. Thompson, and M. Soda. "Cancer incidence in atomic bomb survivors. Part IV: Comparison of

cancer incidence and mortality." *Radiation Research* 137, no. 2 (February 1994): S98–112. https://pubmed.ncbi.nlm.nih.gov/8127954/.

78. Temperton, J. "'Now I am become death, the destroyer of worlds.' The story of Oppenheimer's infamous quote." *WIRED.* July 21, 2023. https://www.wired.co.uk/article/manhattan-project-robert-oppenheimer. Oppenheimer may have misinterpreted the intended meaning of the line.

Chapter 9. In Their Genes: Hereditary Cancer Risk

1. Boland, C. R., and H. T. Lynch. "The history of Lynch syndrome." *Familial Cancer* 12, no. 2 (June 2013): 145–57. https://doi.org/10.1007 /s10689-013-9637-8.

2. Giardiello, F. M., J. I. Allen, J. E. Axilbund, C. R. Boland, C. A. Burke, R. W. Burt, et al. "Guidelines on genetic evaluation and management of Lynch Syndrome: a consensus statement by the US Multi-Society Task Force on Colorectal Cancer." *Gastroenterology* 147, no. 2 (July 18, 2014): 502–26. https://doi.org/10.1053/j.gastro.2014.04.001.

3. Rubenstein, J. H., R. Enns, J. Heidelbaugh, A. Barkun, M. A. Adams, S. D. Dorn, et al. "American Gastroenterological Association Institute Guideline on the Diagnosis and Management of Lynch Syndrome." *Gastroenterology* 149, no. 3 (July 27, 2015): 777–82. https://doi.org/10.1053 /j.gastro.2015.07.036.

4. Zhao, S., L. Chen, Y. Zang, W. Liu, S. Liu, F. Teng, et al. "Endometrial cancer in Lynch syndrome." *International Journal of Cancer* 150, no. 1 (August 16, 2021): 7–17. https://doi.org/10.1002/ijc.33763.

5. National Institutes of Health. "Mary-Claire King, Ph.D." National Cancer Institute, Division of Cancer Prevention. n.d. https://prevention .cancer.gov/about-dcp/history-and-timeline/commemoration-50th/mary -claire-king.

6. Angier, N. "Fierce competition marked fervid race for cancer gene." *New York Times.* September 20, 1994. C1. https://www.nytimes.com/1994/09 /20/science/fierce-competition-marked-fervid-race-for-cancer-gene.html.

7. Kuchenbaecker, K. B., J. L. Hopper, D. R. Barnes, K.-A. Phillips, T. M. Mooij, M.-J. Roos-Blom, et al. "Risks of breast, ovarian, and contralateral breast cancer for BRCA1 and BRCA2 mutation carriers." *JAMA* 317, no. 23 (June 20, 2017): 2402. https://doi.org/10.1001/jama.2017.7112.

8. Li, S., V. Silvestri, G. Leslie, T. R. Rebbeck, S. L. Neuhausen, J. L. Hopper, et al. "Cancer risks associated with *BRCA1* and *BRCA2* pathogenic variants." *Journal of Clinical Oncology* 40, no. 14 (January 25, 2022): 1529–41. https://doi.org/10.1200/jco.21.02112.

9. Li, S., V. Silvestri, G. Leslie, T. R. Rebbeck, S. L. Neuhausen, J. L. Hopper, et al. "Cancer risks associated with *BRCA1* and *BRCA2* pathogenic variants." *Journal of Clinical Oncology* 40, no. 14 (January 25, 2022): 1529–41. https://doi.org/10.1200/jco.21.02112.

10. Nyberg, T., D. Frost, D. Barrowdale, D. G. Evans, E. Bancroft, J. Adlard, et al. "Prostate cancer risks for male BRCA1 and BRCA2 mutation carriers: a prospective cohort study." *European Urology* 77, no. 1 (September 6, 2019): 24–35. https://doi.org/10.1016/j.eururo.2019.08.025.

11. Li, S., V. Silvestri, G. Leslie, T. R. Rebbeck, S. L. Neuhausen, J. L. Hopper, et al. Cancer risks associated with *BRCA1* and *BRCA2* pathogenic variants. *Journal of Clinical Oncology* 40, no. 14 (January 25, 2022): 1529–41. https://doi.org/10.1200/JCO.21.02112.

12. Rubenstein, J. H., R. Enns, J. Heidelbaugh, A. Barkun, M. A. Adams, S. D. Dorn, et al. "American Gastroenterological Association Institute Guideline on the Diagnosis and Management of Lynch Syndrome." *Gastroenterology* 149, no. 3 (July 27, 2015): 777–82. https://doi.org/10.1053/j.gastro.2015.07.036.

13. Whittemore, A. S., G. Gong, E. M. John, V. McGuire, F. P. Li, K. L. Ostrow, et al. "Prevalence of BRCA1 mutation carriers among U.S. non-Hispanic Whites." *Cancer Epidemiology, Biomarkers, & Prevention* 13, no. 12 (December 1, 2004): 2078–83. https://pubmed.ncbi.nlm.nih.gov/15598764.

14. Hartge, P., J. P. Struewing, S. Wacholder, L. C. Brody, and M. A. Tucker. "The Prevalence of common BRCA1 and BRCA2 mutations among Ashkenazi Jews." *American Journal of Human Genetics* 64, no. 4 (April 1, 1999): 963–70. https://doi.org/10.1086/302320.

15. Tobin, A. "Ashkenazi Jews descend from 350 people, study finds." *The Times of Israel.* September 10, 2014. https://www.timesofisrael.com/ashkenazi-jews-descend-from-350-people-study-finds/#:~:text=An%20analysis%20of%20the%20gene,just%20350%20or%20so%20people.

16. Gross, S. J., B. A. Pletcher, K. G. Monaghan, and Professional Practice and Guidelines Committee. "Carrier screening in individuals of Ashkenazi Jewish descent." *Genetics in Medicine* 10, no. 1 (2008): 54–56. https://doi.org/10.1097/GIM.0b013e31815f247c.

17. Hutter, C., and J. C. Zenklusen. "The Cancer Genome Atlas: creating lasting value beyond its data." *Cell* 173, no. 2 (2018): 283–85. https://doi.org/10.1016/j.cell.2018.03.042.

18. MedlinePlus. "Genetics." National Library of Medicine. n.d. https://ghr.nlm.nih.gov/primer/genomicresearch/snp.

19. 23andMe. "See our list of Personalised Genetic Reports." n.d. https://www.23andme.com/dna-reports-list/.

20. SNPedia. "Testing." November 23, 2019. https://www.snpedia.com /index.php/Testing.

21. Jouvenal, J., M. Berman, D. Harwell, and T. Jackman. "Data on a genealogy site led police to the 'Golden State Killer' suspect. Now others worry about a 'treasure trove' of data." *Washington Post.* April 27, 2018. https://www.washingtonpost.com/news/true-crime/wp/2018/04/27 /golden-state-killer-dna-website-gedmatch-was-used-to-identify-joseph -deangelo-as-suspect-police-say/.

22. Associated Press. "Dozens of states sue to block the sale of 23andMe personal genetic data without customer consent." NPR. June 10, 2025. https://www.npr.org/2025/06/10/nx-s1-5429041/23andme-states-lawsuit -genetic-data.

23. "Promethease." n.d. https://promethease.com/.

24. SNPedia. "SNPedia." July 19, 2017. https://www.snpedia.com/index .php/SNPedia.

25. Williams, B. K. "Filtering a Promethease report: one genetic counselor's strategy." Watershed DNA. February 25, 2018. https://www .watersheddna.com/blog-and-news/filtering-a-promethease-report-one -genetic-counselors-strategy.

26. US Equal Employment Opportunity Commission. "Genetic information discrimination." Accessed June 15, 2025. https://www.eeoc.gov /genetic-information-discrimination.

27. Warner, E. "Screening BRCA1 and BRCA2 mutation carriers for breast cancer." *Cancers* 10, no. 12 (November 30, 2018): 477. https://doi.org /10.3390/cancers10120477.

28. Warner, E. "Screening BRCA1 and BRCA2 mutation carriers for breast cancer." *Cancers* 10, no. 12 (November 30, 2018): 477. https://doi.org /10.3390/cancers10120477.

29. Tung, N. M., J. C. Boughey, L. J. Pierce, M. E. Robson, I. Bedrosian, J. R. Dietz, et al. "Management of hereditary breast cancer: American Society of Clinical Oncology, American Society for Radiation Oncology, and Society of Surgical Oncology Guideline." *Journal of Clinical Oncology* 38, no. 18 (April 3, 2020): 2080–2106. https://doi.org/10.1200/jco.20.00299.

30. Manahan, E. R., H. M. Kuerer, M. Sebastian, K. S. Hughes, J. C. Boughey, D. M. Euhus, et al. "Consensus Guidelines on Genetic Testing for Hereditary Breast Cancer from the American Society of Breast Surgeons."

Annals of Surgical Oncology 26, no. 10 (July 24, 2019): 3025–31. https://doi .org/10.1245/s10434-019-07549-8.

31. Collins, J. M., and C. Isaacs. "Management of breast cancer risk in BRCA1/2 mutation carriers who are unaffected with cancer." *The Breast Journal* 26, no. 8 (July 11, 2020): 1520–27. https://doi.org/10.1111/tbj.13970.

32. Doren, A., A. Vecchiola, B. Aguirre, and P. Villaseca. "Gynecological– endocrinological aspects in women carriers of BRCA1/2 gene mutations." *Climacteric* 21, no. 6 (October 8, 2018): 529–35. https://doi.org/10.1080 /13697137.2018.1514006.

33. Rubenstein, J. H., R. Enns, J. Heidelbaugh, A. Barkun, and Clinical Guidelines Committee. "American Gastroenterological Association Institute Guideline on the Diagnosis and Management of Lynch Syn- drome." *Gastroenterology* 149, no. 3 (July 27, 2015): 777–82. https://doi.org /10.1053/j.gastro.2015.07.036.

34. Crosbie, E. J., N. A. J. Ryan, M. J. Arends, J. Wilson, N. Wood, D. G. Evans, et al. "The Manchester International Consensus Group recommen- dations for the management of gynecological cancers in Lynch syndrome." *Genetics in Medicine* 21, no. 10 (2019): 2390–400. https://doi.org/10.1038 /s41436-019-0489-y.

35. Gambini, D., S. Ferrero, and E. Kuhn. "Lynch Syndrome: from carcinogenesis to prevention interventions." *Cancers* 14, no. 17 (August 24, 2022): 4102. https://doi.org/10.3390/cancers14174102.

36. American Pregnancy Association. "Diagnóstico Genético Preim- plantacional: DGP." December 9, 2021. http://americanpregnancy.org /infertility/preimplantation-genetic-diagnosis/.

37. MRCTV. "Advocacy groups condemn Iceland's drive to end Down syndrome by abortion." August 16, 2017. https://cnsnews.com/author /annabel-scott.

38. Sanghavi, D. "Wanting babies like themselves, some parents choose genetic defects." *New York Times.* December 5, 2006. https://www.nytimes .com/2006/12/05/health/wanting-babies-like-themselves-some-parents -choose-genetic-defects.html.

39. Sanghavi, D. "Wanting babies like themselves, some parents choose genetic defects." *New York Times.* December 5, 2006. https://www.nytimes .com/2006/12/05/health/wanting-babies-like-themselves-some-parents -choose-genetic-defects.html.

40. Retassie, R. "Genetic test to screen embryos for low intelligence developed in US." PET. November 19, 2018. https://www.progress.org.uk /genetic-test-to-screen-embryos-for-low-intelligence-developed-in-us/.

41. Retassie, R. "Genetic test to screen embryos for low intelligence developed in US." PET. November 19, 2018. https://www.progress.org.uk/genetic-test-to-screen-embryos-for-low-intelligence-developed-in-us/.

42. Retassie, R. "Genetic test to screen embryos for low intelligence developed in US." PET. November 19, 2018. https://www.progress.org.uk/genetic-test-to-screen-embryos-for-low-intelligence-developed-in-us/.

43. Farber, S. A. "U.S. scientists' role in the eugenics movement (1907–1939): a contemporary biologist's perspective." *Zebrafish* 5, no. 4 (December 1, 2008): 243–45. https://doi.org/10.1089/zeb.2008.0576.

44. National Human Genome Research Institute. "Eugenics: its origin and development (1883 - present)." National Institutes of Health. November 30, 2021. https://www.genome.gov/about-genomics/educational-resources/timelines/eugenics.

45. United States Holocaust Memorial Museum. "Law for the 'Prevention of Offspring with Hereditary Diseases.'" n.d. https://encyclopedia.ushmm.org/content/en/timeline-event/holocaust/1933-1938/law-for-the-prevention-of-offspring-with-hereditary-diseases.

46. Berenbaum, M. "T4 Program: Nazi policy." Encyclopedia Britannica. October 3, 2024. https://www.britannica.com/event/T4-Program.

47. Jewish Virtual Library. "The Nazis and the Jews: the Madagascar Plan." n.d. https://www.jewishvirtuallibrary.org/the-madagascar-plan-2.

Chapter 10. Burning Questions: Inflammation,
the Microbiome, and Cancer

1. Denk, D., and F. R. Greten. "Inflammation: the incubator of the tumor microenvironment." *Trends in Cancer* 8, no. 11 (2022): 901–14. https://doi.org/10.1016/j.trecan.2022.07.002.

2. Rubin, D. T., A. N. Ananthakrishnan, C. A. Siegel, B. G. Sauer, and M. D. Long. "ACG Clinical Guideline: Ulcerative Colitis in Adults." *American Journal of Gastroenterology* 114, no. 3 (February 27, 2019): 384–413. https://doi.org/10.14309/ajg.0000000000000152.

3. Shergill, A. K., J. R. Lightdale, D. H. Bruining, R. D. Acosta, V. Chandrasekhara, K. V. Chathadi, et al. "The role of endoscopy in inflammatory bowel disease." *Gastrointestinal Endoscopy* 81, no. 5 (April 9, 2015): 1101–21. https://doi.org/10.1016/j.gie.2014.10.030.

4. Zhang, M., Y. Wang, Y. Wang, Y. Bai, and D. Gu. "Association between systemic lupus erythematosus and cancer morbidity and mortality: findings from cohort studies." *Frontiers in Oncology* 12 (May 4, 2022). https://doi.org/10.3389/fonc.2022.860794.

5. Rovin, B. H., I. M. Ayoub, T. M. Chan, Z.-H. Liu, J. M. Mejía-Vilet, and J. Floege. "KDIGO 2024 Clinical Practice Guideline for the management of LUPUS NEPHRITIS." *Kidney International* 105, no. 1 (January 1, 2024): S1–69. https://doi.org/10.1016/j.kint.2023.09.002.

6. Chougule, D., M. Nadkar, K. Venkataraman, A. Rajadhyaksha, N. Hase, T. Jamale, et al. "Adipokine interactions promote the pathogenesis of systemic lupus erythematosus." *Cytokine* 111 (August 8, 2018): 20–27. https://doi.org/10.1016/j.cyto.2018.08.002.

7. Diallo, A., M. Deschasaux, P. Latino-Martel, S. Hercberg, P. Galan, P. Fassier, et al. "Red and processed meat intake and cancer risk: Results from the prospective NutriNet-Santé cohort study." *International Journal of Cancer* 142, no. 2 (September 15, 2017): 230–37. https://doi.org/10.1002/ijc.31046.

8. Mayo Clinic. "Metabolic syndrome - Symptoms & causes." May 6, 2021. https://www.mayoclinic.org/diseases-conditions/metabolic-syndrome/symptoms-causes/syc-20351916.

9. Pugliese, N. R., P. Pellicori, F. Filidei, N. De Biase, P. Maffia, T. J. Guzik, et al. "Inflammatory pathways in heart failure with preserved left ventricular ejection fraction: implications for future interventions." *Cardiovascular Research* 118, no. 18 (August 24, 2022): 3536–55. https://doi.org/10.1093/cvr/cvac133.

10. Ho, F. K., C. Celis-Morales, F. Petermann-Rocha, S. L. Parra-Soto, J. Lewsey, D. Mackay, et al. "Changes over 15 years in the contribution of adiposity and smoking to deaths in England and Scotland." *BMC Public Health* 21, no. 169 (2021). https://doi.org/10.1186/s12889-021-10167-3.

11. Parohan, M., A. Sadeghi, S. R. Khatibi, M. Nasiri, A. Milajerdi, M. Khodadost, et al. "Dietary total antioxidant capacity and risk of cancer: a systematic review and meta-analysis on observational studies." *Critical Reviews in Oncology/Hematology* 138 (April 4, 2019): 70–86. https://doi.org/10.1016/j.critrevonc.2019.04.003.

12. Yang, J., S. Qian, X. Na, and A. Zhao. "Association between dietary and supplemental antioxidants intake and lung cancer risk: evidence from a cancer screening trial." *Antioxidants* 12, no. 2 (January 31, 2023): 338. https://doi.org/10.3390/antiox12020338.

13. Lee, K. H., H. J. Seong, G. Kim, G. H. Jeong, J. Y. Kim, H. Park, et al. "Consumption of fish and ω-3 fatty acids and cancer risk: an umbrella review of meta-analyses of observational studies." *Advances in Nutrition* 11, no. 5 (April 22, 2020): 1134–49. https://doi.org/10.1093/advances/nmaa055.

14. Wang, J., Y. Zhang, and L. Zhao. "Omega-3 PUFA intake and the risk of digestive system cancers." *Medicine* 99, no. 19 (May 1, 2020): e20119. https://doi.org/10.1097/md.0000000000020119.

15. Guo, Y., H. Qian, X. Xin, and Q. Liu. "Effects of different exercise modalities on inflammatory markers in the obese and overweight populations: unraveling the mystery of exercise and inflammation." *Frontiers in Physiology* 15 (June 12, 2024). https://doi.org/10.3389/fphys.2024.1405094.

16. Murugathasan, M., A. Jafari, A. Amandeep, S. A. Hassan, M. Chihata, and A. A. Abdul-Sater. "Moderate exercise induces trained immunity in macrophages." *AJP Cell Physiology* 325, no. 2 (June 12, 2023): C429–42. https://doi.org/10.1152/ajpcell.00130.2023.

17. Wang, S., J. Shen, W.-P. Koh, J.-M. Yuan, X. Gao, Y. Peng, et al. "Comparison of race- and ethnicity-specific BMI cutoffs for categorizing obesity severity: a multicountry prospective cohort study." *Obesity* 32, no. 10 (September 3, 2024): 1958–66. https://doi.org/10.1002/oby.24129.

18. Heymsfield, S. B., C. M. Peterson, D. M. Thomas, M. Heo, and J. M. Schuna. "Why are there race/ethnic differences in adult body mass index–adiposity relationships? A quantitative critical review." *Obesity Reviews* 17, no. 3 (December 11, 2015): 262–75. https://doi.org/10.1111/obr.12358.

19. Weeldreyer, N. R., J. C. De Guzman, C. Paterson, J. D. Allen, G. A. Gaesser, and S. S. Angadi. "Cardiorespiratory fitness, body mass index and mortality: a systematic review and meta-analysis." *British Journal of Sports Medicine* 59, no. 5 (November 13, 2024). https://doi.org/10.1136/bjsports-2024-108748.

20. Selickman, J., C. S. Vrettou, S. D. Mentzelopoulos, and J. J. Marini. "COVID-19-related ARDS: key mechanistic features and treatments." *Journal of Clinical Medicine* 11, no. 16 (August 20, 2022): 4896. https://doi.org/10.3390/jcm11164896.

21. Sarma, A., S. A. Christenson, A. Byrne, E. Mick, A. O. Pisco, C. DeVoe, et al. "Tracheal aspirate RNA sequencing identifies distinct immunological features of COVID-19 ARDS." *Nature Communications* 12, no. 1 (August 26, 2021). https://doi.org/10.1038/s41467-021-25040-5.

22. Li, J., H. Bai, H. Qiao, C. Du, P. Yao, Y. Zhang, et al. "Causal effects of COVID-19 on cancer risk: a Mendelian randomization study." *Journal of Medical Virology* 95, no. 4 (April 1, 2023). https://doi.org/10.1002/jmv.28722.

23. Du Plessis, M., C. Fourie, J. Riedemann, W. J. S. De Villiers, and A. M. Engelbrecht. "Cancer and Covid-19: collectively catastrophic."

Cytokine & Growth Factor Reviews 63 (October 25, 2021): 78–89. https://doi
.org/10.1016/j.cytogfr.2021.10.005.

24. Wang, S., N. Zhao, T. Luo, S. Kou, M. Sun, and K. Chen. "Causality
between COVID-19 and multiple myeloma: a two-sample Mendelian
randomization study and Bayesian co-localization." *Clinical and Experimental
Medicine 24,* no. 1 (2024): 42. https://doi.org/10.1007/s10238-024-01299-y.

25. Costa, B. A., K. V. da Luz, S. E. V. Campos, G. S. Lopes, J. P. V. Leitão,
and F. B. Duarte. "Can SARS-CoV-2 induce hematologic malignancies in
predisposed individuals? A case series and review of the literature."
Hematology, Transfusion and Cell Therapy 44, no. 1 (2022): 26–31. https://
doi.org/10.1016/j.htct.2021.11.015.

26. Malagón, T., J. H. E. Yong, P. Tope, W. H. Miller, and E. L. Franco.
"Predicted long-term impact of COVID-19 pandemic-related care delays
on cancer mortality in Canada." *International Journal of Cancer* 150, no. 8
(November 29, 2021): 1244–54. https://doi.org/10.1002/ijc.33884.

27. World Cancer Research Fund, and American Institute for Cancer
Research. "Diet, nutrition, physical activity and stomach cancer." 2016.
https://www.wcrf.org/sites/default/files/Stomach-Cancer-2016-Report.pdf.

28. World Cancer Research Fund, and American Institute for Cancer
Research. "Diet, nutrition, physical activity and stomach cancer." 2016.
https://www.wcrf.org/sites/default/files/Stomach-Cancer-2016-Report.pdf.

29. Graham, D. Y. "*Helicobacter pylori* update: gastric cancer, reliable
therapy, and possible benefits." *Gastroenterology* 148, no. 4 (February 2,
2015): 719–731. https://doi.org/10.1053/j.gastro.2015.01.040.

30. Okada, H., C. Kuhn, H. Feillet, and J.-F. Bach. "The 'hygiene
hypothesis' for autoimmune and allergic diseases: an update." *Clinical &
Experimental Immunology* 160, no. 1 (March 11, 2010): 1–9. https://doi.org
/10.1111/j.1365-2249.2010.04139.x.

31. Bach, J.-F. "The hygiene hypothesis in autoimmunity: the role of
pathogens and commensals." *Nature Reviews Immunology* 18, no. 2 (October 16, 2017): 105–20. https://doi.org/10.1038/nri.2017.111.

32. Versini, M., P.-Y. Jeandel, T. Bashi, G. Bizzaro, M. Blank, and
Y. Shoenfeld. "Unraveling the Hygiene Hypothesis of helminthes and
autoimmunity: origins, pathophysiology, and clinical applications." *BMC
Medicine* 13, no. 1 (April 13, 2015). https://doi.org/10.1186/s12916-015-0306-7.

33. McNeil, D. G. Jr. "Deadly, drug-resistant 'superbugs' pose huge
threat, WHO says." *New York Times*. February 27, 2017. https://www
.nytimes.com/2017/02/27/health/who-bacteria-pathogens-antibiotic
-resistant-superbugs.html.

34. Garabatos, N., and P. Santamaria. "Gut microbial antigenic mimicry in autoimmunity." *Frontiers in Immunology* 13 (April 27, 2022). https://doi.org/10.3389/fimmu.2022.873607.

35. Brown, E. M., D. J. Kenny, and R. J. Xavier. "Gut microbiota regulation of T cells during inflammation and autoimmunity." *Annual Review of Immunology* 37, no. 1 (April 26, 2019): 599–624. https://doi.org/10.1146/annurev-immunol-042718-041841.

36. Mousa, W. K., F. Chehadeh, and S. Husband. "Microbial dysbiosis in the gut drives systemic autoimmune diseases." *Frontiers in Immunology* 13 (October 20, 2022). https://doi.org/10.3389/fimmu.2022.906258.

37. Yang, R., Z. Chen, and J. Cai. "Fecal microbiota transplantation: emerging applications in autoimmune diseases." *Journal of Autoimmunity* 141 (April 26, 2023): 103038. https://doi.org/10.1016/j.jaut.2023.103038.

38. Zeng, L., Y. Deng, K. Yang, J. Chen, Q. He, and H. Chen. "Safety and efficacy of fecal microbiota transplantation for autoimmune diseases and autoinflammatory diseases: a systematic review and meta-analysis." *Frontiers in Immunology* 13 (September 30, 2022). https://doi.org/10.3389/fimmu.2022.944387.

39. Seida, I., M. Al Shawaf, and N. Mahroum. "Fecal microbiota transplantation in autoimmune diseases—an extensive paper on a pathogenetic therapy." *Autoimmunity Reviews* 23, no. 7–8 (April 7, 2024): 103541. https://doi.org/10.1016/j.autrev.2024.103541.

40. Song, M., A. T. Chan, and J. Sun. "Influence of the gut microbiome, diet, and environment on risk of colorectal cancer." *Gastroenterology* 158, no. 2 (October 3, 2019): 322–40. https://doi.org/10.1053/j.gastro.2019.06.048.

41. Sun, J., F. Chen, and G. Wu. "Potential effects of gut microbiota on host cancers: focus on immunity, DNA damage, cellular pathways, and anticancer therapy." *The ISME Journal* 17, no. 10 (August 8, 2023): 1535–51. https://doi.org/10.1038/s41396-023-01483-0.

42. Tilg, H., T. E. Adolph, R. R. Gerner, and A. R. Moschen. "The intestinal microbiota in colorectal cancer." *Cancer Cell* 33, no. 6 (April 12, 2018): 954–64. https://doi.org/10.1016/j.ccell.2018.03.004.

43. Tekle, G. E., N. Andreeva, and W. S. Garrett. "The role of the microbiome in the etiopathogenesis of colon cancer." *Annual Review of Physiology* 86, no. 1 (February 12, 2024): 453–78. https://doi.org/10.1146/annurev-physiol-042022-025619.

44. D'Antonio, D. L., S. Marchetti, P. Pignatelli, A. Piattelli, and M. C. Curia. "The oncobiome in gastroenteric and genitourinary cancers."

International Journal of Molecular Sciences 23, no. 17 (August 26, 2022): 9664. https://doi.org/10.3390/ijms23179664.

45. Kolobaric, A., C. Andreescu, E. Jašarević, C. H. Hong, H. W. Roh, J. Y. Cheong, et al. "Gut microbiome predicts cognitive function and depressive symptoms in late life." *Molecular Psychiatry* 29 (April 25, 2024): 3064–75. https://doi.org/10.1038/s41380-024-02551-3.

46. Luqman, A., M. He, A. Hassan, M. Ullah, L. Zhang, M. R. Khan, et al. "Mood and microbes: a comprehensive review of intestinal microbiota's impact on depression." *Frontiers in Psychiatry* 15 (February 9, 2024). https://doi.org/10.3389/fpsyt.2024.1295766.

47. McCollum, S. E., and Y. M. Shah. "Stressing out cancer: chronic stress induces dysbiosis and enhances colon cancer growth." *Cancer Research* 84, no. 5 (March 4, 2024): 645–47. https://doi.org/10.1158/0008-5472.can-23-3871.

48. Liu, Y., S. Tian, B. Ning, T. Huang, Y. Li, and Y. Wei. "Stress and cancer: the mechanisms of immune dysregulation and management." *Frontiers in Immunology* 13 (October 5, 2022). https://doi.org/10.3389/fimmu.2022.1032294.

49. Zajecka, J. M. "Treating depression to improve survival in coronary heart disease: What have we learned?" *Journal of the American College of Cardiology* 84, no. 3 (2024): 273–75. https://doi.org/10.1016/j.jacc.2024.06.019.

50. Zajecka, J. M. "Treating depression to improve survival in coronary heart disease: What have we learned?" *Journal of the American College of Cardiology* 84, no. 3 (2024): 273–75. https://doi.org/10.1016/j.jacc.2024.06.019.

51. National Cancer Institute. "Stress and cancer." U.S. Department of Health and Human Services. October 21, 2022. https://www.cancer.gov/about-cancer/coping/feelings/stress-fact-sheet.

Chapter 11. To Prevent the Recurrence of Misery: Cancer Relapse and Screening

1. Solzhenitsyn, A. I. *Cancer ward.* Farrar, Straus and Giroux. 1991. 296.

2. Vogelzang, N. J., D. Raghavan, and B. J. Kennedy. "VP-16-213 (etoposide): the mandrake root from Issyk-Kul." *American Journal of Medicine* 72, no. 1 (1982): 136–44. https://doi.org/10.1016/0002-9343(82)90600-3.

3. Division of Cancer Control and Population Sciences. "Statistics and Graphs." n.d. National Institutes of Health, National Cancer Institute. https://cancercontrol.cancer.gov/ocs/statistics#:~:text=As%20of%20

January%202022%2C%20it,approximately%205.4%25%20of%20the%20
population.&text=The%20number%20of%20cancer%20survivors%20
is%20projected%20to%20increase%20by,to%2022.5%20million%2C%
20by%202032.

4. American Society of Clinical Oncology. "Movement is medicine: structured exercise program challenge." December 13, 2024. https://www .asco.org/about-asco/press-center/news-releases/movement-medicine -structured-exercise-program-challenge.

5. Liu, S., and J. Wang. "Current and future perspectives of cell-free DNA in liquid biopsy." *Current Issues in Molecular Biology* 44, no. 6 (June 10, 2022): 2695–709. https://doi.org/10.3390/cimb44060184.

6. American Mathematical Society. "The legend of Abraham Wald." n.d. https://www.ams.org/publicoutreach/feature-column/fc-2016-06.

7. Hsiue, E. H.-C., T. J. Moore, and G. C. Alexander. "Estimated costs of pivotal trials for U.S. Food and Drug Administration–approved cancer drugs, 2015–2017." *Clinical Trials* 17, no. 2 (February 29, 2020): 119–25. https://doi.org/10.1177/1740774520907609.

8. Mole, B. "Big Pharma shells out $20B each year to schmooze docs, $6B on drug ads." Ars Technica. January 11, 2019. https://arstechnica.com /science/2019/01/healthcare-industry-spends-30b-on-marketing-most-of -it-goes-to-doctors/.

9. Surveillance, Epidemiology, and End Results Program. "Cancer Stat Facts: Pancreatic Cancer." National Institutes of Health, National Cancer Institute. n.d. https://seer.cancer.gov/statfacts/html/pancreas.html.

10. Kelly, S.-L. "Two early symptoms of 'silent killer' cancer have been identified." HuffPost UK. May 2, 2023. https://www.huffingtonpost.co.uk /entry/two-early-symptoms-of-silent-killer-cancer-have-been-identified _uk_64511692e4b04997b579f503#:~:text=Early%20Warning%20Signs%20 Of%20Pancreatic%20Cancer&text=Now%2C%20two%20symptoms%20 that%20can,thirst%20and%20dark%20yellow%20urine.

11. Barsouk, A., K. Saginala, J. S. Aluru, P. Rawla, and A. Barsouk. "US cancer screening recommendations: developments and the impact of COVID-19." *Medical Sciences* 10, no. 1 (March 1, 2022): 16. https://doi.org /10.3390/medsci10010016.

12. Kafka, F. *The trial*. Schocken Books. 1999. 1.

13. Kafka, F. *The trial*. Schocken Books. 1999. 55.

14. Naeim, R. M., R. A. Marouf, M. A. Nasr, and M. E. Abd El-Rahman. "Comparing the diagnostic efficacy of digital breast tomosynthesis with full-field digital mammography using BI-RADS scoring." *Egyptian Journal*

of Radiology and Nuclear Medicine 52, no. 1 (February 2, 2021). https://doi
.org/10.1186/s43055-021-00421-4.

15. Keen, J. D., and J. E. Keen. "What is the point: will screening
mammography save my life?" *BMC Medical Informatics and Decision
Making* 9, no. 1 (April 2, 2009). https://doi.org/10.1186/1472-6947-9-18.

16. Hendrick, R. E., J. A. Baker, and M. A. Helvie. "Breast cancer deaths
averted over 3 decades." *Cancer* 125, no. 9 (February 11, 2019): 1482–88.
https://doi.org/10.1002/cncr.31954.

17. Barsouk, A., K. Saginala, J. S. Aluru, P. Rawla, and A. Barsouk. "US
cancer screening recommendations: developments and the impact of
COVID-19." *Medical Sciences* 10, no. 1 (March 1, 2022): 16. https://doi.org
/10.3390/medsci10010016.

18. Cairns, A., V. M. Jones, K. Cronin, M. Yocobozzi, C. Howard,
N. Lesko, et al. "Impact of the COVID-19 pandemic on breast cancer
screening and operative treatment." *American Surgeon* 88, no. 6 (2022):
1051–53. https://doi.org/10.1177/00031348221087920.

19. Tan, S., and Y. Tatsumura. "George Papanicolaou (1883–1962):
discoverer of the Pap smear." *Singapore Medical Journal* 56, no. 10 (October 1, 2015): 586–87. https://doi.org/10.11622/smedj.2015155.

20. Barsouk, A., K. Saginala, J. S. Aluru, P. Rawla, and A. Barsouk. "US
cancer screening recommendations: developments and the impact of
COVID-19." *Medical Sciences* 10, no. 1 (March 1, 2022): 16. https://doi.org
/10.3390/medsci10010016.

21. Roche. "Roche launches a human papillomavirus (HPV) self-
sampling solution, expanding cervical cancer screening options." n.d.
https://diagnostics.roche.com/global/en/news-listing/2022/roche
-launches-a-human-papillomavirus-hpv-self-sampling-solution
-expanding-cervical-cancer-screening-options.html.

22. Powell, A. "Should colon cancer screening start at 40?" *Harvard
Gazette.* July 1, 2024. https://news.harvard.edu/gazette/story/2024/07
/should-colon-cancer-screening-start-at-40/.

23. Ahlquist, D. A. "Stool-based tests vs screening colonoscopy for the
detection of colorectal cancer." August 1, 2019. https://www.ncbi.nlm.nih
.gov/pmc/articles/PMC6771036/.

24. Maringe, C., J. Spicer, M. Morris, A. Purushotham, E. Nolte,
R. Sullivan, et al. "The impact of the COVID-19 pandemic on cancer deaths
due to delays in diagnosis in England, UK: a national, population-based,
modelling study." *Lancet Oncology* 21, no. 8 (July 20, 2020): 1023–34.
https://doi.org/10.1016/s1470-2045(20)30388-0.

25. Maringe, C., J. Spicer, M. Morris, A. Purushotham, E. Nolte, R. Sullivan, et al. "The impact of the COVID-19 pandemic on cancer deaths due to delays in diagnosis in England, UK: a national, population-based, modelling study." *Lancet Oncology* 21, no. 8 (July 20, 2020): 1023–34. https://doi.org/10.1016/s1470-2045(20)30388-0.

26. American Cancer Society. "Lung cancer screening guidelines." January 29, 2024. https://www.cancer.org/health-care-professionals /american-cancer-society-prevention-early-detection-guidelines/lung -cancer-screening-guidelines.html.

27. Carter-Bawa, L. "Shifting the lens on lung cancer screening inequities." *JAMA Network Open* 7, no. 5 (2024): e2412782. https://doi.org/10.1001 /jamanetworkopen.2024.12782.

28. Maringe, C., J. Spicer, M. Morris, A. Purushotham, E. Nolte, R. Sullivan, et al. "The impact of the COVID-19 pandemic on cancer deaths due to delays in diagnosis in England, UK: a national, population-based, modelling study." *Lancet Oncology* 21, no. 8 (July 20, 2020): 1023–34. https://doi.org/10.1016/s1470-2045(20)30388-0.

29. Jacklin, C., Y. Philippou, S. F. Brewster, and R. J. Bryant. 'More men die with prostate cancer than because of it' - an old adage that still holds true in the 21st century." *Cancer Treatment and Research Communications* 26 (2021): 100225. https://doi.org/10.1016/j.ctarc.2020 .100225.

30. Branca, M. "GC Genome Corp. releases results on liquid biopsy study." Inside Precision Medicine. August 22, 2023. https://www .insideprecisionmedicine.com/topics/molecular-dx-topic/liquid-biopsies /gc-genome-corp-releases-results-on-liquid-biopsy-study/.

31. Research and Markets. "Cell free DNA (cfDNA) testing market outlook to 2028 & 2033: projected to generate revenues of $20.63 billion by 2028, fueled by advances in liquid biopsy and personalized medicine." GlobeNewswire. December 13, 2024. https://www.globenewswire.com /news-release/2024/12/13/2996876/28124/en/Cell-Free-DNA-cfDNA -Testing-Market-Outlook-to-2028-2033-Projected-to-Generate -Revenues-of-20-63-Billion-by-2028-Fueled-by-Advances-in-Liquid -Biopsy-and-Personalized-Medicine.html:contentReference {index=2}.

32. WTOP News. "Breast cancer vaccine results promising: moves to next stage in clinical trials." Accessed May 16, 2025. https://wtop.com /health-fitness/2025/03/breast-cancer-vaccine-results-promising-moves -to-next-stage-in-clinical-trials/.

33. Park, A., and E. Solano. "The race to make a vaccine for breast cancer." *TIME*. October 6, 2022. https://time.com/6220114/breast-cancer -vaccine-development/.

34. American Cancer Society. "Immune checkpoint inhibitors and their side effects." n.d. https://www.cancer.org/cancer/managing-cancer /treatment-types/immunotherapy/immune-checkpoint-inhibitors .html#:~:text=PD%2D1%20and%20PD%2DL1%20inhibitors,-PD%2D1%20 is&text=It%20normally%20acts%20as%20a,leave%20the%20other%20 cell%20alone.

35. Das, S., and D. B. Johnson. "Immune-related adverse events and anti-tumor efficacy of immune checkpoint inhibitors." *Journal for Immuno-Therapy of Cancer* 7, no. 1 (2019): 306. https://doi.org/10.1186/s40425-019 -0805-8.

36. Kuah, C. Y., R. Monfries, M. Quartagno, M. J. Seckl, and E. Gho-rani. "What is the optimal duration, dose and frequency for anti-PD1 therapy of non-small cell lung cancer?" *Therapeutic Advances in Medical Oncology* 15 (2023): 17588359231210271. https://doi.org/10.1177 /17588359231210271.

37. Penn Medicine. "What is CAR T therapy?" December 13, 2024. https://www.pennmedicine.org/cancer/navigating-cancer-care/treatment -types/immunotherapy/what-is-car-t-therapy.

38. Chesney, J. A., A. Ribas, G. V. Long, J. M. Kirkwood, R. Dummer, I. Puzanov, et al. "Randomized, double-blind, placebo-controlled, global phase III Trial of talimogene laherparepvec combined with pembroli-zumab for advanced melanoma." *Journal of Clinical Oncology* 41, no. 3 (August 23, 2022): 528–40. https://doi.org/10.1200/jco.22.00343.

Chapter 12. Some Are More Equal: Cancer Disparities and Health Care Reform

1. KFF. "Key data on health and health care by race and ethnicity." June 11, 2024. https://www.kff.org/key-data-on-health-and-health-care-by -race-and-ethnicity/?entry=executive-summary-key-takeaways.

2. Tong, M., L. Hill, and S. Artiga. "Racial disparities in cancer out-comes, screening, and treatment." KFF. February 3, 2022. https://www.kff .org/racial-equity-and-health-policy/issue-brief/racial-disparities-in -cancer-outcomes-screening-and-treatment/.

3. Tuskegee University. "About the USPHS syphilis study." n.d. https:// www.tuskegee.edu/about-us/centers-of-excellence/bioethics-center/about -the-usphs-syphilis-study.

4. Tuskegee University. "About the USPHS syphilis study." n.d. https://www.tuskegee.edu/about-us/centers-of-excellence/bioethics-center/about-the-usphs-syphilis-study.

5. BBC News. "Henrietta Lacks: 'mother' of modern medicine honoured." October 13, 2021. https://www.bbc.com/news/world-us-canada-58903934.

6. Barsouk, A., O. Elghawy, J. H. Sussman, J. Xu, R. Mamtani, and L. Mei. "Survival disparities by race in advanced urothelial carcinoma (aUC): A real-world analysis." Supplement, *Journal of Clinical Oncology* 43, no. 5 (February 18, 2025): 668. https://doi.org/10.1200/JCO.2025.43.5_suppl.668.

7. Dehal, A., A. Abbas, and S. Johna. "Racial disparities in clinical presentation, surgical treatment and in-hospital outcomes of women with breast cancer: analysis of nationwide inpatient sample database." *Breast Cancer Research and Treatment* 139, no. 2 (May 20, 2013): 561–69. https://doi.org/10.1007/s10549-013-2567-1.

8. Darden, M., G. Parker, D. Monlezun, E. Anderson, and J. F. Buell. "Race and gender disparity in the surgical management of hepatocellular cancer: analysis of the Surveillance, Epidemiology, and End Results (SEER) program registry." *World Journal of Surgery* 45, no. 8 (April 23, 2021): 2538–45. https://doi.org/10.1007/s00268-021-06091-7.

9. Bliton, J. N., M. Parides, P. Muscarella, K. T. Papalezova, and H. In. "Understanding racial disparities in gastrointestinal cancer outcomes: lack of surgery contributes to lower survival in African American patients." *Cancer Epidemiology, Biomarkers & Prevention* 30, no. 3 (December 10, 2020): 529–38. https://doi.org/10.1158/1055-9965.epi-20-0950.

10. Pellini, B., and A. A. Chaudhuri. "Racial disparities in early-stage NSCLC treatment: a call for action." *Cancer Epidemiology, Biomarkers & Prevention* 33, no. 6 (April 8, 2024): 769–70. https://doi.org/10.1158/1055-9965.epi-24-0339.

11. Torres, J. M., M. O. Sodipo, M. F. Hopkins, P. D. Chandler, and E. T. Warner. "Racial differences in breast cancer survival between black and white women according to tumor subtype: a systematic review and meta-analysis." *Journal of Clinical Oncology* 42, no. 32 (September 17, 2024). https://doi.org/10.1200/jco.23.02311.

12. White, A., D. Joseph, S. H. Rim, C. J. Johnson, M. P. Coleman, and C. Allemani. "Colon cancer survival in the United States by race and stage (2001–2009): findings from the CONCORD-2 study." *Cancer* 123, no. S24 (December 5, 2017): 5014–36. https://doi.org/10.1002/cncr.31076.

13. Alberg, A. J., M. V. Brock, J. G. Ford, J. M. Samet, and S. D. Spivack. "Epidemiology of lung cancer." *CHEST* 143, no. 5 (May 1, 2013): e1S–e29S. https://doi.org/10.1378/chest.12-2345.

14. Giaquinto, A. N., K. D. Miller, K. Y. Tossas, R. A. Winn, A. Jemal, and R. L. Siegel. "Cancer statistics for African American/Black people 2022." *Cancer Journal for Clinicians* 72, no. 3 (February 10, 2022): 202–29. https://doi.org/10.3322/caac.21718.

15. Din, N. U., O. C. Ukoumunne, G. Rubin, W. Hamilton, B. Carter, S. Stapley, et al. "Age and gender variations in cancer diagnostic intervals in 15 cancers: analysis of data from the UK Clinical Practice Research Datalink." *PLoS ONE* 10, no. 5 (May 15, 2015): e0127717. https://doi.org/10.1371/journal.pone.0127717.

16. Huebschmann, A., and A. Regensteiner. "Women are at a higher risk of dying from heart disease, in part because doctors don't take major sex and gender differences into account." The Conversation. October 22, 2024. https://theconversation.com/women-are-at-a-higher-risk-of-dying-from-heart-disease-in-part-because-doctors-dont-take-major-sex-and-gender-differences-into-account-233861.

17. Toren, P., A. Wilkins, K. Patel, A. Burley, T. Gris, R. Kockelbergh, et al. "The sex gap in bladder cancer survival—a8 missing link in bladder cancer care?" *Nature Reviews Urology* 21, no. 3 (August 21, 2023): 181–92. https://doi.org/10.1038/s41585-023-00806-2.

18. Stewart, S. L., R. Harewood, M. Matz, S. H. Rim, S. A. Sabatino, K. C. Ward, et al. "Disparities in ovarian cancer survival in the United States (2001–2009): findings from the CONCORD-2 study." *Cancer* 123, no. S24 (December 5, 2017): 5138–59. https://doi.org/10.1002/cncr.31027.

19. Plug, I., S. van Dulmen, W. Stommel, T. C. olde Hartman, and E. Das. "Physicians' and patients' interruptions in clinical practice: a quantitative analysis." *Annals of Family Medicine* 20, no. 5 (September 1, 2022): 423–29. https://doi.org/10.1370/afm.2846.

20. Takeshita, J., S. Wang, A. W. Loren, N. Mitra, J. Shults, D. B. Shin, et al. "Association of racial/ethnic and gender concordance between patients and physicians with patient experience ratings." *JAMA Network Open* 3, no. 11 (November 9, 2020): e2024583. https://doi.org/10.1001/jamanetworkopen.2020.24583.

21. Victor, R. G., K. Lynch, N. Li, C. Blyler, E. Muhammad, J. Handler, et al. "A cluster-randomized trial of blood-pressure reduction in Black barbershops." *New England Journal of Medicine* 378, no. 14 (March 12, 2018): 1291–1301. https://doi.org/10.1056/nejmoa1717250.

22. Sizer, W., and Y. Conyers. "BarberED then screened: disrupting the colorectal cancer disparity in urban Black men." *Journal of the American Association of Nurse Practitioners* 34, no. 6 (May 16, 2022): 859–65. https://doi.org/10.1097/jxx.0000000000000725.

23. Hart, A., S. M. Underwood, W. R. Smith, D. J. Bowen, B. M. Rivers, R. A. Jones, et al. "Recruiting African-American barbershops for prostate cancer education." *Journal of the National Medical Association* 100, no. 9 (September 1, 2008): 1012–20. https://doi.org/10.1016/s0027-9684(15) 31437-1.

24. "Historical." n.d. https://www.cms.gov/data-research/statistics -trends-and-reports/national-health-expenditure-data/historical#:~:text =U.S.%20health%20care%20spending%20grew,trillion%20or%20 %2413%2C493%20per%20person.

25. Worldometer. "Life expectancy by country and in the world (2024)." n.d. https://www.worldometers.info/demographics/life-expectancy/.

26. Rosenthal, E. "Survey: 79 million Americans have problems with medical bills or debt." The Commonwealth Fund. June 16, 2022. https:// www.commonwealthfund.org/publications/newsletter-article/survey-79 -million-americans-have-problems-medical-bills-or-debt.

27. Rakshit, S., M. McGough, L. Cotter, and G. Claxton "The burden of medical debt in the United States." Peterson-KFF Health System Tracker. February 12, 2024. Retrieved from https://www.healthsystemtracker.org /brief/the-burden-of-medical-debt-in-the-united-states/.

28. Smith, E. R. "A two-tiered health care system: is there anything new?" *Canadian Journal of Cardiology* 23, no. 11 (2007): 915–16. https://doi .org/10.1016/s0828-282x(07)70852-8.

29. Wallace, L. S. "A view of health care around the world." *Annals of Family Medicine* 11, no. 1 (2013): 84. https://doi.org/10.1370/afm.1484.

30. Soril, L. J. J., T. Adams, M. Phipps-Taylor, U. Winblad, and F. Clement. "Is Canadian healthcare affordable? A comparative analysis of the Canadian healthcare system from 2004 to 2014." *Health Policy* 13, no. 1 (2017): 43–58. https://doi.org/10.12927/hcpol.2017.25192.

31. Marshall, E. G., L. Miller, and L. R. Moritz. "Challenges and impacts from wait times for specialist care identified by primary care providers: results from the MAAP study cross-sectional survey." *Healthcare Management Forum* 36, no. 5 (202): 340–46. https://doi.org/10.1177/08404704231182671.

32. Stevens, A. J., Y. Boukari, S. English, A. Kadir, B. N. Kumar, and D. Devakumar. "Discriminatory, racist and xenophobic policies and practice against child refugees, asylum seekers and undocumented

migrants in European health systems." *Lancet Regional Health - Europe* 41 (2024): 100834. https://doi.org/10.1016/j.lanepe.2023.100834.

33. Scott, Dylan. "Medicaid is a hassle for doctors. That's hurting patients." Vox. June 7, 2021. https://www.vox.com/2021/6/7/22522479/medicaid-health-insurance-doctors-billing-research.

34. Bryan, A. F., and T. C. Tsai. "Health insurance profitability during the COVID-19 pandemic." *Annals of Surgery* 273, no. 3 (2021): e88–e90. https://doi.org/10.1097/SLA.0000000000004696.

35. Lo, J., M. Long, R. Wallace, M. Salaga, and K. Pestaina. (January 27, 2025). "Claims denials and appeals in ACA Marketplace plans in 2023." KFF. https://www.kff.org/private-insurance/issue-brief/claims-denials-and-appeals-in-aca-marketplace-plans-in-2023/.0.

36. Lopes, L., A. Montero, M. Presiado, and L. Hamel. "Americans' challenges with health care costs." KFF. May 7, 2024. https://www.kff.org/health-costs/issue-brief/americans-challenges-with-health-care-costs/.

37. Suozzo, A., A. Glassford, A. Ngu, and B. Roberts. "Upmc." ProPublica. May 9, 2013. https://projects.propublica.org/nonprofits/organizations/208295721.

38. Landman, K. "The profit-obsessed monster destroying American emergency rooms." Vox. October 3, 2024. https://www.vox.com/health-care/374820/emergency-rooms-private-equity-hospitals-profits-no-surprises.

39. Martin-Misener, R., P. Harbman, F. Donald, K. Reid, K. Kilpatrick, N. Carter, et al. "Cost-effectiveness of nurse practitioners in primary and specialised ambulatory care: systematic review." *BMJ Open* 5, no. 6 (June 1, 2015): e007167. https://doi.org/10.1136/bmjopen-2014-007167.

40. Antkowiak, P. S., S.-Y. Lai, R. C. Burke, M. Janes, T. Zawi, N. I. Shapiro, et al. "Characterizing malpractice cases involving emergency department advanced practice providers, physicians in training, and attending physicians." *Academic Emergency Medicine* 30, no. 12 (September 8, 2023): 1237–45. https://doi.org/10.1111/acem.14800.

41. Mafi, J. N., A. Chen, R. Guo, K. Choi, P. Smulowitz, C.-H. Tseng, et al. "US emergency care patterns among nurse practitioners and physician assistants compared with physicians: a cross-sectional analysis." *BMJ Open* 12, no. 4 (April 1, 2022): e055138. https://doi.org/10.1136/bmjopen-2021-055138.

42. Carranza, A. N., P. J. Munoz, and A. J. Nash. "Comparing quality of care in medical specialties between nurse practitioners and physicians." *Journal of the American Association of Nurse Practitioners* 33, no. 3 (May 6, 2020): 184–93. https://doi.org/10.1097/jxx.0000000000000394.

43. AAMC. "New AAMC report shows continuing projected physician shortage." March 26, 2024. https://www.aamc.org/news/press-releases/new-aamc-report-shows-continuing-projected-physician-shortage.

44. Jena, A. B. "Is an 80-hour workweek enough to train a doctor?" *Harvard Business Review.* July 12, 2019. https://hbr.org/2019/07/is-an-80-hour-workweek-enough-to-train-a-doctor.

45. Ledley, F. D., S. S. McCoy, G. Vaughan, and E. G. Cleary. "Profitability of large pharmaceutical companies compared with other large public companies." *JAMA* 323, no. 9 (2020): 834–43. https://doi.org/10.1001/jama.2020.0442.

46. The White House. "FACT SHEET: Biden-Harris administration announces new, lower prices for first ten drugs selected for Medicare price negotiation to lower costs for millions of Americans." August 15, 2024. https://www.whitehouse.gov/briefing-room/statements-releases/2024/08/15/fact-sheet-biden-harris-administration-announces-new-lower-prices-for-first-ten-drugs-selected-for-medicare-price-negotiation-to-lower-costs-for-millions-of-americans/.

47. Health Resources and Services Administration. "340B Drug Pricing Program." October 1, 2024. https://www.hrsa.gov/opa.

48. American Medical Association. "New AMA analysis of consolidation in PBM markets." September 9, 2024. Press release. https://www.ama-assn.org/press-center/ama-press-releases/new-ama-analysis-consolidation-pbm-markets.

49. ProPublica. "Upmc." May 9, 2013. https://projects.propublica.org/nonprofits/organizations/208295721.

Chapter 13. The Art of Living and Dying Well: Palliative and End-of-Life Care

1. Tolstoy, L. *The Death of Ivan Ilyich.* https://www.goodreads.com/quotes/7865258-what-tormented-ivan-ilyich-most-was-the-deception-the-lie.

Conclusion

1. Islami, F., E. C. Marlow, B. Thomson, M. L. McCullough, H. Rumgay, S. M. Gapstur, et al. "Proportion and number of cancer cases and deaths attributable to potentially modifiable risk factors in the United States, 2019." *CA: A Cancer Journal for Clinicians* 74, no. 5 (July 11, 2024): 405–32. https://doi.org/10.3322/caac.21858.

Bibliography

AAMC. "New AAMC Report Shows Continuing Projected Physician Shortage," March 26, 2024. https://www.aamc.org/news/press-releases /new-aamc-report-shows-continuing-projected-physician-shortage.

Ahmed, Niyaz. "23 years of the discovery of *Helicobacter pylori*: Is the debate over?" *Annals of Clinical Microbiology and Antimicrobials* 4, no. 1 (October 31, 2005). https://doi.org/10.1186/1476-0711-4-17.

Alberg, Anthony J., Malcolm V. Brock, Jean G. Ford, Jonathan M. Samet, and Simon D. Spivack. "Epidemiology of Lung Cancer." *CHEST Journal* 143, no. 5 (May 1, 2013): e1S-e29S. https://doi.org/10.1378/chest.12-2345.

American Cancer Society. "Lifetime Risk of Developing or Dying From Cancer," n.d. https://www.cancer.org/cancer/risk-prevention /understanding-cancer-risk/lifetime-probability-of-developing-or -dying-from-cancer.html

Arif, Irtaqa, Matthew D. Adams, and Marc T.J. Johnson. "A meta-analysis of the carcinogenic effects of particulate matter and polycyclic aromatic hydrocarbons." *Environmental Pollution*, April 1, 2024, 123941. https:// doi.org/10.1016/j.envpol.2024.123941.

Arnold, Melina, Suzanne P. Moore, Sven Hassler, Lis Ellison-Loschmann, David Forman, and Freddie Bray. "The burden of stomach cancer in indigenous populations: a systematic review and global assessment." *Gut* 63, no. 1 (October 23, 2013): 64–71. https://doi.org/10.1136/gutjnl -2013-305033.

Attanoos, Richard L., Andrew Churg, Francoise Galateau-Salle, Allen R. Gibbs, and Victor L. Roggli. "Malignant Mesothelioma and Its Non-Asbestos Causes." *Archives of Pathology & Laboratory Medicine* 142, no. 6 (February 26, 2018): 753–60. https://doi.org/10.5858/arpa.2017 -0365-ra.

Bagnardi, V., M. Rota, E. Botteri, I. Tramacere, F. Islami, V. Fedirko, L. Scotti, et al. "Alcohol consumption and site-specific cancer risk: a comprehensive dose–response meta-analysis." *British Journal of Cancer* 112, no. 3 (November 25, 2014): 580–93. https://doi.org/10.1038/bjc .2014.579.

Behrens, Thomas, Calvin Ge, Roel Vermeulen, Benjamin Kendzia, Ann Olsson, Joachim Schüz, Hans Kromhout, et al. "Occupational exposure to nickel and hexavalent chromium and the risk of lung cancer in a pooled analysis of case-control studies (SYNERGY)." *International Journal of Cancer* 152, no. 4 (September 2, 2022): 645–60. https://doi.org /10.1002/ijc.34272.

Bibbins-Domingo, K., D. C. Grossman, S. J. Curry, K. W. Davidson, M. Ebell, J. W. Epling, F. A. R. García, M. W. Gillman, A. R. Kemper, A. H. Krist, et al. "Screening for skin cancer US preventive services task force recommendation statement." *JAMA-J. Am. Med. Assoc.* 2016, *22*, 652–665.

Bliton, John N., Michael Parides, Peter Muscarella, Katia T. Papalezova, and Haejin In. "Understanding Racial Disparities in Gastrointestinal Cancer Outcomes: Lack of Surgery Contributes to Lower Survival in African American Patients." *Cancer Epidemiology Biomarkers & Prevention* 30, no. 3 (December 10, 2020): 529–38. https://doi.org/10.1158 /1055-9965.epi-20-0950.

Cao, Yin, Walter C. Willett, Eric B. Rimm, Meir J. Stampfer, and Edward L. Giovannucci. "Light to moderate intake of alcohol, drinking patterns, and risk of cancer: results from two prospective US cohort studies." *BMJ*, August 18, 2015, h4238. https://doi.org/10.1136/bmj.h4238.

de Nie, I., C. J. M. de Blok, T. M. van der Sluis, et al. "Prostate Cancer Incidence under Androgen Deprivation: Nationwide Cohort Study in Trans Women Receiving Hormone Treatment." *J Clin Endocrinol Metab.* 2020;105(9):e3293–e3299. doi:10.1210/clinem/dgaa412.

Dehal, Ahmed, Ali Abbas, and Samir Johna. "Racial disparities in clinical presentation, surgical treatment and in-hospital outcomes of women with breast cancer: analysis of nationwide inpatient sample database." *Breast Cancer Research and Treatment* 139, no. 2 (May 20, 2013): 561–69. https://doi.org/10.1007/s10549-013-2567-1.

Denk, D., F. R. Grete. "Inflammation: the incubator of the tumor microenvironment." *Trends Cancer.* 2022;8(11):901–914. doi:10.1016/j .trecan.2022.07.002.

Diallo, Abou, Mélanie Deschasaux, Paule Latino-Martel, Serge Hercberg, Pilar Galan, Philippine Fassier, Benjamin Allès, Françoise Guéraud, Fabrice H. Pierre, and Mathilde Touvier. "Red and processed meat intake and cancer risk: Results from the prospective NutriNet-Santé cohort study." *International Journal of Cancer* 142, no. 2 (September 15, 2017): 230–37. https://doi.org/10.1002/ijc.31046.

Din, Nafees U., Obioha C. Ukoumunne, Greg Rubin, William Hamilton, Ben Carter, Sal Stapley, and Richard D. Neal. "Age and Gender Variations in Cancer Diagnostic Intervals in 15 Cancers: Analysis of Data from the UK Clinical Practice Research Datalink." *PLoS ONE* 10, no. 5 (May 15, 2015): e0127717. https://doi.org/10.1371/journal.pone.0127717.

Doll, R., and A. B. Hill. "Smoking and Carcinoma of the Lung: Preliminary Report." *British Medical Journal*, 2(4682), (1950): 739–748.

Dryson, Evan, Andrea 't Mannetje, Chris Walls, Dave McLean, Fiona McKenzie, Milena Maule, Soo Cheng, et al. "Case-control study of high-risk occupations for bladder cancer in New Zealand." *International Journal of Cancer* 122, no. 6 (November 20, 2007): 1340–46. https://doi.org/10.1002/ijc.23194.

Du Plessis, M., C. Fourie, J. Riedemann, W.J.S. de Villiers, and A.M. Engelbrecht. "Cancer and Covid-19: Collectively catastrophic." *Cytokine & Growth Factor Reviews* 63 (October 25, 2021): 78–89. https://doi.org/10.1016/j.cytogfr.2021.10.005.

Eidy, Mountaha, Angela C. Regina, and Kevin Tishkowski. "Radon Toxicity." StatPearls - NCBI Bookshelf. January 26, 2024. https://www.ncbi.nlm.nih.gov/books/NBK562321/.

Floud, Sarah, Carol Hermon, Rachel F. Simpson, and Gillian K. Reeves. "Alcohol consumption and cancer incidence in women: interaction with smoking, body mass index and menopausal hormone therapy." *BMC Cancer* 23, no. 1 (August 16, 2023). https://doi.org/10.1186/s12885-023-11184-8.

Fortner, Renée T., Kathryn L. Terry, Noemi Bender, Nicole Brenner, Katrin Hufnagel, Julia Butt, Tim Waterboer, and Shelley S. Tworoger. "Sexually transmitted infections and risk of epithelial ovarian cancer: results from the Nurses' Health Studies." *British Journal of Cancer* 120, no. 8 (March 21, 2019): 855–60. https://doi.org/10.1038/s41416-019-0422-9.

Frisch, Morten, Bengt Glimelius, Adriaan J.C. van den Brule, Jan Wohlfahrt, Chris J.L.M. Meijer, Jan M.M. Walboomers, Sven Goldman, Christer Svensson, Hans-Olov Adami, and Mads Melbye. "Sexually Transmitted Infection as a Cause of Anal Cancer." *New England Journal of Medicine* 337, no. 19 (November 6, 1997): 1350–58. https://doi.org/10.1056/nejm199711063371904.

Fu, Shiting, Hao Ke, Huozhong Yuan, Huaimeng Xu, Wenyan Chen, and Limin Zhao. "Dual role of pregnancy in breast cancer risk." *General and Comparative Endocrinology* 352 (March 26, 2024): 114501. https://doi.org/10.1016/j.ygcen.2024.114501.

Goodman, Elizabeth, Marisa Felsher, Dong Wang, Lixia Yao, and Ya-Ting Chen. "Early Initiation of HPV Vaccination and Series Completion in

Early and Mid-Adolescence." *Pediatrics* 151, no. 3 (February 27, 2023). https://doi.org/10.1542/peds.2022-058794.

Gordon, L. G., A. J. Rodriguez-Acevedo, B. Køster, G. P. Guy, Jr., C. Sinclair, E. Van Deventer, A. C. Green "Association of Indoor Tanning Regulations With Health and Economic Outcomes in North America and Europe." *JAMA Dermatol. 156*, 2020: 401–410.

Goswami, Sohini, Satadal Adhikary, Suchandra Bhattacharya, Ruchika Agarwal, Abhratanu Ganguly, Sayantani Nanda, and Prem Rajak. "The alarming link between environmental microplastics and health hazards with special emphasis on cancer." *Life Sciences* 355 (August 3, 2024): 122937. https://doi.org/10.1016/j.lfs.2024.122937.

Guo, Chong, Bo Zhan, Meng-Yuan Li, Li Yue, and Chao Zhang. "Association between oral contraceptives and cervical cancer: A retrospective case–control study based on the National Health and Nutrition Examination Survey." *Frontiers in Pharmacology* 15 (July 17, 2024). https://doi.org/10.3389/fphar.2024.1400667.

Hart, Alton, Sandra M. Underwood, Wally R. Smith, Deborah J. Bowen, Brian M. Rivers, Randy A. Jones, Dennis Parker, and Johnnie Allen. "Recruiting African-American Barbershops for Prostate Cancer Education." *Journal of the National Medical Association* 100, no. 9 (September 1, 2008): 1012–20. https://doi.org/10.1016/s0027-9684(15)31437-1.

Hashibe, Mia, Hal Morgenstern, Yan Cui, Donald P. Tashkin, Zuo-Feng Zhang, Wendy Cozen, Thomas M. Mack, and Sander Greenland. "Marijuana Use and the Risk of Lung and Upper Aerodigestive Tract Cancers: Results of a Population-Based Case-Control Study." *Cancer Epidemiology Biomarkers & Prevention* 15, no. 10 (October 1, 2006): 1829–34. https://doi.org/10.1158/1055-9965.epi-06-0330.

Heymsfield, S. B., C. M. Peterson, D. M. Thomas, M. Heo, and J. M. Schuna. "Why are there race/ethnic differences in adult body mass index–adiposity relationships? A quantitative critical review." *Obesity Reviews* 17, no. 3 (December 11, 2015): 262–75. https://doi.org/10.1111/obr.12358.

Husby, Anders, Jan Wohlfahrt, and Mads Melbye. "Pregnancy duration and ovarian cancer risk: A 50-year nationwide cohort study." *International Journal of Cancer* 151, no. 10 (June 25, 2022): 1717–25. https://doi.org/10.1002/ijc.34192.

Iversen, Lisa, Selvaraj Sivasubramaniam, Amanda J. Lee, Shona Fielding, and Philip C. Hannaford. "Lifetime cancer risk and combined oral contraceptives: the Royal College of General Practitioners' Oral

Contraception Study." *American Journal of Obstetrics and Gynecology* 216, no. 6 (February 8, 2017): 580.e1-580.e9. https://doi.org/10.1016/j .ajog.2017.02.002.

Iyengar N. M., A. Gucalp, A. J. Dannenberg, and C. A. Hudis. "Obesity and Cancer Mechanisms: Tumor Microenvironment and Inflammation." *Journal of Clinical Oncology: Official Journal of the American Society of Clinical Oncology.* 2016 Dec;34(35):4270–4276. DOI: 10.1200/ jco.2016.67.4283. PMID: 27903155; PMCID: PMC5562428.

Jepsen, Peter, Frederik Kraglund, Joe West, Gerda E. Villadsen, Henrik Toft Sørensen, and Hendrik Vilstrup. "Risk of hepatocellular carcinoma in Danish outpatients with alcohol-related cirrhosis." *Journal of Hepatology* 73, no. 5 (June 5, 2020): 1030–36. https://doi.org/10.1016/j.jhep .2020.05.043.

Kamolratanakul, Supitcha, and Punnee Pitisuttithum. "Human Papillomavirus Vaccine Efficacy and Effectiveness against Cancer." *Vaccines* 9, no. 12 (November 30, 2021): 1413. https://doi.org/10.3390/vaccines9121413.

Karlsson, Torgny, Therese Johansson, Julia Höglund, Weronica E. Ek, and Åsa Johansson. "Time-Dependent Effects of Oral Contraceptive Use on Breast, Ovarian, and Endometrial Cancers." *Cancer Research* 81, no. 4 (February 15, 2021): 1153–62. https://doi.org/10.1158/0008-5472.can-20 -2476.

Kimanya, Martin E., Michael N. Routledge, Emmanuel Mpolya, Chibundu N. Ezekiel, Candida P. Shirima, and Yun Yun Gong. "Estimating the risk of aflatoxin-induced liver cancer in Tanzania based on biomarker data." *PLoS ONE* 16, no. 3 (March 11, 2021): e0247281. https:// doi.org/10.1371/journal.pone.0247281.

Knoops, Kim T. B., Lisette C. P. G. M. de Groot, Daan Kromhout, Anne-Elisabeth Perrin, Olga Moreiras-Varela, Alessandro Menotti, and Wija A. van Staveren. "Mediterranean Diet, Lifestyle Factors, and 10-Year Mortality in Elderly European Men and Women." *JAMA* 292, no. 12 (September 21, 2004): 1433. https://doi.org/10.1001/jama.292.12.1433.

Kolobaric, A., C. Andreescu, E. Jašarević, C. H. Hong, H. W. Roh, J. Y. Cheong, Y. K. Kim, et al. "Gut microbiome predicts cognitive function and depressive symptoms in late life." *Molecular Psychiatry*, April 25, 2024. https://doi.org/10.1038/s41380-024-02551-3.

Larson, Heidi J., Emmanuela Gakidou, and Christopher J.L. Murray. "The Vaccine-Hesitant Moment." *New England Journal of Medicine* 387, no. 1 (June 29, 2022): 58–65. https://doi.org/10.1056/nejmra2106441.

Leonard, Sophie V. L., Catriona R. Liddle, Charlotte A. Atherall, Emma Chapman, Matthew Watkins, Simon D. J. Calaminus, and Jeanette M. Rotchell. "Microplastics in human blood: Polymer types, concentrations and characterisation using μFTIR." *Environment International* 188 (May 14, 2024): 108751. https://doi.org/10.1016/j.envint.2024.108751.

Li, Jia, Haocheng Bai, Hao Qiao, Chong Du, Peizhuo Yao, Yu Zhang, Yifan Cai, et al. "Causal effects of COVID-19 on cancer risk: A Mendelian randomization study." *Journal of Medical Virology* 95, no. 4 (April 1, 2023). https://doi.org/10.1002/jmv.28722.

Li, Na, Zhen Zhai, Yi Zheng, Shuai Lin, Yujiao Deng, Grace Xiang, Jia Yao, et al. "Association of 13 Occupational Carcinogens in Patients With Cancer, Individually and Collectively, 1990–2017." *JAMA Network Open* 4, no. 2 (February 18, 2021): e2037530. https://doi.org/10.1001/jamanetworkopen .2020.37530.

Li, Wenjie, and Wei Wang. "Causal effects of exposure to ambient air pollution on cancer risk: Insights from genetic evidence." *The Science of the Total Environment* 912 (February 1, 2024): 168843. https://doi.org/10.1016 /j.scitotenv.2023.168843.

Liu, Yixin, Sheng Tian, Biao Ning, Tianhe Huang, Yi Li, and Yongchang Wei. "Stress and cancer: The mechanisms of immune dysregulation and management." *Frontiers in Immunology* 13 (October 5, 2022). https://doi.org/10.3389/fimmu.2022.1032294.

Ma, Yanlei, Yongzhi Yang, Feng Wang, Peng Zhang, Chenzhang Shi, Yang Zou, and Huanlong Qin. "Obesity and Risk of Colorectal Cancer: A Systematic Review of Prospective Studies." *PLoS ONE* 8, no. 1 (January 17, 2013): e53916. https://doi.org/10.1371/journal.pone.0053916.

Mannetje, Andrea 't, Vladimir Bencko, Paul Brennan, David Zaridze, Neonila Szeszenia-Dabrowska, Peter Rudnai, Jolanta Lissowska, et al. "Occupational exposure to metal compounds and lung cancer. Results from a multi-center case–control study in Central/Eastern Europe and UK." *Cancer Causes & Control* 22, no. 12 (September 29, 2011): 1669–80. https://doi.org/10.1007/s10552-011-9843-3.

Marks, Dustin H., Sarah Tuttleton Arron, and Matthew Mansh. "Skin Cancer and Skin Cancer Risk Factors in Sexual and Gender Minorities." *Dermatologic Clinics* 38, no. 2 (November 23, 2019): 209–18. https://doi .org/10.1016/j.det.2019.10.005.

Martin-Misener, Ruth, Patricia Harbman, Faith Donald, Kim Reid, Kelley Kilpatrick, Nancy Carter, Denise Bryant-Lukosius, et al. "Cost-effectiveness of nurse practitioners in primary and specialised ambulatory care: systematic review." *BMJ Open*5, no. 6 (June 1, 2015): e007167. https://doi.org/10.1136/bmjopen-2014-007167.

Mauri, Gianluca, Andrea Sartore-Bianchi, Antonio-Giampiero Russo, Silvia Marsoni, Alberto Bardelli, and Salvatore Siena. "Early-onset colorectal cancer in young individuals." *Molecular Oncology* 13, no. 2 (December 6, 2018): 109–31. https://doi.org/10.1002/1878-0261.12417.

Mørch, Lina Steinrud, Amani Meaidi, Giulia Corn, Marie Hargreave, and Charlotte Wessel Skovlund. "Breast Cancer in Users of Levonorgestrel-Releasing Intrauterine Systems." *JAMA*, October 16, 2024. https://doi .org/10.1001/jama.2024.18575.

Murugathasan, Mayoorey, Ardavan Jafari, Amandeep Amandeep, Syed A. Hassan, Matthew Chihata, and Ali A. Abdul-Sater. "Moderate exercise induces trained immunity in macrophages." *AJP Cell Physiology* 325, no. 2 (June 12, 2023): C429–42. https://doi.org/10.1152/ajpcell.00130 .2023.

Nielsen, Kristoffer Juul, Kathrine Kronberg Jakobsen, Jakob Schmidt Jensen, Christian Grønhøj, and Christian Von Buchwald. "The Effect of Prophylactic HPV Vaccines on Oral and Oropharyngeal HPV Infection—A Systematic Review." *Viruses* 13, no. 7 (July 11, 2021): 1339. https://doi.org/10.3390/v13071339.

Okamoto, Katie. "Black Plastic Kitchen Tools Might Expose You to Toxic Chemicals. Here's What to Use Instead." Wirecutter: Reviews for the Real World. November 23, 2024. https://www.nytimes.com/wirecutter /reviews/toxic-black-plastic-kitchen-alternatives/.

Pellini, Bruna, and Aadel A. Chaudhuri. "Racial disparities in early-stage NSCLC treatment: A call for action." *Cancer Epidemiology Biomarkers & Prevention* 33, no. 6 (April 8, 2024): 769–70. https://doi.org/10.1158/1055 -9965.epi-24-0339.

Rider, Jennifer R., Kathryn M. Wilson, Jennifer A. Sinnott, Rachel S. Kelly, Lorelei A. Mucci, and Edward L. Giovannucci. "Ejaculation Frequency and Risk of Prostate Cancer: Updated Results with an Additional Decade of Follow-up." *European Urology* 70, no. 6 (March 28, 2016): 974–82. https://doi.org/10.1016/j.eururo.2016.03.027.

Saginala, Kalyan, Adam Barsouk, John Sukumar Aluru, Prashanth Rawla, Sandeep Anand Padala, and Alexander Barsouk. "Epidemiology of Bladder Cancer." *Medical Sciences* 8, no. 1 (March 13, 2020): 15. https:// doi.org/10.3390/medsci8010015.

Schaal, Courtney, and Srikumar P. Chellappan. "Nicotine-Mediated Cell Proliferation and Tumor Progression in Smoking-Related Cancers."

Molecular Cancer Research 12, no. 1 (January 8, 2014): 14–23. https://doi
.org/10.1158/1541-7786.mcr-13-0541.

Selickman, John, Charikleia S. Vrettou, Spyros D. Mentzelopoulos, and
John J. Marini. "COVID-19-Related ARDS: Key Mechanistic Features
and Treatments." *Journal of Clinical Medicine* 11, no. 16 (August 20,
2022): 4896. https://doi.org/10.3390/jcm11164896.

Shergill, Amandeep K., Jenifer R. Lightdale, David H. Bruining, Ruben D.
Acosta, Vinay Chandrasekhara, Krishnavel V. Chathadi, G. Anton
Decker, et al. "The role of endoscopy in inflammatory bowel disease."
Gastrointestinal Endoscopy 81, no. 5 (April 9, 2015): 1101–1121.e13.
https://doi.org/10.1016/j.gie.2014.10.030.

Shi, Jingyi, Kui Zhang, Tianshu Xiao, Jingxuan Yang, Yanan Sun, Chan
Yang, Hao Dai, and Wenxing Yang. "Exposure to disinfection byproducts and risk of cancer: A systematic review and dose-response
meta-analysis." *Ecotoxicology and Environmental Safety* 270 (January 1,
2024): 115925. https://doi.org/10.1016/j.ecoenv.2023.115925.

Song, Mingyang, Andrew T. Chan, and Jun Sun. "Influence of the Gut
Microbiome, Diet, and Environment on Risk of Colorectal Cancer."
Gastroenterology 158, no. 2 (October 3, 2019): 322–40. https://doi.org/10
.1053/j.gastro.2019.06.048.

Starr, P. "Oral Nicotinamide Prevents Common Skin Cancers in High-Risk
Patients, Reduces Costs." *Am Health Drug Benefits*. 2015;8(Spec Issue):13–14.

Stevens A. J., Y. Boukari, S. English, A. Kadir, B. N. Kumar, D. Devakumar.
"Discriminatory, racist and xenophobic policies and practice against
child refugees, asylum seekers and undocumented migrants in
European health systems." *Lancet Reg Health Eur*. 2024;41:100834.
Published 2024 May 28. doi:10.1016/j.lanepe.2023.100834.

Sun, Jiaao, Feng Chen, and Guangzhen Wu. "Potential effects of gut
microbiota on host cancers: focus on immunity, DNA damage, cellular
pathways, and anticancer therapy." *The ISME Journal* 17, no. 10 (August 8, 2023): 1535–51. https://doi.org/10.1038/s41396-023-01483-0.

Szabo E., J. T. Mao, S. Lam, M. E. Reid, R. L. Keith. "Chemoprevention of
lung cancer: Diagnosis and management of lung cancer, 3rd ed: American College of Chest Physicians evidence-based clinical practice guidelines." *Chest*. 2013;143(5 Suppl):e40S-e60S. doi:10.1378/chest.12-2348.

Takkouche, B., C. Regueira-Mendez, and A. Montes-Martinez. "Risk of
cancer among hairdressers and related workers: a meta-analysis."
International Journal of Epidemiology 38, no. 6 (September 14, 2009):
1512–31. https://doi.org/10.1093/ije/dyp283.

Tang, Moon-Shong, Xue-Ru Wu, Hyun-Wook Lee, Yong Xia, Fang-Ming Deng, Andre L. Moreira, Lung-Chi Chen, William C. Huang, and Herbert Lepor. "Electronic-cigarette smoke induces lung adenocarcinoma and bladder urothelial hyperplasia in mice." *Proceedings of the National Academy of Sciences* 116, no. 43 (October 7, 2019): 21727–31. https://doi.org/10.1073/pnas.1911321116.

Tanne, Janice Hopkins. "US consumer group names 'dirty dozen' dietary supplements." *BMJ* 328, no. 7446 (April 22, 2004): 975.4. https://doi.org/10.1136/bmj.328.7446.975-c.

Tekle, Geniver El, Natalia Andreeva, and Wendy S. Garrett. "The Role of the Microbiome in the Etiopathogenesis of Colon Cancer." *Annual Review of Physiology* 86, no. 1 (February 12, 2024): 453–78. https://doi.org/10.1146/annurev-physiol-042022-025619.

Terushkin, V., E. Ng, J. A. Stein, S. Katz, D. E. Cohen, S. Meehan, D. Polsky. "A prospective study evaluating the utility of a 2-mm biopsy margin for complete removal of histologically atypical (dysplastic) nevi." *J. Am. Acad. Dermatol. 77*, (2017): 1096–1099.

Tilg, Herbert, Timon E. Adolph, Romana R. Gerner, and Alexander R. Moschen. "The Intestinal Microbiota in Colorectal Cancer." *Cancer Cell* 33, no. 6 (April 12, 2018): 954–64. https://doi.org/10.1016/j.ccell.2018.03.004.

Tomlinson, Ian, Peter Sasieni, and Walter Bodmer. "How Many Mutations in a Cancer?" *American Journal of Pathology* 160, no. 3 (March 1, 2002): 755–58. https://doi.org/10.1016/s0002-9440(10)64896-1.

Tong, Michelle, Latoya Hill, and Samantha Artiga. "Racial Disparities in Cancer Outcomes, Screening, and Treatment | KFF." KFF. February 3, 2022. https://www.kff.org/racial-equity-and-health-policy/issue-brief/racial-disparities-in-cancer-outcomes-screening-and-treatment/.

Toren, Paul, Anna Wilkins, Keval Patel, Amy Burley, Typhaine Gris, Roger Kockelbergh, Taha Lodhi, Ananya Choudhury, and Richard T. Bryan. "The sex gap in bladder cancer survival—a missing link in bladder cancer care?" *Nature Reviews Urology* 21, no. 3 (August 21, 2023): 181–92. https://doi.org/10.1038/s41585-023-00806-2.

Torres-Duque, C., D. Maldonado, R. Perez-Padilla, M. Ezzati, and G. Viegi. "Biomass Fuels and Respiratory Diseases: A Review of the Evidence." *Proceedings of the American Thoracic Society* 5, no. 5 (July 14, 2008): 577–90. https://doi.org/10.1513/pats.200707-100rp.

Torres, Juliana M., Michelle O. Sodipo, Margaret F. Hopkins, Paulette D. Chandler, and Erica T. Warner. "Racial Differences in Breast Cancer Survival Between Black and White Women According to Tumor

Subtype: A Systematic Review and Meta-Analysis." *Journal of Clinical Oncology*, September 17, 2024. https://doi.org/10.1200/jco.23.02311.

US Surgeon General's Report (1964). *Smoking and Health: Report of the Advisory Committee to the Surgeon General of the Public Health Service.*

Umar, Sheikh Ahmad, and Sheikh Abdullah Tasduq. "Ozone Layer Depletion and Emerging Public Health Concerns - An Update on Epidemiological Perspective of the Ambivalent Effects of Ultraviolet Radiation Exposure." *Frontiers in Oncology* 12 (March 10, 2022). https://doi.org/10.3389/fonc.2022.866733.

Wang L., R. Xu, D. C. Kaelber, N. A. Berger. "Glucagon-Like Peptide 1 Receptor Agonists and 13 Obesity-Associated Cancers in Patients With Type 2 Diabetes." *JAMA Netw Open.* 2024;7(7):e2421305. Published 2024 Jul 1. doi:10.1001/jamanetworkopen.2024.21305.

White, Arica, Djenaba Joseph, Sun Hee Rim, Christopher J. Johnson, Michel P. Coleman, and Claudia Allemani. "Colon cancer survival in the United States by race and stage (2001-2009): Findings from the CONCORD-2 study." *Cancer* 123, no. S24 (December 5, 2017): 5014–36. https://doi.org/10.1002/cncr.31076.

World Health Organization. "Shortages impacting access to glucagon-like peptide 1 receptor agonist products; increasing the potential for falsified versions." *WHO.* January 29, 2024. https://www.who.int/news/item/29-01-2024-shortages-impacting-access-to-glucagon-like-peptide-1-receptor-agonist-products--increasing-the-potential-for-falsified-versions.

World Health Organization. "Cost-effectiveness of radon control." WHO Handbook on Indoor Radon - NCBI Bookshelf. 2009. https://www.ncbi.nlm.nih.gov/books/NBK143215/.

Yang, Jiaqi, Sicheng Qian, Xiaona Na, and Ai Zhao. "Association between Dietary and Supplemental Antioxidants Intake and Lung Cancer Risk: Evidence from a Cancer Screening Trial." *Antioxidants* 12, no. 2 (January 31, 2023): 338. https://doi.org/10.3390/antiox12020338.

Zhao, Jianhui, Liying Xu, Jing Sun, Mingyang Song, Lijuan Wang, Shuai Yuan, Yingshuang Zhu, et al. "Global trends in incidence, death, burden and risk factors of early-onset cancer from 1990 to 2019." *BMJ Oncology* 2, no. 1 (July 1, 2023): e000049. https://doi.org/10.1136/bmjonc-2023-000049.

Index

abortions, 138, 201

acetaldehyde, 145, 147

acquired immunodeficiency syndrome (AIDS): epidemic, 134, 135; in gay community, 134–35; Kaposi sarcoma, 135; preventive measures, 136; related cancers, 134; symptoms, 135; transmission mode, 136

acquired immunodeficiency syndrome treatment: antiretroviral drugs, 137; AZT or zidovudine, 137; cost effective, 137; HAART, 137

acral melanoma, 170

actinic cheilitis, 169

actinic keratosis, 169

acute respiratory distress syndrome (ARDS), 215

addiction: and autonomy, 151–56; medicine service, 153; opioid, 153; and poverty, 150–51; psychological and societal ills, 150; public health epidemic, 155; root cause of, 150; smoking, 18; sugar, 72, 81

advanced practice providers (APPs): appointment, 263; cost-conscious health care delivery, 264; and doctors, 263, 266; online training, 263; purposes, 263

Affordable Care Act, 198, 260

aflatoxins, 41–42, 59–60, 69

Agent Orange, 99

AIDS Coalition to Unleash Power (ACT UP), 136

alcohol consumption: in American culture, 149; binge drinking, 149; cirrhosis, 148; dependency and addiction, 149; excessive drinking, 149; Great Depression, 151; heavy drinking, 149; liver disease, 37–38; no

safe level consumption, 148–49; per day, 148–49; preventive measures, 151; psychological and societal ills, 150; for relaxation, 149

alcohol consumption as cancer cause, 90; acetaldehyde damage, 147–48; breast, 148, 282; colorectal, 148, 282; endometrial, 148; head and neck, 148; liver, 148, 282; lung, 148; pancreatic, 148; risks, 147

alcohol use disorder, 155

allergies, 207, 218

alpha radiation, 171

ALS (Lou Gehrig's disease), 90

American Association of Medical Colleges, 264–65

American Cancer Society (ACS), 65, 233, 263, 237, 240, 241

American Indian and Alaska Native (AIAN), 247

American Institute for Cancer Research (AICR), 54

American Society of Clinical Oncology, 199

anal cancer: human papillomavirus, 128, 130, 134, 283; vaccine, 131

angiogenesis, 208

anti-aging supplements, 90

antibiotics, 25–26, 31, 47, 218–19

antidepressant medicines, 89, 223

anti-inflammatory medicines, 223, 224

anti-inflammatory nutrients, 212

antioxidants, 211–13, 225; lower risk of heart disease, 85; sources of, 85

antioxidant supplements: beta-carotene, 86; selenium, 86; vitamin A, C, or E, 85–86

anti-parasitic medications, 49

anxiety, 222, 223

2008, 198; medical-grade germline tests, 197–98; patient-driven decision, 199; Promethease, 196–97; protecting individual genetic information, 198; single nucleotide polymorphisms, 195–96
Genomic Prediction, 201
Georgine v. Amchem Products, Inc., 101
Gibbs, Lois, 108, 109
glioblastoma, 1, 2, 4
glucagon-like peptide 1 (GLP-1) agonists, 82, 83, 91–93; Alzheimer disease, 80; loss of facial fat, 80–81; medullary thyroid cancer risk, 81; obesity-related cancers, 80
gonorrhea, 129, 133
Guillain-Barre syndrome, 133
Guinea worms, 28
gut microbiome: beneficial gut bacteria, 220, 221, 222, 224; definition, 219; dysbiosis, 220–21; function, 220; immune system and, 220; leaky gut, 220; mental health, stress, and dementia, 222–24; role, 219–20; SCFAs, 220, 222; slow burn, chronic inflammation, 223–24

Hashimoto's thyroiditis, 221
head and neck cancer: alcohol consumption risk, 148; areca nut, 61; human papillomavirus, 130; lymphoma to HPV, 27; tobacco cause, 157; ultra-processed foods, 66
health care delivery, 261–62, 264
health care reform: affordable medicines, 255; costs, 255; cultural competency, 252–54; health care delivery, monopolization of, 261–62; principles, 267–68; single-payer health care (*see* single-payer health care); strategies, 254–55; US health care, 255, 268–69. *See also* pharmaceutical companies

health care reform and cancer care stakeholders: cost-cutting hospital administrators, 256; doctors and research institutions, 255; government or insurance companies, 255; patients, 255; pharmaceutical industry, 255–56
health care reform and medical training and practice, 262–66; advanced practice providers, 263–64; collaborative work, 266; lifestyle, 265; medical education and, 265–66; in residency, 265; underpaid apprentice, 265
heart attack, 71–72; avoiding red meat to reduce risk, 55; Black people with higher BMI, 76; cholesterol plaque deposits, 73; exercise reduce, 77; obesity risk, 72; oxygen free radicals, 85; stenting techniques, 77; tobacco risk, 142; vegan diet lower risk of, 55
heart failure with preserved ejection fraction (HFpEF), 211
Helicobacter pylori, 24–25, 27–32, 49, 51–52, 217; antibiotics, 25–26, 31, 218–19; associated stomach inflammation, 24–26, 30, 31; cause of gastritis, 25; complications, 31–32; culture growth, 24–25; gastric cancer, 29, 57–58; gastritis symptoms, 25; high-incidence, 30; hygiene hypothesis, 30–31; lymph node, 27–28; microscopic structure, 24; noncardia stomach cancer, 218; risk factors, 30; stomach ulcers by, 28; strains, 30; vagotomy, 31
hemophilia, 136
hepatitis A virus, 35
hepatitis B virus, 36; adult vaccination, 39–40; antiviral drugs, 39; estimated cases, 38; follow-up screening, 40; global vaccination program, 39; immunosuppressive medications,

40; infant vaccination, 39; inflammation, 36; liver cancer, 38, 39; liver cirrhosis, 38–39; prevalence, 39; primary source, 39; public health initiatives, 39; screening, 39; symptoms, 38; transmission mode, 38

hepatitis C virus, 49; blood samples test, 35; estimated cases, 38; infection spread, 35–36; oral treatment, 35; screening for, 37, 38; sterilization techniques, 35; victim blaming, 40–41

hepatitis D virus, 36

hepatitis E virus, 35

hepatitis virus: chronic liver disease, 37; inflammation of, 36; life-threatening blood loss, 36; types, 35–36

hepatocellular carcinoma, 37

hereditary nonpolyposis colorectal cancer (HNPCC). See Lynch syndrome

highly active antiretroviral therapy (HAART), 134, 137

high-sensitivity guaiac fecal occult blood test (HSgFOBT), 239

homosexual men: AIDS in (see acquired immunodeficiency syndrome (AIDS)); vs. heterosexual men, 128; skin cancer risk, 128

Hooker Chemical Company, 107

hot beverages, 62–63

Human Genome Project (HGP), 193–94

human immunodeficiency virus (HIV), 283; AIDS and (see acquired immunodeficiency syndrome (AIDS)); and HPV, 134; immunosuppressive drugs, 168; mortality, 137

human papillomavirus (HPV), 283; anal cancer, 130; anal sex, 130; cervical cancer, 130; head and neck cancer, 130; high-risk strains, 129–30; HIV

and, 134; low-risk strains, 129; molecular testing for, 237; oral sex, 130; p53, 130; pap smears and HPV test, 130; penile cancer, 130; self-sampling tests, 238; symptoms, 129; types, 129

HPV vaccine, 130, 244; administration, 131; age recommendation, 132; cause autism, 132; high-risk strains, 131; optimal age to receive, 132; for pre-adolescent children, 131–32; for preventing cancer, 131; side effects, 133; smallpox vaccine, 131

hygiene hypothesis, 217–19

hyperthermic intraperitoneal chemotherapy, 126

ibuprofen, 224

increased intestinal permeability, 220

infectious disease, 47, 48

inflammation: characteristics, 207; condition, 206; COVID-19 (see coronavirus disease (COVID-19)); defence mechanism, 207; definition, 206; fat and, 74–77, 92; goal of, 207; hepatitis B and, 36; immune system activation, 207–8; occurrence, 207; stomach, 24–26, 30, 31

inflammation, chronic: microenvironment tumor growth, 208; poor diet and obesity, 211; role in atherosclerosis, 221; slow burn, 223; stomach, 217 (see also stomach cancer). See also chronic inflammatory diseases

integrated delivery networks (IDNs), 261–62

intellectual disability, 202

International Agency for Research on Cancer (IARC), 53, 147

International Nuclear Event (INE) Scale, 178

International Workers' Day, 178–79

preventing methods, 173; spas,
172–73; State Indoor Radon Grants
program, 174; testing costs, 173–74
testicular cancer, 146, 227
T4 Program, 203–4
thalassemia, 26
Thomas, Brian, 260
3D mammography, 235
Three Mile Island nuclear power
plant, 181
throat cancer: radiation therapy,
158–59; smoking/chewing tobacco,
282; tobacco and areca nut, 61
thyroid cancer, 179, 181
tobacco: addiction, 150, 156; alcohol and,
141; global usage, 142; heart attack
risk, 142; history, 140; industrial
revolution, 140–41; psychological and
societal ills, 150; smokers vs. marijuana smokers, 146; stroke risk, 142;
successful quitting, 142
tobacco and cancer: carcinogens
inhalation, 141; DNA damage, 141;
esophagus, 142; gastrointestinal, 142;
head and neck cancer, 157; KRAS
gene mutation, 141; lung cancer, 171,
282; mouth, 142; nicotine, 141, 142;
oral, 142; p53 gene mutation, 141;
throat, 142
tobacco and companies deception on
smoking, 157; Big Tobacco, 143–45;
corporate influence, 145; cultural
norm, 143; danger of, 143; funded
research on dangers of, 144; heart
disease, 143; internal tobacco
industry documents, 144, 145;
Kohlberg Kravis Roberts & Co, 145;
legal fees and taxes on, 145; lobbying
efforts, 144; Master Settlement
Agreement, 144–45; public relations
campaigns, 144; safer cigarettes,
falsely advertised, 144; Tobacco
Industry Research Committee, 143

toxic waste: birth defects, 108; chemical
waste in abandoned canal, 107;
childhood illnesses, 108; government
action against, 108–9; health risks,
108; industrial waste, 107; Love
Canal disaster, 108, 109; miscarriages, 108; Superfund program, 109;
Teflon (see Teflon)
transgender men: ovarian or uterine
cancer in, 128; pap smears for, 128
transgender women: breast cancer, 128;
prostate cancer, 128; prostate
screening for, 128
trichomonas, 133
Troisier, Charles Emile, 28
Trump, Donald, 255
Tru-Niagen, 90
type 1 diabetes, 218, 221
type 2 diabetes, 221

ulcerative colitis, 209, 221
ultra-processed foods, 70; air-popped
popcorn, 66; associated with cancer
risk, 66, 68; cookie or cake, 66;
dietary recommendations, 67–68;
high consumption of, 66; junk foods,
65–66; sparkling water, 66; sugars
and, 66, 68
ultraviolet protective factor (UPF), 166
ultraviolet radiation (UV): African and
non-African people, 162; carbon
dioxide emissions, 163; causes, 161;
climate variations, 162–63; DNA
damage and mutations, 161–62; due
to sun exposure, 160–61; melanin,
162; Montreal Protocol, 163; ozone
layer depletion, 163; preventing
measures, 163; public health
initiatives, 163–64; and skin cancer,
184, 283; SunSmart program, 164;
SunWise program, children education, 164–65; UV-A, 160–61; UV-B,
160, 161; UV-C, 160

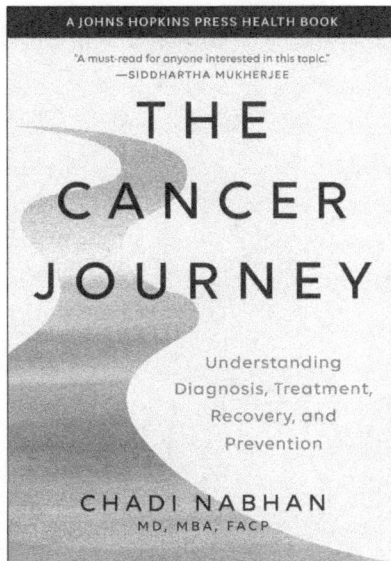

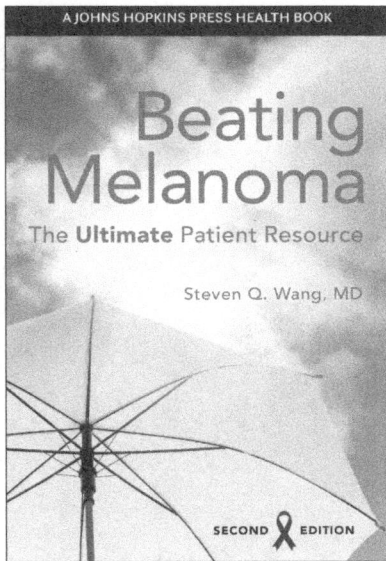

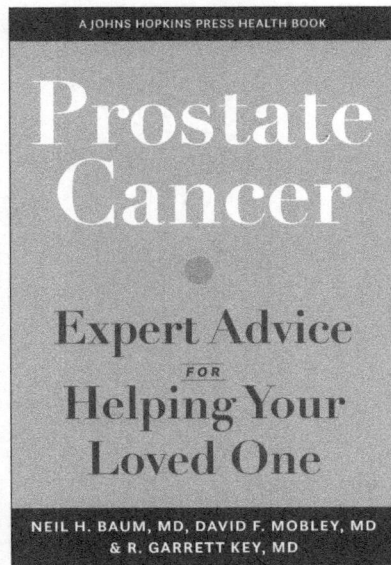

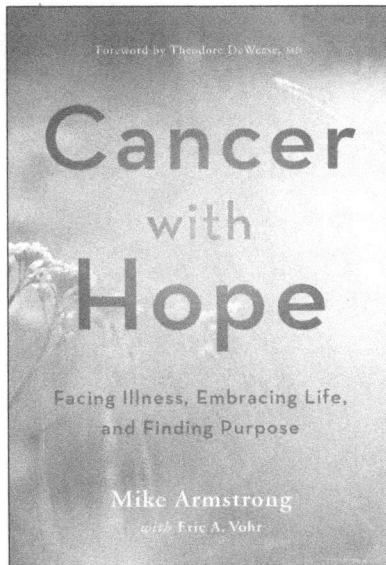